PRACTICAL MANAGEMENT OF CHRONIC VIRAL HEPATITIS

Edited by **Gaetano Serviddio**

Practical Management of Chronic Viral Hepatitis

http://dx.doi.org/10.5772/46043
Edited by Gaetano Serviddio

Contributors

Zahid Hussain, Ahmad Ali Asadi Noghabi, Mitra Zandi, Fatameh Bahramnejad, Helen Reeves, Rajiv Lochan, Derek Manas, Yukihiro Shimizu, Hadi Parsian, Gianfranco Lauletta, Gaetano Scotto, Rosa Prato, Luca Macarini, Luca Stoppino, Teresa Santantonio, Giuseppe Valerio Torres, Emanuela Apicella, Elisa D'Alterio, Angela Chiara Cecere, Antonello Bellomo, Gianluigi Vendemiale, Antonino D. Romano, Mario Mastrolonardo, Gaetano Serviddio, Rosanna Villani, Francesco Bellanti

Published by InTech

Janeza Trdine 9, 51000 Rijeka, Croatia

Publishing Process Manager Danijela Duric
Technical Editor InTech DTP team
Cover InTech Design team

Additional hard copies can be obtained from orders@intechopen.com

Practical Management of Chronic Viral Hepatitis, Edited by Gaetano Serviddio
p. cm.
ISBN 978-953-51-1109-2

For EU product safety concerns:
IN TECH d.o.o., Prolaz Marije Krucifikse Kozulić 3, 51000 Rijeka, Croatia,
info@intechopen.com or visit our website at intechopen.com.

Meet the editor

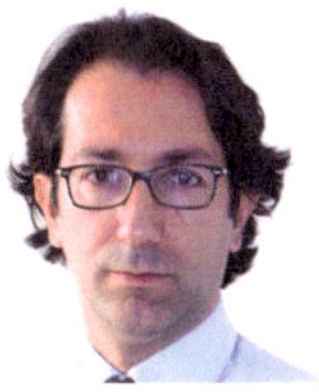

Gaetano Serviddio is professor of Internal Medicine at the University of Foggia. He has been working in the research field of redox biology in liver diseases at the University of Turin (Italy) and Valencia (Spain) from 1999 to 2003 when he moved to the University of Foggia where he founded the University Centre for the Research and treatment of liver diseases (C.U.R.E.). The centre encompasses the management of acute and chronic viral hepatitis and encourages and supports research in nonalcoholic fatty liver diseases (NAFLD). He has been awarded as investigator from the Italian Society of Internal Medicine and from the European Association for the Study of Liver disease and in 2012 he was granted from the Society for Free Radical Research Europe with the prestigious "Catherine Pasquier Award" for his research in liver diseases.
He is editorial board of international journals and member of the SFRR-E council. He has an extensive publication record in Liver disorders.

Contents

Preface

Continuous acquisition of new knowledge in Medicine is essential to ensure progression in diagnostics and therapeutics.

In the last decade the discipline of Hepatology has achieved important results in the treatment of viral hepatitis. A global success of hepatitis A and B vaccinations has been observed, and we are now following the clinical application of new generations of anti-HCV drugs that will provide more effective and less toxic anti-HCV therapies.

Moroever, hepatocellular carcinoma, which is one of the most important complications of end-stage liver disease, has become an area for innovative targeted anti-cancer therapies.

This book has been realized by a team of experts daily facing clinical problems in the prevention and management of liver diseases and has been designed for a global readership to offer some practical tips to physicians who want update their level of practice in the field.

It's a practical volume for daily reference but also an instrument for improving expertise in viral hepatology and discovering the unresolved issues.

Management of HBV and HCV hepatitis in young and elderly, HEV hepatitis, evaluation of liver fibrosis, hepatocellular carcinoma, vaccine and prevention of viral hepatitis are some of the most important topics covered by the authors.

The book is organized in three different sections containing 14 chapters. The first deals with the epidemiology and the development of vaccine in viral hepatitis.

The second covers the practical management of viral hepatitis, the skin involvement of liver diseases and the impact of the treatment on the skin physiopathology and the modern interpretation of non-invasive scores of liver fibrosis and the psychiatric disorders related to antiviral therapy.

The third section analyses the hepatocellular carcinoma, the malignant lymphoproliferative diseases and the cryoglobulinemia as the most important complications of viral infection. A specific chapter has been dedicated to patient education.

I want to thank all the authors who have shared the project with me from all over the world for their efforts in the realization of the final book.

Dr. Gaetano Serviddio
Assistant Professor of Internal Medicine,
Department of Medical Sciences,
University of Foggia, Italy

Section 1

From the Virus to the Vaccine

Chapter 1

Epidemiology and Prevention of Viral Hepatitis B and C

Domenico Martinelli, Francesca Fortunato,
Gulsun Simsek and Rosa Prato

Additional information is available at the end of the chapter

http://dx.doi.org/10.5772/55870

1. Introduction

Viral hepatitis is a family of viral infections that affect the liver caused by at least five distinct viruses: hepatitis A virus (HAV), hepatitis B virus (HBV), hepatitis C virus (HCV), hepatitis D virus (HDV), and hepatitis E virus (HEV). Hepatitis A and E appear as acute self-limiting diseases and do not become chronic; occasionally, a fulminant form of hepatitis develops (acute liver failure), which can lead to death. In contrast, HBV and HCV infections can evolve as serious chronic diseases that often remain clinically silent for decades. Fulminant hepatitis B develops in 0.1–0.6% of acute cases; rarely, it also have been reported among perinatally infected infants. People with chronic hepatitis B and C are infectious to others [1, 2, 3]. HDV is a "defective virus" that requires co-infection with HBV for its own replication. Infection with HDV is associated with the most severe forms of acute and chronic hepatitis in many HBsAg-positive patients [4].

Subjects affected by chronic HBV and/or HCV infection are at increased risk for liver cirrhosis and hepatocellular carcinoma (HCC) later in life. About 5% of all acute HBV infections progress to chronic active infection (persistence of HBsAg for more than 6 months). The risk of developing a chronic hepatitis B decreases with age of infection [5], dropping from 90% in infants <1 years old to 30%-50% in children 1-5 years old and to 5%-10% in adults [1, 6, 7]. Chronic active hepatitis B develops in more than 25% of carriers and often results in cirrhosis; approximately the same proportion of cases dies prematurely from cirrhosis or liver cancer [5]. About 75%-85% of subjects affected by HCV develop a chronic infection, 5%-20% develop cirrhosis and 1%-5% die for cirrhosis or liver cancer [8].

2. Burden of HBV infection

Diseases caused by hepatitis B virus have a worldwide distribution. About one third of the world's population has been exposed to HBV with more than 2 billion people infected worldwide. Approximately 350 million subjects develop a chronic form and about 600,000 die every year for acute or chronic consequences of hepatitis B [6, 9, 10].

The prevalence of HBV infection varies all around the world. In Western countries, it is relatively rare and acquired primarily in adulthood with a prevalence of HBsAg positive <2% (low endemicity areas). In Asia and most of Africa, HBV infection is common and usually acquired perinatally or in childhood with a prevalence of HBsAg positive 2%-7% in intermediate endemicity areas and ≥8% in high endemicity areas [9, 11].

A general decrease of new cases of acute disease was observed in North America in the last decades. Between 1987 and 2004 in the United States, the incidence declined 80%, falling from 10.7 per 100,000 (25,916 cases reported) to 2.1 per 100,000 (6,212 cases reported) in all age groups, and the largest proportional decrease among 0-15 years (-95%) and 15-24 years (-87%) [12]. In 2009, 3,371 new cases were reported to Centre for Diseases Control and Prevention (CDC). Prevalence of HBsAg-positive individuals – chronic infection was generally low (0.33% in 1976-1980, 0.42% in 1988-1994 and 0.30% in 2005-2006). Between 2004 and 2009, 800,000 to 1.4 million persons developed a chronic Hepatitis B, with about 3,000 deaths / year [12,13].

In the European Union, 7,000-8,000 newly diagnosed cases of hepatitis B occurr each year. The incidence per 100,000 population has declined over the past ten years from 6.7 cases per 100,000 in 1995 to 1.5 cases per 100,000 in 2007. The prevalence of HBsAg-positives in the general population of European countries reported from ECDC – European Centre for Disease Prevention and Control range from 0.1% to 7%. The higher rates are registered in the southern Europe, being Romania the country with the highest prevalence (>4%), followed by medium prevalence countries (> 1-2%) as Spain, Italy, and Greece. Belgium, Czech Republic, Finland, Germany, Ireland, Netherlands, Slovakia and Sweden reported the lowest prevalence (<1%) [2,14].

Among developing areas, the highest prevalence are described in sub-Saharan regions of Africa (≥10%) [15]. In 2005, North Africa and the Middle Eastern region showed lower intermediate HBsAg endemicity across all age groups [16]. China and other countries of East Asia are at high/intermediate endemicity for Hepatitis B. Most people in those regions become infected during childhood and up-to 8–10% of the adult population is chronically infected. There, liver cancer caused by chronic hepatitis B is among the first three causes of death from cancer in men and a major cause of cancer in women [6]. Central Asia and the Caucasus are at intermediate HBsAg endemicity too, with 2–5% of the general population chronically infected by HBV. High HBV prevalence is reported also in the Amazon area (South America), in the north regions of Canada and in Greenland [17].

3. Burden of HCV infection

Every year, 3-4 million people in the world are newly infected with the hepatitis C virus [8]. WHO estimates that approximately 3% (170 million persons) of the world's population has been infected with HCV [18] and about 150 million are chronically infected and at risk of developing liver cirrhosis and/or liver cancer. More than 350,000 people die from related liver diseases every year [8].

The prevalence of HCV infection is higher (up to 15%) in some countries in Africa and Asia. Countries with higher rates of chronic infection are Egypt (15%), Pakistan (4.8%) and China (3.2%).

For most developed countries, the prevalence of HCV infection is <3%.

In the United States, the more recent estimates amount to 17,000 new Hepatitis C virus infections and 2.7-3.9 million chronic infections (prevalence: 1.3%-1.9%) [13, 19]. With an HCV antibody prevalence of 3.25%, persons born during 1945–1965 account for approximately three fourths of all chronic HCV infections among adults [20].

In the European Union, hepatitis C showed a significant increase over the past ten years. The number of newly reported cases incidence raised from 4.3 per 100,000 population in 1995 to 6.9 cases per 100,000 in 2007 (27,000-29,000 newly diagnoses /year). This trend may reflect changes in testing practices and reporting rather than a real increase [14]. The highest prevalence rates (more than 2%) are reported in the southern Europe countries, including Italy, Romania and Spain. Medium prevalence was observed in Bulgaria, France, Greece, and Poland. Countries with low prevalence (less than 1%) include Belgium, Germany, the Netherlands, Sweden, and the United Kingdom [14].

4. Cirrhosis and hepatocellular carcinoma attributable to HBV or HCV

With more than 5% of all cancers worldwide, hepatocellular carcinoma is one of the most common malignant tumors. More than 500,000 cases are estimated every year [21], with a mean annual incidence of around 3-4% [22]. In 2008, WHO estimated that cirrhosis and primary liver cancer caused 849,000 and 695,000 deaths, respectively. These conditions, together, account for approximately one of every forty deaths (2.7%) worldwide [23].

HBV and HCV chronic infection represents the main cause of cirrhosis and is the major contributor to HCC in many parts of the world. Alcohol abuse is a critical risk factor for these diseases, with some evidence for a synergistic effect in the presence of viral infection [24, 25].

The annual risk of HBV-related HCC is 0.5% for asymptomatic HBsAg carriers and 0.8% for chronic hepatitis B cases [26]. Patients with related-HBV cirrhosis present a risk of developing HCC 1,000 times higher than HBsAg-negative controls [27]. The HBV replication status may play an important role in the development of HCC [28-30]. The relative risk of HCC among HBsAg positive subjects could be about ten times higher than those without HBsAg, with approximately a sixty-fold increase in the risk when they are positive for both HBsAg and HBeAg [29].

Whereas liver cancer represents a rare occurrence during the first 10–15 years after HCV-infection [31-35], the risk of HCC increases with the establishment of cirrhosis (yearly incidence between 3–8%) [36-41]. The risk of cirrhosis is <10% in women infected at a young age and >30% in men infected after the age of 40 over a 20 year period [42,43]. Genotype 1b, the most prevalent in Europe and in Japan, could be associated with a higher incidence of HCC than other genotypes [44,45]. Co-infection of both HBV and HCV has been found in more severe liver diseases than either infection alone [46].

The incidence of HCC reflects the global distribution of HBV and HCV infections with approximately 80% of HCC cases occurring in developing countries. Eastern Asia, Middle Africa and some Western African countries show age-adjusted incidence rates (AAIR) of 27.6-36.6 per 100,000 (in men), 20.8–31.1 per 100,000 and 30–48 per 100,000, respectively. Northern Europe, Australia, New Zealand and the Caucasian populations of North and Latin America (AAIR 1.5–3.0) represent the areas at lowest risk. The AAIR raises to about 10 per 100,000 in men in Southern Europe [47].

In a study published in 2006, Perz et al. estimated that, globally, 57% of cirrhosis cases were attributable to either HBV (30%, ranging from 5% in North America to 57% in WHO Western Pacific Region B) or HCV (27%, ranging from 16% in WHO Africa Regions D/E to 62% in Western Pacific Region A). About three-quarters (78%) of HCC were attributable to HBV (53%) or HCV (25%). The attributable fractions of HCC due to HBV or HCV ranged from 16% in North America to 65% in Western Pacific Region B (China, Cambodia, etc.), and from 13% in Eastern Mediterranean Region (Bahrain, Cyprus, Iran, Jordan, etc.) to 66% in Western Pacific Region A, respectively. The two viruses taken together accounted for >50% of HCC in all of the regions and for >50% of cirrhosis in 8 of 11 regions [48].

5. Risk factors for hepatitis B and C

HBV is transmitted by percutaneous or mucous membrane contact with infected blood or other body fluids of an infected person.

In developing countries the transmission routes are perinatal, early childhood exposure, unsafe injections or needle stick in health care settings, unsafe blood transfusions, unprotected sexual contact [6].

In developed countries infections are mainly transmitted during young adulthood by sexual activity and injecting drug use. Historically, male homosexual contacts have been associated with an high risk for HBV infection [6]. More recently, heterosexual transmission is recognised as the most common cause of acute HBV infection in adults [12]. The risk of sexual transmission is mostly related with multiple sex partners and history of a sexually transmitted infections [7]. In some countries, transmission via household contacts (persons who have prolonged but non sexual interpersonal contacts with someone), has also been demonstrated [1, 6]. Sharing items such as razors or toothbrushes with an infected person also give rises to HBV transmission [10].

HBV is a common cause of occupational disease transmitted from patients to health care workers and also to health care workers' families. The risk of transmission depends on the viral load and exposure frequency but the most important factors in the exposure are health care workers skill levels and expertise and the specific hospital departments environment (e.g., dentists, dental hygienists, emergency medical technicians, first responders, laboratory technologists/technicians, nurses, nurse practitioners, phlebotomists, physicians, physician assistants, and students entering these professions). In contrast, transmission from health care workers to patients is rare [49]. Dentists and dental staff are the category at the highest risk of infection and transmission of HBV to their patients [50].

Several studies showed that tattooing, acupuncture and beauty treatments are associated with hepatitis B transmission when sterilization or disinfection procedures are unavailable [51-53].

In many contexts, the risk of HBV transmission via transfusion of blood and plasma-derived products has been eliminated through donor screening but in some developing countries it can continue to occur in heath care settings by not-adherence to guidelines [12].

Travellers to developing countries with high rates of hepatitis B are considered at high risk, especially subjects who engage in unprotected sex with local commercial sex workers [6, 54].

HCV is a blood borne pathogen, most commonly transmitted through exposure to infectious blood [8].

In the past, blood transfusion represented one of the most serious risk factor for HCV infection. In the late 1980s and early 1990s, specific donor screening for HCV was implemented and the risk of HCV infection from a unit of transfused blood was drastically reduced. As of 2001, the risk is less than one per million transfused blood units [55]. Currently, in Europe, the estimated residual risk for acquiring HCV via blood products ranges from 1 to 40 per 10 million transfusions [7].

Nosocomial transmission of HCV via contaminated substances or multiple dose vials as well as via haemodialysis, is still a concern [7]. Especially in developing countries, the incidence of hepatitis C virus infection among patients on hemodialysis was significantly higher [56].

Although in many developing countries unsafe medical injections and transfusions are still predominant sources of infection, at global level HCV transmission is increasingly driven by injected drugs use [57]. In 2010, about 10.0 million injection drug users (IDUs, range 6.0–15.2 million) could have been anti-HCV positive with a midpoint prevalence of 67.0% among all IDUs globally [58]. Individuals who injected drugs, even if they did so on occasionally in the past, are at highest risk for HCV infection that is rapidly acquired following the initiation of injection drug use and occurs from the sharing of needles, syringes, or other equipment associated with drug use [55]. Increasing age, increasing duration of injecting drug use and imprisonment were identified as risk factors [2, 59, 60].

Less commonly, hepatitis C may be transmitted through sex with an infected person. In 2001, sexual exposures accounted for about 15% of cases of hepatitis C in USA [55]. High-risk sexual behaviour among men who have sex with men (predominantly HIV-positive) may predispose to HCV infection probably via permucosal route and mucosal damage rather than by sexual contact [7].

Together with HBV, HCV is considered a common cause of occupational hazard for health care workers, significantly correlated with factors such as the type of procedure (replacing a hollow-bore needle in a patient's vein or artery, needle recapping, the use of sharp, etc), the severity of percutaneous injury, the gender of the personnel, expertise levels and hospital wards [49].

Other parenteral exposures such as body piercing and tattooing in potentially nonsterile settings [61], or being born to a hepatitis C infected mother [8] have to be considered important risk factors for HCV transmission. Nevertheless, in 2001 CDC estimated that in USA about 10% of people with HCV infection have no recognized source for their infection [55].

6. Prevention of hepatitis B and C

The hepatitis B vaccine, the first vaccine against a major human cancer, is the milestone in hepatitis B prevention [6].

A plasma-derived vaccine was licensed in the early 1980s. It derived from HBsAg particles purified from the plasma of chronic patients. The vaccine was safe and effective but not well accepted because of fears of transmission of live HBV and other bloodborne pathogens, such as HIV [5].

Since the mid 1980s, a new recombinant hepatitis B vaccine has gradually replaced the plasma-derived vaccine. HBsAg in the vaccine is produced in yeast or mammalian cells into which the HBsAg gene or HBsAg/pre-HBsAg genes are inserted using plasmids [9].

The vaccine has an outstanding record of safety and results really effective in preventing infection and its chronic consequences [6, 7]. After three intramuscular doses, more than 95% of infants, children, and adolescents (0-19 years) and more than 90% of healthy adults develop adequate antibody responses. By 60 years of age, 75% of immunised subjects develop protective antibody titers.

Hepatitis B vaccine is available as monovalent formulations or in combination with diphtheria–tetanus–pertussis, Haemophilus influenzae type b, hepatitis A and inactivated polio vaccines [9].

The recommended doses vary with the different formulations of vaccine and the age of the vaccinees. From 2 to 4 times the normal adult dose or an increased number of doses may be necessary in hemodialysis patients or in other immunocompromised subjects to induce protective antibodies [5]. A recombinant vaccine using alum and lipid A as adjuvants is available for adult patients with renal insufficiency [62].

Conventionally, the primary hepatitis B immunization infancy series consists of 3 doses; 4 doses may be administered for programmatic reasons according to the schedules of national routine immunization programmes. For older children and adults, the primary series of 3 doses with appropriate intervals applies [9]. The use of routine booster doses does not appear necessary to maintain long-term protection in successfully vaccinated immunocompetent children [9, 63, 64].

Although some studies suggest that a universal infant vaccination may be more cost-effective in intermediate- and high-endemicity regions, WHO strongly recommends that all newborn infants receive the hepatitis B vaccine at birth [7, 9, 65-69, 75]. Universal immunization beginning at birth and other successful hepatitis B vaccination strategies have drastically reduced HBV transmission in many high endemicity countries. In recent years, the significantly reduced price of hepatitis B vaccine in developing countries has facilitated its introduction into many more countries [6, 9]. As of 2011, 179 countries had incoporated hepatitis B vaccine as a part of their national infant immunization schedules, and an estimated 69% of the 2008 birth cohort received 3 doses of hepatitis B vaccine [6]. In 2006, approximately 27% of newborns worldwide received a birth dose of hepatitis B vaccine [70].

In areas where HBV is mainly spread from mother to infant at birth, the first dose of vaccine should be given as soon as possible after birth, preferably within 24 hours. The need for catch-up vaccination in cohorts of children with low coverage should be considered to increase the number of protected children since the risk for chronic infection is highest in younger age groups [9].

In intermediate/low endemicity countries target groups for catch-up vaccination can include adolescents and people with risk factors for acquiring HBV infection, such as subjects frequently requiring blood or blood products, dialysis patients, people with chronic liver disease, recipients of solid organ transplantations, people interned in prisons, injecting drug users, household and sexual contacts of people with chronic HBV infection, people with multiple sexual partners, men who have sexual contact with other men, HIV positives [7, 71, 76]. Healthcare workers, staff of facilities for developmentally disabled persons and others subjects exposed to blood and blood products must be vaccinated. Immunization remains the best defence not only for the workers themselves, but also to prevent transmission of infectious agents to the their patients [9, 76]. Also unvaccinated or incompletely vaccinated travellers to high endemicity countries should be offered the vaccine before leaving for endemic areas [6].

Prevaccination serological tests are not recommended routinely. Though routine postvaccination testing for immunity is not necessary, it is recommended 1-2 months after the last dose of the vaccine series for high-risk individuals, such as people at risk of occupationally acquired infection, infants born to HBsAg-positive mothers, chronic haemodialysis patients, HIV positives and other immunocompromised people, sex partners or needle-sharing partners of HBsAg positive subjects [9].

In several European countries and in USA, routine prenatal screening of pregnant women for HBsAg to identify newborns who require postexposure immunoprophylaxis has been introduced or recommended [2, 75] and some developing countries are considering this opportunity in order to prevent perinatal hepatitis B virus infection [72-74]. In some European countries, screening programmes for high-risk groups (inject drug users, men having sex with men, contacts of HBsAg-positive individuals, health care workers) have also been carried out [2].

Temporary immunity (3-6 months) may be obtained by administering hepatitis B immunoglobulin (HBIG) for postexposure prophylaxis [9]. HBIG is prepared from the plasma of donors with high concentrations of anti-HBs. The plasma is screened to eliminate positives for HBsAg, antibodies to HIV and hepatitis C virus, and HCV RNA [75]. HBIG is typically used as an adjunct to hepatitis B vaccine for postexposure immunoprophylaxis or as the primary means of protection after an HBV exposure for non-responders to hepatitis B vaccination [75]. HBIG prophylaxis in conjunction with HBV vaccination may be of additional benefit for infants born to HBsAg-positive mothers, particularly if they are HBeAg positive, subjects exposed to HBsAg-positive blood or body fluids, people sexually exposed to an HBsAg-positive person, and patients who need protection from recurrent HBV infection following liver transplantation [9].

A vaccine against HCV is not yet available [8, 77], and immunoglobulin does not provide protection [18]. The primary prevention is aimed to reduce the risk for HCV transmission [78] and includes:

- avoiding unnecessary and unsafe injections, unsafe sharps waste collection and disposal;
- screening of blood, plasma, organ, tissue, and semen donors;
- controlling use of illicit drugs and preventing the sharing of injection equipment among drug users;
- promoting protected sex with hepatitis C-infected subjects;
- advising household contacts of HCV infects about the risk related to share of sharp personal items;
- avoiding tattoos, piercings and acupuncture performed with not sterilized equipment [8, 79-81].

Identifying persons at risk but not yet infected with HCV provides opportunity for counseling on how to reduce their risk [78].

Travelers should be advised against the use of medical, surgical, and dental equipments not adequately sterilized or disinfected and they should consider the risks about getting a tattoo or body piercing in areas where adequate sterilization or disinfection procedures might not be available or practiced [18].

Secondary prevention aims to reduce risks for liver chronic diseases in HCV-infected persons by identification, counseling, and testing and by providing appropriate medical management and antiviral therapy [78, 82].

The determination of which risk groups to recommend for routine testing should be based on the knowledge of the epidemiologic link between a risk factor and acquiring HCV infection, prevalence of risk factors or behavior for infection in the population, and prevalence of infection among those with a risk factors or behavior [78].

Risk groups to test routinely shoud be injected illegal drugs users; subjects who received (i) clotting factor concentrates produced before the late 1980s, (ii) blood from a donor who later tested positive for HCV infection, (iii) transfusion of blood / blood components or an organ transplant before the early 1990s; patients on long-term hemodialysis or with persistently abnormal alanine aminotransferase levels [78, 83].

Based on a recognized exposure, healthcare, emergency medical and public safety workers after needle sticks, sharps, or mucosal exposures to HCV-positive blood and children born to

http://dx.doi.org/10.5772/55870

HCV-positive mothers should be tested routinely. Immunoglobulin and antiviral agents are not recommended for postexposure prophylaxis of hepatitis C.

In USA, CDC strongly recommends that adults of all ages at risk for HCV infection should be tested; particularly, those born during 1945–1965 without prior ascertainment of HCV risk should receive one-time testing for HCV [20].

Counselling directed to HCV positives must include messages on how to protect the liver from further harm by receiving hepatitis A and B vaccination if susceptible, reducing alcohol consumption, avoiding new medicines (including over-the-counter and herbal agents) without first checking with their health-care provider, and obtaining HIV risk testing [20]. Persons overweight/obese must loose weight and follow an healthy diet and a physically active health-style [20, 84].

First of all, HCV positives must not donate blood, tissue, or semen and/or share devices that come into contact with blood, such as toothbrushes, dental appliances, razors, and nail clippers, to minimize the risk of transmission to others [20].

Epidemiological surveillance represents the mainstay in the prevention of viral hepatitis since it provides the information for determining new infections and trends in incidence, changing patterns of transmission and persons at highest risk for infection, and for evaluating effectiveness or missed opportunities for prevention [78].

In USA, each week, state and territorial health departments report cases of acute, symptomatic viral hepatitis to CDC's [1].

Most of European countries have a passive mandatory surveillance system for acute hepatitis having clinicians as the main source of data, using an electronic format at the national level, and collecting a similar set of basic data. Underreporting is common, but the exact extent is unknown [8].

Chronic hepatitis B and C, although accounting for the greatest burden of disease, are not reported by most states.

Serologic surveys carried out periodically can add information on geographical variations in prevalence of infections, populations at high risk, trends, and prevention programs [78].

Author details

Domenico Martinelli[1], Francesca Fortunato[1], Gulsun Simsek[2] and Rosa Prato[1*]

*Address all correspondence to: r.prato@unifg.it

1 Sector of Hygiene, Department of Medical and Surgical Sciences, University of Foggia, Foggia, Italy

2 Medico Social Unit, Merkez Health Center, Hacettepe University, Ankara, Turkey

References

[1] Centers for Disease Control and Prevention. CDC: Viral hepatitis surveillance, United States, 2009–2011. http://www.cdc.gov/hepatitis/Statistics/2010Surveillance/Commentary.htm#bkgrndB (accessed 28 September 2012).

[2] European Center for Disease Prevention and Control. ECDC: The report on hepatitis B and C in the EU neighbourhood: prevalence, burden of disease and screening policies. EU neighbourhood: prevalence, burden of disease and screening policies. ecdc.europa.eu/en/publications/Publications/TER_100914_Hep_B_C%20_EU_neighbourhood.pdf (accessed 28 September 2012).

[3] Centers for Disease Control and Prevention. CDC: Hepatitis B FAQs for the Public. http://www.cdc.gov/hepatitis/B/bFAQ.htm#statistics (accessed 28 September 2012).

[4] World Health Organization. WHO: Hepatitis D. http://www.who.int/csr/disease/hepatitis/whocdscsrncs20011/en/index1.html (accessed 1 October 2012).

[5] Centers for Disease Control and Prevention. CDC: Hepatitis B. Epidemiology and Prevention of Vaccine. Preventable Diseases. The Pink Book: Course Textbook - 12th Edition Second Printing (May 2012). http://www.cdc.gov/vaccines/pubs/pinkbook/hepb.html (accessed 1 October 2012).

[6] World Health Organization. WHO: Hepatitis B. Fact Sheet No. 204. http://www.who.int/mediacentre/factsheets/fs204/en/ (accessed 28 September 2012).

[7] European Centre for Disease Prevention and Control. ECDC: Technical Report. Surveillance and prevention of hepatitis B and C in Europe. Stockholm October 2010. http://ecdc.europa.eu/en/press/news/Lists/News/ECDC_DispForm.aspx?List=32e43ee8-e230-4424-a78385742124029a&ID=391 (accessed 1 October 2012).

[8] World Health Organization. WHO: Hepatitis C. Fact Sheet No. 164. http://www.who.int/mediacentre/factsheets/fs164/en/index.html (accessed 28 September 2012).

[9] World Health Organization. WHO: Hepatitis B Vaccines. Weekly epidemiological record, 2 october 2009. www.who.int/wer/2009/wer8440.pdf (accessed 28 September 2012).

[10] Centers for Disease Control and Prevention. CDC: Hepatitis B FAQs for the Public. http://www.cdc.gov/hepatitis/B/bFAQ.htm#statistics (accessed 28 September 2012).

[11] Lavanchy D. Hepatitis B virus epidemiology, disease burden, treatment, and current and emerging prevention and control measures. Journal of Viral Hepatitis 2004 Mar; 11(2):97-107.

[12] Kim WR. Epidemiology of Hepatitis B in the United States. Hepatology 2009 May; 49(5 Suppl):S28-34.

[13] Centers for Disease Control and Prevention. CDC: Disease Burden from Viral Hepatitis A, B, and C in the United States. National Center for HIV/AIDS, Viral Hepatitis, STD & TB Prevention. Division of Viral Hepatitis. http://www.cdc.gov/hepatitis/statistics/index.htm (accessed 1 October 2012).

[14] European Center for Disease Prevention and Control. ECDC: Read the info sheet on hepatitis B and C: current situation in EU/EEA. http://ecdc.europa.eu/en/press/news/Lists/News/ECDC_DispForm.aspx?List=32e43ee8-e230-4424-a78385742124029a&ID=391 (accessed 28 September 2012).

[15] Rossi C, Shrier I, Marshall L, Cnossen S, Schwartzman K, Klein MB, Schwarzer G, Greenaway C. Seroprevalence of chronic hepatitis B virus infection and prior immunity in immigrants and refugees: a systematic review and meta-analysis. PLoS One 2012;7(9):e44611. Epub 2012 Sep 5.

[16] Ott JJ, Stevens GA, Groeger J, Wiersma ST. Global epidemiology of hepatitis B virus infection: new estimates of age-specific HBsAg seroprevalence and endemicity. Vaccine 2012 Mar 9;30(12):2212-9. Epub 2012 Jan 24.

[17] Centers for Disease Control and Prevention. CDC: Infectious Diseases Related To Travel. Hepatitis B. http://wwwnc.cdc.gov/travel/yellowbook/2012/chapter-3-infectious-diseases-related-to-travel/hepatitis-b.htm (accessed 28 September 2012).

[18] Centers for Disease Control and Prevention. CDC: Infectious Diseases Related To Travel. Hepatitis C. http://wwwnc.cdc.gov/travel/yellowbook/2012/chapter-3-infectious-diseases-related-to-travel/hepatitis-c.htm (accessed 28 September 2012).

[19] Centers for Disease Control and Prevention. CDC: Hepatitis C FAQs for the Public. http://www.cdc.gov/knowmorehepatitis/HepC-FAQ.htm#cFAQ04. (accessed 28 September 2012).

[20] Centers for Disease Control and Prevention. CDC: Recommendations for the Identification of Chronic Hepatitis C Virus Infection Among Persons Born During 1945–1965. MMWR / August 17, 2012 / Vol.61 / No.4.

[21] Bruix J, Sherman M, Llovet JM, Beaugrand M, Lencioni R, Burroughs AK, Christensen E, Pagliaro L, Colombo M, Rodes J, EASL Panel of Experts on HCC. Clinical management of hepatocellular carcinoma. Conclusions of the Barcelona-2000 EASL conference. Journal of Hepatology 2001, 35:421-430.

[22] Llovet JM, Beaugrand M. Hepatocellular carcinoma: present status and future prospects. Journal of Hepatology. 2003, 38(Suppl 1):136-149

[23] World Health Organization. WHO: Hepatitis D. http://apps.who.int/ghodata/?vid=10012 (accessed 1 October 2012).

[24] Donato F, Tagger A, Gelatti U, et al. Alcohol and hepatocellular carcinoma: the effect of lifetime intake and hepatitis virus infections in men and women. American Journal of Epidemiology 2002;155:323–331.

[25] Hassan MM, Hwang LY, Hatten CJ, et al. Risk factors for hepatocellular carcinoma: synergism of alcohol with viral hepatitis and diabetes mellitus. Hepatology 2002;36:1206–1213.

[26] Liaw YF, Tai DI, Chu CM, Lin DY, Sheen IS, Chen TJ, Pao CC. Early detection of hepatocellular carcinoma in patients with chronic type B hepatitis. A prospective study. Gastroenterology 1986, 90:263-267.

[27] Beasley RP, Hwang LY, Lin CC, Chien CS. Hepatocellular carcinoma and hepatitis B virus. A prospective study of 22707 men in Taiwan. Lancet 1981, 2:1129-1133.

[28] Sakuma K, Saitoh N, Kasai M, Jitsukawa H, Yoshino I, Yamaguchi M, Nobutomo K, Yamumi M, Tsuda F, Komazawa T. Relative risks of death due to liver disease among Japanese male adults having various statuses for hepatitis B s and e antigen/antibody in serum: a prospective study. Hepatology 1988, 8:1642-1646.

[29] Yang HI, Lu SN, Liaw YF, You SL, Sun CA, Wang LY, Hsiao CK, Chen PJ, Chen DS, Chen CJ, Taiwan Community-Based Cancer Screening Project Group. Hepatitis B e antigen and the risk of hepatocellular carcinoma. The New England Journal Medicine 2002, 347:168-174.

[30] Ohkubo K, Kato Y, Ichikawa T, Kajiya Y, Takeda Y, Higashi S, Hamasaki K, Nakao K, Nakata K, Eguchi K. Viral load is a significant prognostic factor for hepatitis B virus-associated hepatocellular carcinoma. Cancer 2002, 94:2663-2668.

[31] Hopf U, Moller B, Kuther D, Stemerowicz R, Lobeck H, Ludtke-Hand- jery A, Walter E, Blum HE, Roggendorf M, Deinhardt F. Long-term follow-up of posttransfusion and sporadic chronic hepatitis non-A, non-B and frequency of circulating antibodies to hepatitis C virus (HCV). Journal of Hepatology 1990, 10:69-76.

[32] Di Bisceglie AM, Goodman ZD, Ishak KG, Hoofnagle JH, Melpolder JJ, Alter HJ. Long-term clinical and histopathological follow-up of chronic posttransfusion hepatitis. Hepatology 1991, 14:969-974.

[33] Tremolada F, Casarin C, Alberti A, Drago C, Tagger A, Ribero ML, Realdi G. Long-term follow-up of non-A, non-B (type C) post- transfusion hepatitis. Journal of Hepatology 1992, 6:273-281.

[34] Koretz RL, Abbey H, Coleman E, Gitnick G. Non-A, non-B post-transfusion hepatitis. Looking back in the second decade. Annals of Internal Medicine 1993, 119:110-115.

[35] Mattsson L, Sonnerborg A, Weiland O. Outcome of acute symptomatic non-A, non-B hepatitis: a 13-year follow-up study of hepatitis C virus markers. Liver 1993, 13:274-278.

[36] Colombo M, de Franchis R, Del Ninno E, Sangiovanni A, De Fazio C, Tommasini M, Donato MF, Piva A, Di Carlo V, Dioguardi N. Hepatocellular carcinoma in Italian patients with cirrhosis. The New England Journal Medicine 1991, 325:675-680.

[37] Tsukuma H, Hiyama T, Tanaka S, Nakao M, Yabuuchi T, Kitamura T, Nakanishi K, Fujimoto I, Inoue A, Yamazaki H, Kawashima T. Risk factors for hepatocellular carcinoma among patients with chronic liver disease. The New England Journal Medicine 1993, 328:1797-1801.

[38] Bolondi L, Sofia S, Siringo S, Gaiani S, Casali A, Zironi G, Piscaglia F, Gramantieri L, Zanetti M, Sherman M. Surveillance programme of cirrhotic patients for early diagnosis and treatment of hepatocellular carcinoma: a cost effectiveness analysis. An International Journal of Gastroenterology & Hepatology 2001, 48:251-259.

[39] Bruno S, Silini E, Crosignani A, Borzio F, Leandro G, Bono F, Asti M, Rossi S, Larghi A, Cerino A, Podda M, Mondelli MU. Hepatitis C virus genotypes and risk of hepatocellular carcinoma in cirrhosis: a prospective study. Hepatology 1997, 25:754-758.

[40] Ikeda K, Saitoh S, Koida I, Arase Y, Tsubota A, Chayama K, Kumada H, Kawanishi M. A multivariate analysis of risk factors for hepatocellular carcinogenesis: a prospective observation of 795 patients with viral and alcoholic cirrhosis. Hepatology 1993, 18:47-53.

[41] Degos F, Christidis C, Ganne-Carrie N, Farmachidi JP, Degott C, Guettier C, Trinchet JC, Beaugrand M, Chevret S. Hepatitis C virus related cirrhosis: time to occurrence of hepatocellular carcinoma and death. An International Journal of Gastroenterology & Hepatology 2000, 47:131-136.

[42] Crowe J, Doyle C, Fielding JF, Holloway H, Keegan M, Kelleher D, Kelly P, Leader M, Little M, McDonald G, McCarthy CF, McWeeney J, O'Keane C, Rajan E. Presentation of hepatitis C in a unique uniform cohort 17 years from inoculation [abstract]. Gastroenterology 1995, 108:1054.

[43] Poynard T, Bedossa P, Opolon P. Natural history of liver fibrosis progression in patients with chronic hepatitis C. Lancet 1997, 349:825-832.

[44] Pozzato G, Kaneko S, Moretti M, Croce LS, Franzin F, Unoura M, Bercich L, Tiribelli C, Crovatto M, Santini G, Kobayashi S, Crovatto M, Santini G, Kobayashi S. Different genotypes of hepatitis C virus are associated with different severity of chronic liver disease. Journal of Medical Virology 1994, 43:291-296.

[45] Bruno S, Silini E, Crosignani A, Borzio F, Leandro G, Bono F, Asti M, Rossi S, Larghi A, Cerino A, Podda M, Mondelli MU. Hepatitis C virus genotypes and risk of hepatocellular carcinoma in cirrhosis: a prospective study. Hepatology 1997, 25:754-758.

[46] Sato S, Fujiyama S, Tanaka M, Yamasaki K, Kuramoto I, Kawano S, Sato T, Mizuno K, Nonaka S: Coinfection of hepatitis C virus in patients with chronic hepatitis B infection. Jounal of Hepatology 1994, 21:159-166.

[47] Bosch FX, Ribes J, Borras J. Epidemiology of primary liver cancer. Seminars in Liver Disease 1999, 19:271-285.

[48] Perz JF, Armstrong GL, Farrington LA, Hutin YJ, Bell BP. The contributions of hepatitis B virus and hepatitis C virus infections to cirrhosis and primary liver cancer worldwide. Journal of Hepatology 2006 Oct;45(4):529-38. Epub 2006 Jun 23.

[49] Askarian M, Yadollahi M, Kuochak F, Danaei M, Vakili V, Momeni M. Precautions for health care workers to avoid hepatitis B and C virus infection. International Journal Occupational and Environmental Medicine 2011 Oct;2(4):191-8.

[50] Mahboobi N, Agha-Hosseini F, Mahboobi N, Safari S, Lavanchy D, Alavian SM. Hepatitis B virus infection in dentistry: a forgotten topic. Journal of Viral Hepatitis 2010 May;17(5):307-16.

[51] Jafari S, Buxton JA, Afshar K, Copes R, Baharlou S. Tattooing and Risk of Hepatitis B: A Systematic Review And Meta-Analysis. Canadian Journal of Public Health 2012 May-Jun;103(3):207-12.

[52] Mele A, Corona R, Tosti ME, et al. Beauty treatments and risk of parenterally transmitted hepatitis: results from the hepatitis surveillance system in Italy. Scandinavian Journal of Infectious Diseases 1995;27(5):441–444.

[53] Mariano A, Mele A, Tosti ME, et al. Role of beauty treatment in the spread of parenterally transmitted hepatitis viruses in Italy. Journal of Medical Virology 2004;74(2): 216–220.

[54] Memish ZA, Osoba AO. International travel and sexually transmitted diseases. Travel Medicine and Infectious Disease 2006 Mar;4(2):86-93.

[55] Centers for Disease Control and Prevention. CDC: National Prevention Strategy - A Comprehensive Strategy for the Prevention and Control of Hepatitis C Virus Infection and its Consequences. http://www.cdc.gov/hepatitis/HCV/Strategy/NatHepC-PrevStrategy.htm (accessed 1 October 2012).

[56] Su Y, Norris JL, Zang C, Peng Z, Wang N. Incidence of hepatitis C virus infection in patients on hemodialysis: A systematic review and meta-analysis. Hemodialysis International 2012 Oct 16.

[57] Alter MJ. Epidemiology of hepatitis C virus infection. World Journal of Gastroenterology 2007; 13(17):2436.

[58] Nelson PK, Mathers BM, Cowie B, Hagan H, Des Jarlais D, Horyniak D, Degenhardt L. Global epidemiology of hepatitis B and hepatitis C in people who inject drugs: results of systematic reviews. Lancet 2011 Aug 13;378(9791):571-83.

[59] Roy K, Hay G, Andragetti R, Taylor A, Goldberg D, Wiessing L. Monitoring hepatitis C virus infection among injecting drug users in the European Union: a review of the literature. Epidemiology and Infection 2002;129:577-85.

[60] Mathei C, Buntinx F, van Damme P. Seroprevalence of hepatitis C markers among intravenous drug users in western European countries: a systematic review. Journal of Viral Hepatitis 2002;9:157-73.

[61] Tohme RA, Holmberg SD. Transmission of hepatitis C virus infection through tattooing and piercing: a critical review. Clinical Infectious Disease 2012 Apr;54(8):1167-78.

[62] Amirzargar AA et al. HLA-DRB1, DQA1 and DQB1 alleles and haplotypes frequencies in Iranian healthy adult responders and non-responders to recombinant epatitis B vaccine. Iranian Journal of Immunology 2008, 5:92–99.

[63] Aypak C, Yüce A, Yıkılkan H, Görpelioğlu S. Persistence of protection of hepatitis B vaccine and response to booster immunization in 2- to 12-year-old children. European Journal of Pediatrics 2012 Aug 16.

[64] Zanetti AR, Mariano A, Romanò L, D'Amelio R, Chironna M, Coppola RC, Cuccia M, Mangione R, Marrone F, Negrone FS, Parlato A, Zamparo E, Zotti C, Stroffolini T, Mele A; Study Group. Long-term immunogenicity of hepatitis B vaccination and policy for booster: an Italian multicentre study. Lancet 2005 Oct 15-21;366(9494):1379-84.

[65] Siddiqui MR, Gay N, Edmunds WJ, Ramsay M. Economic evaluation of infant and adolescent hepatitis B vaccination in the UK. Vaccine 2011 Jan 10;29(3):466-75.

[66] Rots NY, Wijmenga-Monsuur AJ, Luytjes W, Kaaijk P, de Graaf TW, van der Zeijst BA, Boog CJ. Hepatitis B vaccination strategies tailored to different endemicity levels: some considerations. Vaccine 2010 Jan 22;28(4):893-900.

[67] Harris A, Yong K, Kermode M. An economic evaluation of universal infant vaccination against hepatitis B virus using a combination vaccine (Hib-HepB): a decision analytic approach to cost effectiveness. Australian and New Zealand Journal of Public Health 2001, 25:222–229.

[68] Verma R, Khanna P, Prinja S, Rajput M, Chawla S, Bairwa M. Hepatitis B Vaccine in national immunization schedule: a preventive step in India. Human Vaccines. 2011 Dec;7(12):1387-8.

[69] Stroffolini T, Guadagnino V, Rapicetta M, Menniti Ippolito F, Caroleo B, De Sarro G, Focà A, Liberto MC, Giancotti A, Barreca GS, Marascio N, Lombardo F, Staltari O; "Sersale's Study" Collaborating Group. The impact of a vaccination campaign against hepatitis B on the further decrease of hepatitis B virus infection in a southern Italian town over 14years. European Journal of Internal Medicine 2012 Sep 13.

[70] Dumolard L at al. Implementation of newborn hepatitis B vaccination – worldwide, 2006. Morbidity and Mortality Weekly Report, 2008, 57:1249–1252.

[71] Rimšelienė G, Nilsen Ø, Kløvstad H, Blystad H, Aavitsland P. Epidemiology of acute and chronic hepatitis B virus infection in Norway, 1992-2009. BMC Infectious Disease 2011 May 26;11:153.

[72] Cho Y, Bonsu G, Akoto-Ampaw A, Nkrumah-Mills G, Nimo JJ, Park JK, Ki M. The prevalence and risk factors for hepatitis B surface ag positivity in pregnant women in eastern region of ghana. Gut and Liver 2012 Apr;6(2):235-40.

[73] El-Raziky MS, El-Hawary MA, Salama KM, El-Hennawy AM, Helmy HM, Fahmy ME, Hassanin FM, El-Karaksy HM. Patterns of hepatitis B infection in Egyptian children in the era of obligatory hepatitis B vaccination. Arab Journal of Gastroenterology 2012 Mar;13(1):1-3.

[74] Narayanswamy K. Hepatitis B and pregnancy: challenges in India. Journal of Indian Medical Association 2011 Oct;109(10):766-7.

[75] Centers for Disease Control and Prevention. CDC: A Comprehensive Immunization Strategy to Eliminate Transmission of Hepatitis B Virus Infection in the United States. Recommendations of the Advisory Committee on Immunization Practices (ACIP) Part 1: Immunization of Infants, Children, and Adolescents. December 23, 2005 / Vol. 54 / No. RR-16.

[76] Centers for Disease Control and Prevention. CDC: A Comprehensive Immunization Strategy to Eliminate Transmission of Hepatitis B Virus Infection in the United States. Recommendations of the Advisory Committee on Immunization Practices (ACIP) Part II: Immunization of Adults. December 8, 2006 / Vol. 55 / No. RR-16.

[77] Halliday J, Klenerman P, Barnes E. Vaccination for hepatitis C virus: closing in on an evasive target. Expert Review of Vaccines. 2011 May;10(5):659-72.

[78] Centers for Disease Control and Prevention. CDC: Recommendations for Prevention and Control of Hepatitis C Virus (HCV) Infection and HCV-Related Chronic Disease. MMWR/October 16, 1998 / Vol. 47 / No. RR-19

[79] Simonsen L, Kane A, Lloyd J, Zaffran M, Kane M. Unsafe injections in the developing world and transmission of bloodborne pathogens: a review. Bulletin of the World Health Organization 1999;77(10):789-800.

[80] Wright NM, Tompkins CN. A review of the evidence for the effectiveness of primary prevention interventions for hepatitis C among injecting drug users. Harm Reduction Journal. 2006 Sep 6;3:27.

[81] Zanetti AR, Romanò L, Bianchi S. Primary prevention of hepatitis C virus infection. Vaccine. 2003 Jan 30;21(7-8):692-5.

[82] De Flora S, Bonanni P. The prevention of infection-associated cancers. Carcinogenesis. 2011 Jun;32(6):787-95.

[83] Albeldawi M, Ruiz-Rodriguez E, Carey WD. Hepatitis C virus: Prevention, screening, and interpretation of assays. Cleveland Clinic Journal of Medicine. 2010 Sep; 77(9):616-26.

[84] Montella M, Crispo A, Giudice A. HCC, diet and metabolic factors: Diet and HCC. Hepatitis Monthly. 2011 Mar;11(3):159-62

Chapter 2

Genomic Heterogeneity of Hepatitis Viruses (A-E): Role in Clinical Implications and Treatment

Zahid Hussain

Additional information is available at the end of the chapter

http://dx.doi.org/10.5772/55231

1. Introduction

Hepatitis is an inflammation of the liver. There are at least five different viruses causing hepatitis. Each of the five major hepatitis viruses, hepatitis A virus (HAV), hepatitis B virus (HBV), hepatitis C virus (HCV), delta hepatitis virus (HDV) and hepatitis E virus (HEV) belong to a separate family. Currently, all these viral hepatitis (A-E) have been classified into different genotypes and subgenotypes. Several factors, including viral genotypes have been reported to be associated with disease progression and treatment response. Consequently, documentation of genotype recently have been proved to be a valuable tool not only for epidemiological reasons but also for clinical implications and treatment.

2. Hepatitis A virus

HAV is a member of the *Hepatovirus* genus of *Picornaviridae* family. HAV is a non-enveloped (naked), linear, single stranded RNA virus of an icosahedral symmetry measuring 27-32 nm in diameter [1]. HAV infection is hyper-endemic in vast areas of the world, with approximately 1.5 million clinical cases per year [2]. The worldwide distribution is uneven and is based on determinants such as socioeconomic conditions and geographic factors [3-5]. In developing countries, the incidence of disease in adults is relatively low because of exposure to the virus in childhood. Most adults in these areas show prevalence of antibodies against hepatitis A. In developed world endemicity is usually very low and clinical cases occur almost exclusively in adults [6,7]. The variable age distribution among hepatitis A patients in developing and developed countries is a consequence of differing standards of hygiene and sanitation. In many developing countries, improved hygiene standards and socio-economic conditions have led to a reduction in exposure to HAV in childhood and hence large non-immune adult population in the community. This leads to a shift or transition from asymptomatic childhood infections to an increased incidence of symptomatic or clinical disease in adults [8]. The persistence of circulating HAV may lead to hepatitis A outbreaks in susceptible non-immune adult population [8,9].

2.1. Disease severity

HAV causes an acute self-limited illness. The vast majority of hepatitis A patients make a full recovery and fatality rate is low. The estimated mortality rate is 0.1% for children less than 15 years old, 0.3% for adults ages 15 to 39, and 2.1% for adults ages 40 and old [10,11]. HAV does not lead to chronic hepatitis or a carrier state and only rarely leads to fulminant hepatic failure (FHF) [12]. FHF occurs during the first 4-6 weeks of illness which is characterized by sudden onset of high fever, marked abdominal pain, vomiting and jaundice followed by development of hepatic encephalopathy associated with deep coma and seizures [13,14]. Mortality is highly correlated with increasing age, survival being rare over the age 45 years [15]. The acute HAV super infection with chronic liver disease is also associated with severity and high mortality [16,17].

2.2. Genomic organization

Like all picornaviral genomes, HAV is divided into three parts: (i) 5′ non-coding region (NCR) that comprises approximately 10% of the genome (ii) single open reading frame (ORF) of 2227 amino acids, that encode all the viral proteins, with regions designated as P1 for capsid proteins, P2 and P3 for non-structural proteins and (iii) short 3′ non-coding region (Fig. 1).

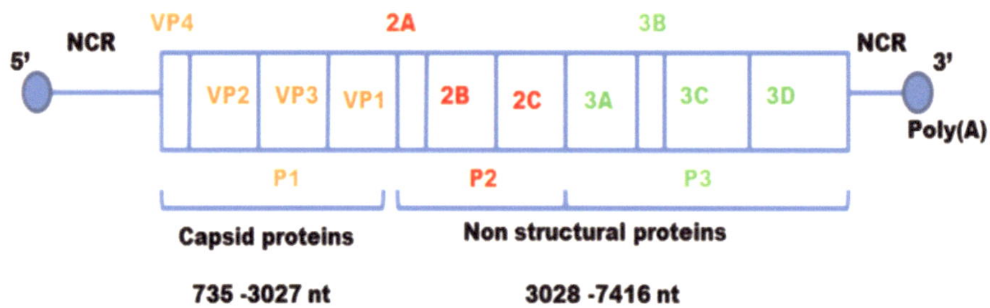

Figure 1. Genomic organization of hepatitis A virus: HAV genome is divided into a 5′ non-coding region (5′ NCR), a giant open reading frame, and a 3' non-coding region (3′ NCR). The coding region is subdivided into regions P1, P2 and P3. (Adapted from: Ref. 20)

HAV RNA genomes lack the cap assembly found at the 5′ end of mRNA species that normally guides the ribosomal complex to the translation start site [18]. Instead, an internal ribosome entry site (IRES) formed by the 5′NCR functions to initiate translations in HAV including other picornaviruses [19, 20]. However, unlike other picornavirus IRESes, the HAV IRES requires an intact eukaryotic initiation factor 4G for its optimal activity [20]. Several other host proteins

http://dx.doi.org/10.5772/55231

are found to be associated with synthetic RNAs representing segments of the 5′ NCR [21]. The viral capsid protein (P1) is further divided into VP4, VP2, VP3 and VP1 regions. The non-structural P2 and P3 polyproteins are divided into 2A, 2B, 2C and 3A, 3B, 3C, 3D respectively (Fig. 1). HAV polyprotein is processed into precursor intermediates and mature proteins by the proteolytic activities of encoded viral proteins. HAV 2A, 2B, 2C protein encodes 45, 251 and 335 amino acids respectively. The 2A and 3C are identified as processing enzyme in hepatitis A virus. The translated 2A regions function as intermediary, partially located on the surface (VP1) and some are assembled inside the virion [20]. Both 2B and 2C proteins play an important role in the replication of the viral RNA. P3 polyproteins encodes 3A, 3B, 3C and 3D proteins with 74, 23, 219 and 489 amino acids respectively. 3C protein acts as sole protease for HAV protein processing, while 3D is the RNA dependent RNA polymerase [22].

2.3. HAV genotypes and geographic distribution

Genetic heterogeneity of hepatitis A has been revealed by sequencing different genome regions, including VP3 carboxyl terminus, the VP1 amino terminus and the VP1/2A junction [23-25] (Fig. 2). The VP3 C-terminal region is relatively conserved, the VP1 amino acid terminus presents an intermediate variability, while VP1/2A junction is more variable and is used to distinguish one strain from another [25]. The genetic variability observed within the putative VP1/2A junction (168 nucleotides) initially defined seven (I-VII) genotypes [26-29]. However, recently new classification of HAV has been done based on the complete sequences of the 900 nucleotides of VP1 region [30] (Fig. 2).

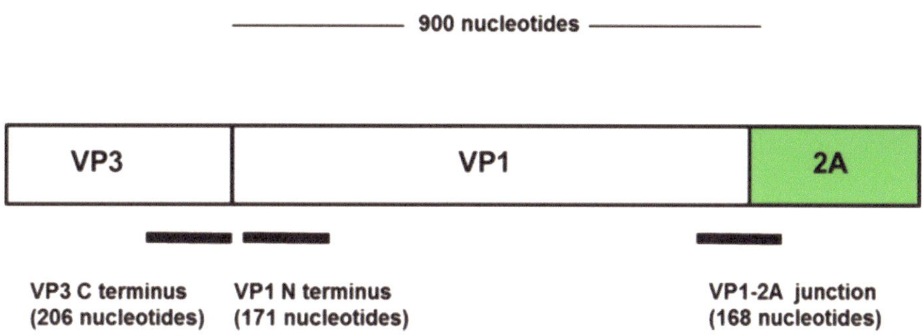

Figure 2. The genomic organization of VP3 C-terminal, the VP1 amino acid terminal and VP1/2A junction region of hepatitis A virus. The complete sequence of the 900 nucleotides of the VP1 gene has been used for new classification of HAV. (Adapted from: Ref. 30)

The phylogenetic analyses of VP1 sequences identified six genotypes (I-VI) that differ among themselves 15-25%. Three isolated from humans (I-III) and three from a simian origin (IV-VI). The genotypes I, II and III were further subdivided into sub-genotypes A and B, which differ in approximately 7.5% of base positions. The worldwide genotype distribution showed genotype I and III comprise the vast majority of human strains within the studied population (Fig. 3). Sub-genotype IA comprises the majority of the human strains studied and constitutes major virus population in North and South America, China, Japan, Russia and Thailand. The sub-genotype IB contains strains from Jordan, North Africa, Australia, Europe, Japan and South America. Most of the remaining human HAV strains segregate into genotype III that is further divided into two sub-genotypes, IIIA, and IIIB [23,27,29]. The sub-genotype IIIA have been subsequently identified in specimens collected from humans with hepatitis A in India, Sri Lanka, Nepal, Malaysia, Sweden and the U.S.A [26,31].The IIIB sub-genotype is responsible for cases of HAV infection in Japan and Denmark.

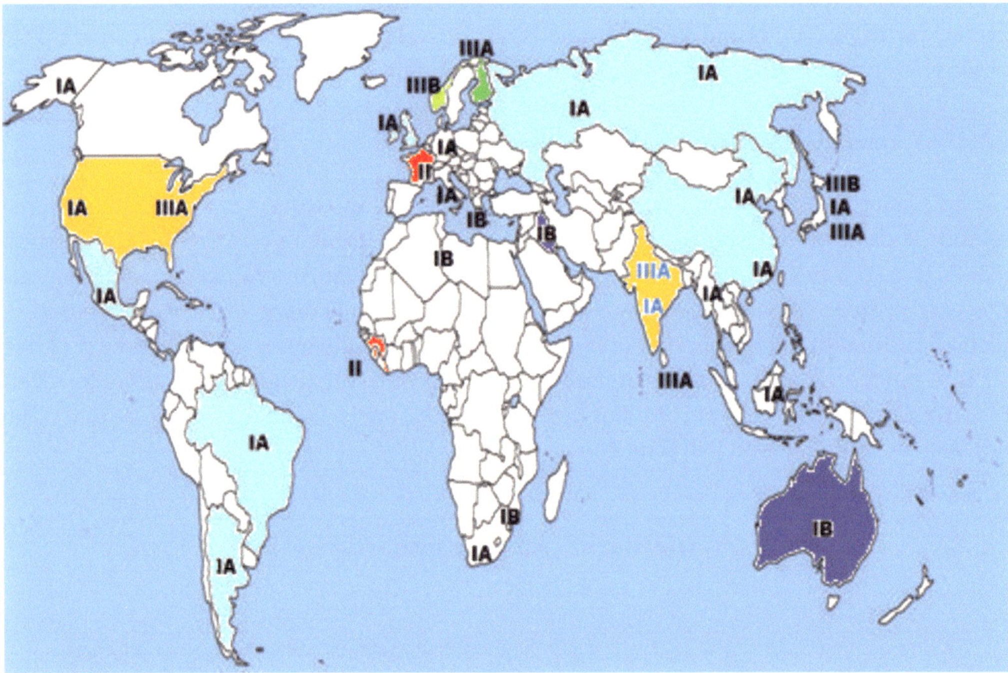

Figure 3. Worldwide distribution of hepatitis A virus genotype(s) according to the VP3 carboxyl terminus, the VP1 amino terminus and the VP1/P2A junction. (Adapted from: Ref. 4, 23, 26, 27, 29, 30 & 31)

2.4. Effect of HAV genotype on disease severity

Although, HAV causes an acute self-limited illness but rarely, it also involved in severe course such as fulminant hepatitis, relapsing hepatitis, prolonged and cholestatic hepatitis. The question arises, if genetic heterogeneity/ genotypes play any role in self-limiting or severe course of the disease. There are contradictory reports regarding the role of HAV genotype in disease severity. Fujiwara *et al.,* [32], reported an association between the severity of hepatitis A and nucleotide variations in the central portion of the 5' NCR of Japanese HAV RNA. Similar study from South Korea reported no association between 5'NCR sequence variations and disease severity [33]. Several other studies also reported no association between genotype or nucleotide changes with disease severity [34-37]. Recently, a comparative analysis of disease severity between genotype 1A and IIIA revealed that the patients with genotype IIIA were older and had high alanine aminotransferase (ALT) levels, prolonged prothrombin times and lower serum albumin level [38]. Another study indicated that co-infection of 2 sub-genotypes (1a and 1b) in a patient with acute hepatitis accounted for the prolonged and severe course of illness [39]. Therefore, additional studies are needed to define the precise role of viral genotypes in the severity of hepatitis A.

2.5. HAV genotype and antiviral treatment response

Since most of the cases are self-limiting, acute HAV does not require antiviral therapy in immunocompetent patients related to any genotype. The immunosuppressed patients should be recommended ribavirin, so that these patients should not progressed to cirrhosis. Liver transplantation is the only treatment option for patients with fulminant hepatic failure due to HAV. Since hepatitis A exists as a single serotype and human is the only host, it is possible to eradicate by selective vaccination against individuals who are susceptible and sero-negative for HAV-IgM.

3. Hepatitis B virus

HBV is a member of the *Hepadnaviridae* family and is known to be one of the smallest human DNA virus [40,41]. HBV infection is very common worldwide with more than 350 million (5%) of the world's population is chronic carriers [42-44]. Most acute infections with hepatitis B virus are self-limited with clearance of virus and development of immunity [45,46]. However, an estimated 5% to 10% of adults and 85% to 95% of children develop chronic hepatitis B virus infection [47].The prevalence of HBV infection varies throughout the world [44,48]. The prevalence of HBV infection in Asia and Africa is high (8%), with perinatal and early childhood transmission resulting in a high rate of chronicity [44,46,48]. The Mediterranean and Eastern Europe have an intermediate (3-5%) endemicity and maintained mainly through sexual, household, nosocomial and perinatal transmission [44,46,48]. The prevalence of chronic infection in some areas of Europe, North America and Australia is less than 1% and disease is mostly transmitted via sexual contact or through intravenous drug use [46].

3.1. Disease severity

Chronic hepatitis B (CHB) is responsible for 1 million deaths per year globally [49]. It is a major cause of cirrhosis of the liver and hepatocellular carcinoma (HCC) worldwide [50,51].The integrity of the host immunological system, viral replication and probably the genetic heterogeneity (genotypes and mutations) of the (HBV) play an important role in the determination of the natural history [52,53]. However, the high morbidity and mortality associated with chronic HBV results in a substantial medical and economic burden on healthcare systems, marking HBV as an international health problem [52,53].

3.2. Genomic organization

HBV is an enveloped virus (42-47 nm in diameter) with an inner icosahedral nucleocapsid containing DNA genome [54]. The viral genome is approximately about 3.2 kb long, partially double-stranded relaxed circular (rc-dsDNA) structure and covalently bond to the viral encoded DNA polymerase [50,55-57]. The HBV genome has a highly compact coding structure consisting of four overlapping reading frames (ORF) designated as P (polymerase), S (surface/envelope), Pre-C/C (core) and X (HBx protein) (Fig. 4) [55,56,58].The polymerase ORF is the largest and it overlaps the X, the core and the pre-S/S. The pre-S/S ORF has 3 initiation codons encoding the small hepatitis B surface protein (SHBs), middle hepatitis B surface protein (preS2 + S) and large hepatitis B surface protein(pre-S1 + pre-S2 + S) proteins. C ORF encodes the core protein (HBcAg) and pre-core or e′ antigen (HBeAg) and it contains an N-terminal extension of 29 amino acids [55,56,58,59].

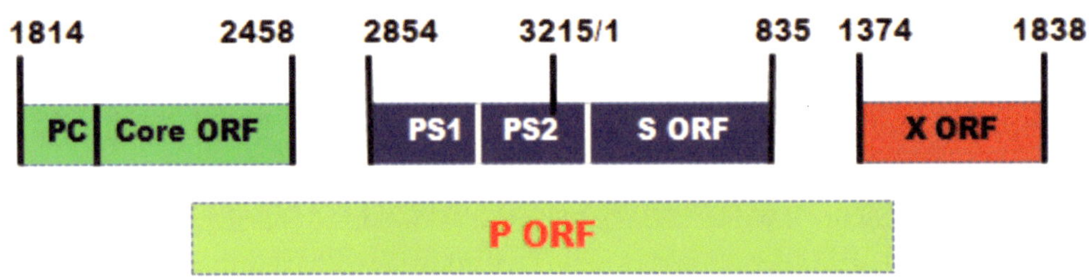

Figure 4. The schematic representation of HBV genome. The circular HBV genome is presented as a linear form. The coding regions for e/core, surface, polymerase and X proteins are designated as Pc/C, S, P and X respectively. (Adapted from: Ref. 59, 55 & 58)

3.3. HBV genotypes and geographic distribution

HBV can be classified into 10 genotypes A to J, based on the comparison of complete HBV genomes [60-64]. These genotypes are based on a divergence of 8% or more in the complete nucleotide sequence of the entire viral genome [61-64]. There are numerous subgenotypes (currently approximately 24) has been identified based on genetic diversity of HBV [65,66]. These subgenotypes were differentiated by a sequence divergence by at least 4% [65,66]. Since genotypic variation of HBV is reflected in a partial sequence of HBV, therefore genotyping of HBV is possible without determining the entire genomic sequence [60,67,68]. As shown in Fig. 5, the S gene is more conserved than the pre-S region, therefore the analysis of the S gene is much more suitable for genotyping. Recently, a fragment of 1306 bp partially comprising HBsAg and polymerase coding regions(S/POL) has also been used for genotyping (Fig. 5) [69]. Several methods have been employed to genotype hepatitis B virus; (a) Direct sequencing [70] (b) Restriction fragment length polymorphism (RFLP) [71] (c) Line Probe Assay (LiPA) [72] (d) Genotype specific PCR [73].

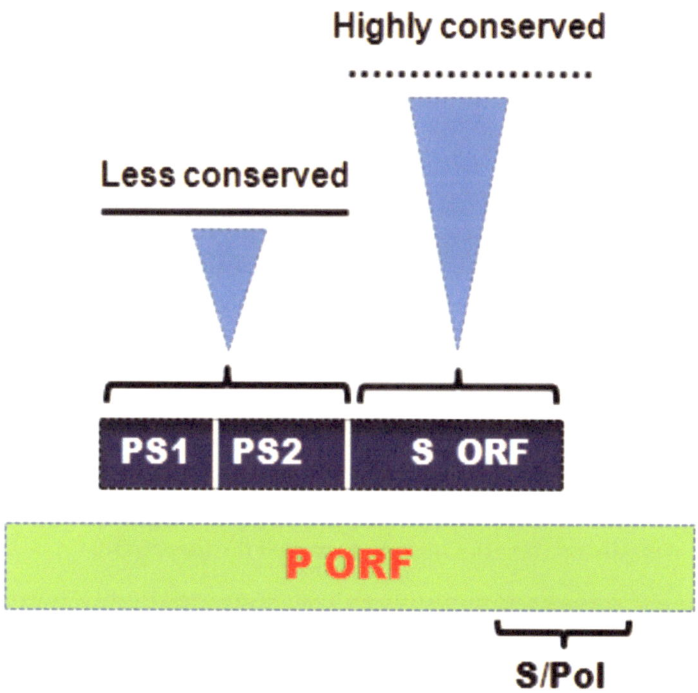

Figure 5. Common genotyping region of HBV genome. The most suitable region for genotyping is S and S/Pol indicated by dotted line (…). (Adapted from: Ref. 60, 67, 68 & 69)

The distribution of HBV genotypes varies across different geographical regions (Fig. 6). HBV Genotype A is most commonly found in the Americas, Africa, India and Western Europe [74, 75]. Genotype B is most common in Asia including Japan, Taiwan, Indonesia, China and Vietnam [76-79]. Genotype C is predominant in East Asia and countries of the Pacific Rim [68], while genotype D most commonly found in the Mediterranean, India, Middle East [75,80-82]. HBV genotype E is mainly identified in sub-Saharan Africa, genotype F in South and Central America as well as Alaska, and genotype G in Central and North America as well as Europe [83-85]. The most recent HBV genotype identified, genotype H, has been found in the United States, Mexico and Central America [86,87]. The genotype F is the most distantly related genetically of the other HBV genotypes (12.8-15.5%) [88]. Recently, genotype I, a novel inter-genotypic recombination among genotypes A, C and G was isolated in Vietnam and Laos [89]. The newest HBV genotype J, was identified in the Ryukyu island in Japan, and this genotype has a close relationship with gibbon, orangutan and human genotype C [90]. The epidemiology of HBV infection is still shifting and the apparent variations in geographical distribution of genotypes is effect of migration from countries with a high prevalence of HBV infection to countries with a lower prevalence.

3.4. Effect of HBV genotypes on disease severity

There are conflicting report about the role of HBV genotypes and severity of the disease. Recent study from Japan demonstrated that genotype B is associated with slower progression to cirrhosis of the liver compared to genotype C [91]. Another study suggested that acute infection with HBV genotype A increases the risk of progression to chronic infection [79,92]. In China, the patients contracted with HBV subtype C2 develops chronic infection more often than those infected with subtype B2 [78,93]. There are conflicting reports from India; one study found that patients infected with genotype D strains had severe chronic liver disease, while another study could not find genotype D strains to be involved in severity [75,94]. Study from East Asia indicated, genotype C as a predominant genotype in subjects with advanced chronic hepatitis (CH), liver cirrhosis (LC) and hepatocellular carcinoma (HCC) [95]. Taiwanese study demonstrated association of genotype C as a risk factor for HCC than genotype B [93,96]. A study from Hong-Kong found that patients infected with genotype B had a higher rate of hepatic decompensation compared to genotype C patients [97]. The HBV patients contracted fulminant hepatitis are more often associated with genotype B [98]. The characteristics of other genotypes (E-J) with disease severity has not been well documented.

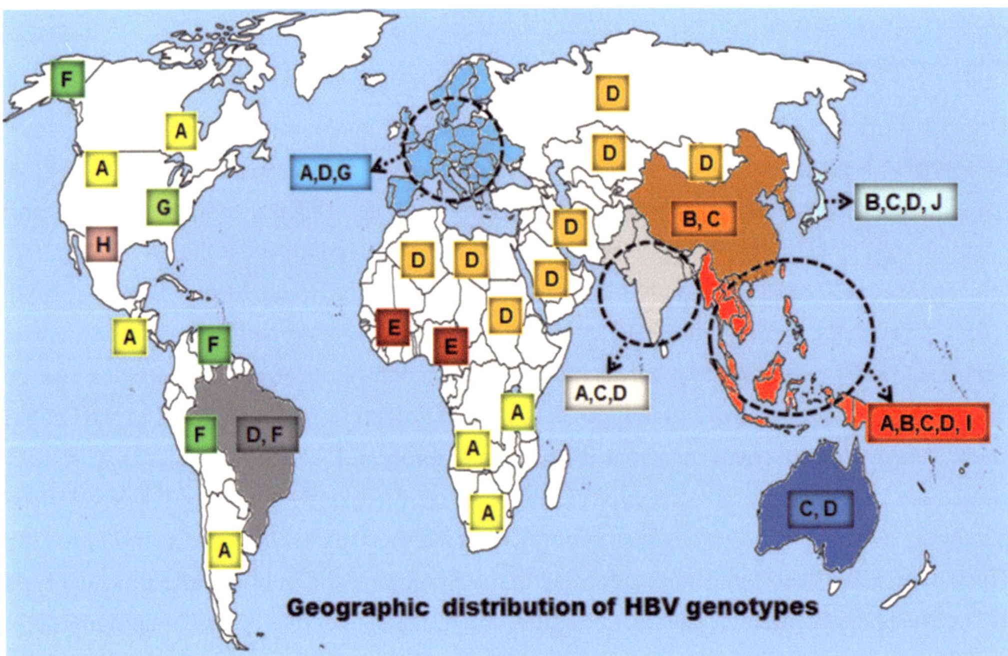

Figure 6. Worldwide geographic distribution of HBV genotypes. (Adapted from: Ref. 68, 74, 75, 77, 79, 81, 82, 83, 84, 86, 87, 88, 89 & 90)

3.4.1. Do genotypes influence seroconversion and seroclearance?

The seroconversion of e' antigen (HBeAg) and seroclearance of surface antigen (HBsAg) are important steps in the natural history of chronic HBV infection [99-102]. Early HBeAg seroconversion typically confers a favorable outcome, while late or absent HBeAg seroconversion after multiple hepatitis flares may accelerate the progression of chronic hepatitis to cirrhosis and hence a poor clinical outcome [99-102]. How these events are influenced by HBV genotypes are subject to a proper understanding and research? Taiwanese study demonstrated that genotype C infection was associated with lower rates of spontaneous HBeAg seroconversion than genotype B [101]. In case of HBsAg seroclearance, the HBV genotypes A and B patients had high frequency compared to genotypes C and D patients [83, 103].

3.4.2. Do genotypes influence frequency of viral mutations?

Several studies revealed that genotypes do influence the frequency of mutations in HBV genetic make-up. The HBV genotype C infections conferred a higher frequency of basal core promoter (BCP) A1762T/G1764A mutation than genotype B [104,105]. Similarly, patients with genotype D infection had a higher prevalence of BCP A1762T/G1764A mutation than those with genotype A infection [106]. The nucleotide(s) deletion within pre-S region is reported to be associated with genotypic variations. The pre-S deletion was higher in genotype C than genotype B patients [107]. In addition, the presence of pre-S deletion was an independent risk factor associated with disease progression as well as HCC development [108-110].

3.5. HBV Genotype and antiviral treatment response

According to different investigators, the nucleotide sequence diversity among different isolates of the virus may play a significant role in response to therapy. The impact of HBV genotype on therapeutic response has been reported in several studies [111,112]. HBV genotype plays a vital role in sustained response (i.e. normalization of serum ALT level and HBeAg seroconversion post treatment) rate. The HBeAg positive patients treated with standard IFN-a, the sustained response rate is significantly better in genotype A and B patients than for genotype C and D [113-116]. Contrary to genotype A-D, patients infected with genotype E–J are rarer and their responses to IFN-based therapy remain largely unknown. In patients treated with nucleos (t) ide analogues, sustained response rate was contradictory in relation to genotype [117,118].

4. Hepatitis C virus

HCV is a small size (55-65 nm), enveloped virus, belong to a member of the family *Flaviviridae* [119,120]. It is mainly transmitted by exposure to contaminated blood or blood products [121,122]. This virus is target specific and replicates in the hepatocytes (liver cells). The initial phase of hepatitis C is called the acute infection [123]. The symptoms of acute HCV infection includes fatigue, jaundice, appetite loss, abdominal pain, nausea and vomiting, joint pain, dark urine and clay-colored stool [124]. Sixty to seventy percent of people in the acute stage have no symptoms and hence most of HCV cases often goes undiagnosed [123,125]. On the other hand, patients who develop symptoms, the average time period between exposure and symptom onset is 4-12 weeks. Fifteen to twenty percent of acute cases spontaneously clear this virus within 2-12 weeks. However, up to 80% of people initially infected with HCV do not clear the virus from their bodies, and continue to have liver disease with 55% develops chronic liver disease [126,127]. Chronic hepatitis C is often silent, most of the times discovered only by routine serological, biochemical and radiological testing [128].

4.1. Disease severity

HCV is a major cause of liver associated disease all over the world with an estimated 3% of the world's populations are chronically infected [129,130]. In some endemic areas, such as the Middle East, North-East Asia and South Africa, the prevalence of HCV infection is as high as 20-30% [122]. Chronic infection often progresses to liver fibrosis, cirrhosis and hepatocellular carcinoma (HCC) in a substantial number of patients [126-128]. The rate of disease progression is variable and several factors have been identified as important in predicting the outcome of progression such as age at infection, gender, genotype/subtype, viral load, and mode of infection.

4.2. Genome organization

HCV viral genome is positive sense RNA with approximately 9.4 kb in length containing a poly (A) tail at the 3'end (Fig. 7). The sequence contained a 5'untranslated region (5'ÚTR) of 341 bases and 3'UTR of about 27 bases [120,131, 132]. The HCV genome has a single open reading frame coding for a polyprotein of 3010 amino acids. The poly-protein is cleaved after translation into structural and non-structural proteins necessary for viral replication and virion formation. The structural proteins situated towards the N-terminus of the genome and non-structural genes located near C-terminal. The 5'UTR is most conserved region of HCV and is pivotal for the initiation of translation and ribosomal binding [133-135]. The structural genes code for the capsid (core) protein (C) and envelope glycoproteins (E1, E2) [133,134]. The first 27 amino acids of the E2 gene constitute the hyper-variable region 1 (HVR1) of the genome and seems to be involved in virus evasion of the immune system and disease progression [136]. The non-structural genes code for a protease (NS2, NS3) and its cofactor (NS4A), a helicase (NS3), a protein of unknown function (NS4B), a phosphoprotein (NS5A), and an RNA-dependent RNA polymerase (NS5B) [137].

The virus replicates in the cytoplasm using an RNA-dependent RNA polymerase that lacks general proofreading ability [138]. This error-prone RNA polymerase is responsible for the genetic variability exhibited by HCV isolates and high spontaneous nucleotide substitution rate with a frequency of 10^{-2} to 10^{-3} substitutions per nucleotide site per year [139]. HCV circulates as a heterogeneous population or quasispecies which differ by 1-5%in nucleotide sequence diversity [140]. Quasispecies permits rapid adaptability of the virus in the event of environmental changes and a clever strategy utilized by the virus to escape selective forces such as nucleotide antiviral agents or the immune system [139,140].

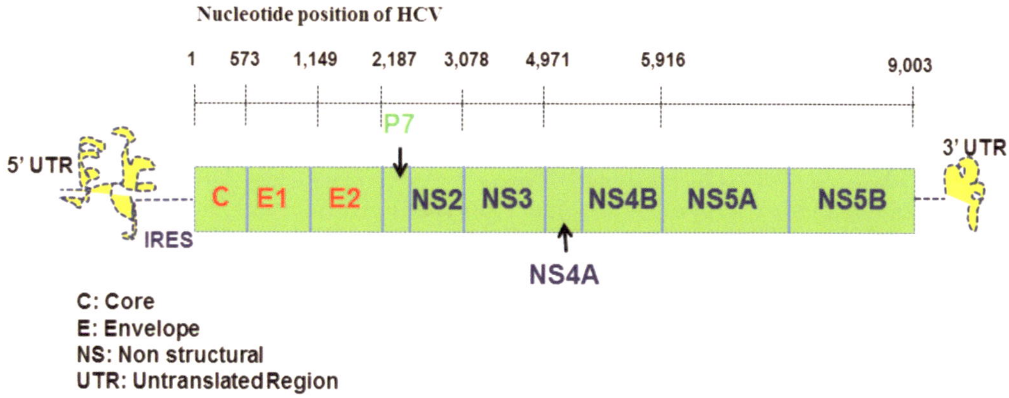

Figure 7. Genomic organization of HCV: The HCV genome contains a single open reading frame (ORF). The genes for structural proteins (C, E1, E2, P7) are situated towards the N-terminus of the ORF. Genes coding for proteins necessary for viral replication are found towards the C-terminus of the ORF. (Adapted from: Ref. 120, 131 & 133)

4.3. HCV genotypes and geographic distribution

The HCV genotype has been determined primarily based on analysis of partial genome sequences. Investigators have typically used sequence analysis of NS5B, core, E1, and 5'UTRs for HCV genotyping (Fig. 8). The most widely accepted classification system of HCV genotyping is that of Simmonds *et al.* 1993 [137]. This system is based on the sequence variability of the 222 base pairs of the NS5B region and it divides HCV isolates into six phylogenetically distinct groups, and more than 80 subtypes. However, following the description of the new genotypes 7-11, Robertson et al., 1998, measured that it was more accurate for the genotypes 7, 8, 9 and 11 to be assigned as subtypes of genotype 6 and the genotype 10 to be a subtype of the genotype 3 [141]. Several methods have been employed to genotype hepatitis C virus; (a) Direct sequencing [140] (b) Restriction fragment length polymorphism (RFLP) [142] (c) Line Probe Assay (LiPA) [143] (d) Genotype specific PCR [144].

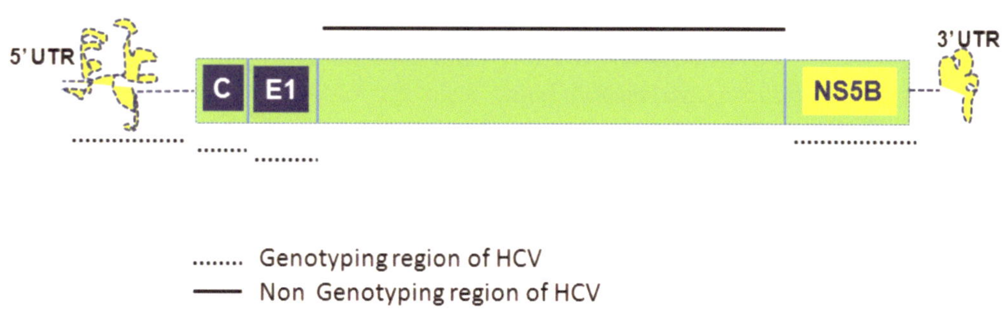

Figure 8. Genotyping region of HCV: The most suitable region for genotyping are 5' UTR, Core (C), E1 and NS5B indicated by dotted (...) line. (Adapted from: Ref. 138, 140, 141, 146 & 147)

At least 6 major genotypes of HCV, each comprising multiple subtypes have been identified worldwide [138,145-147]. Each genotype is separated by sequence divergence in the entire genome exceeding 30%. Substantial regional differences appear to exist in the distribution of HCV genotypes (Fig. 9). Although HCV genotypes 1, 2, and 3 appear to have a worldwide distribution, their relative prevalence varies from one geographic area to another [145]. HCV subtypes 1a and 1b are the most common genotypes in the United States [145]. These subtypes also are predominant in Europe [148]. In Japan, subtype 1b is responsible for up to 73% of cases of HCV infection [149]. Although HCV subtypes 2a and 2b are relatively common in North America, Europe, and Japan, subtype 2c commonly found in northern Italy [146]. HCV genotype 3a is particularly prevalent in intravenous drug abusers in Europe and the United States [150]. HCV genotype 4 appears to be prevalent in North Africa and the Middle East [151, 152], type 5 mainly in South Africa and type 6 principally in Hong Kong and Southeast Asia [137,153]. Mixed genotype infections from a major and a minor HCV population accounts for 4-17% of HCV patients [154].

4.4. Effect of genotype on disease severity

In recent years, substantial evidence has emerged indicating the role of HCV genotypes in disease severity and sensitivity to the antiviral therapy [140,146]. Importantly, patients infected with any of the 6 genotype can develop advanced liver disease, including cirrhosis and HCC. However, some genotypes appear to be more severe compared to the other. For example, Chronic HCV patients infected with genotype 1b is reported to be associated with a more severe liver disease and a more aggressive course compared to genotype 2 (146,155-157]. HCV genotype 1b has also been reported to be associated with the development of advanced liver disease including cirrhosis and hepatocellular carcinoma (HCC) compared to other genotypes (157,158]. However, other investigators failed to arrive at the same conclusions for genotype 1b and therefore further studies are required to elucidate any role of HCV genotype in disease progression or severity [159-162]. A study from India, indicate that most of the chronic hepatitis patients related to genotype 3 is associated with significant steatosis (accumulation of fat within hepatocytes) and fibrosis [163]. Another study report steatosis regardless of genotypes, but resolution of viral infection from genotype 3a patients is associated with disappearance of steatosis and hence genotype 3a and steatosis are interlinked [164]. According to latest statistics 15% of Egyptians are infected with HCV and most of these patients have genotype 4 [165,166]. Genotype 4 has also been associated with a severe disease and increased development of HCC [165]. HCV Genotype 5 is associated with higher mean age compared to other HCV genotype infection [167]. Report from Hong Kong suggested prominence of genotype 6 in patients with thalassemia major and intravenous drug abusers [168].

4.5. HCV genotype and antiviral treatment response

The main objective of therapy administered to patients with chronic hepatitis C is to achieve a Sustained Virological Response (SVR). SVR is characterized by the clearance of serum HCV RNA at the end of therapy and maintained throughout the 6-month follow up period after completion of treatment [169]. The current treatment for HCV infection is two daily doses of

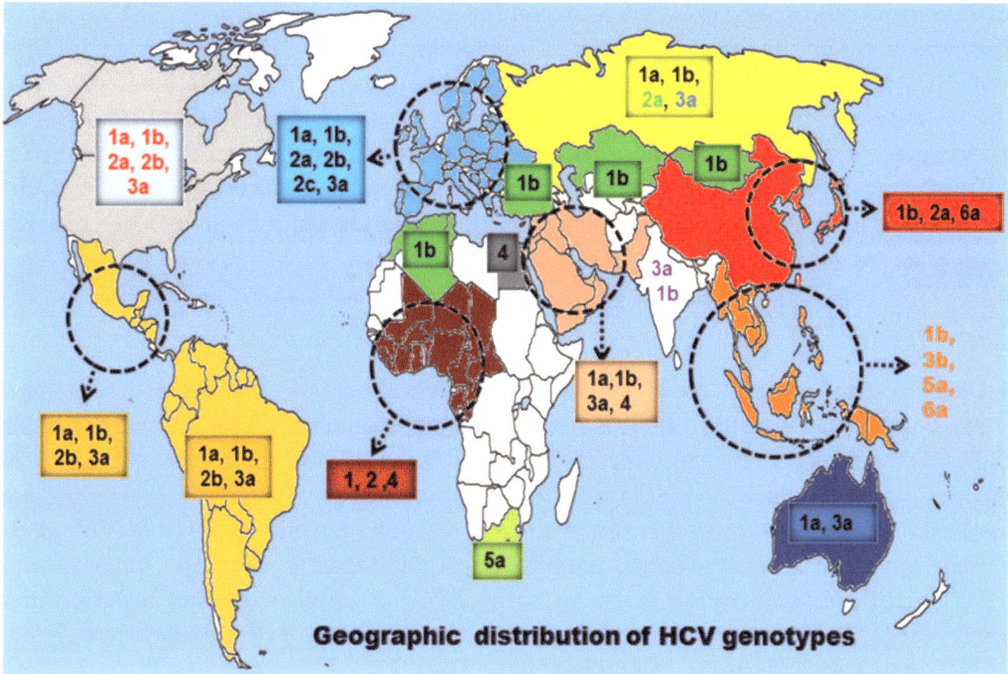

Figure 9. Worldwide geographic distribution of HCV genotypes. (Adapted from: Ref. 138,146,147 & 152)

ribavirin (non-specific anti-viral agent) combined with a weekly injection of interferon-α (standard or pegylated) [170]. The recommended treatment length depends on the virus genotype. Patients with genotypes 2 and 3 are almost three times more likely than patients with genotype 1 to respond to the combination of alpha interferon and ribavirin therapy [129, 164, 171, 172]. Notably, patients with genotype 2 and 3, a 24 week course of combination treatment is adequate, whereas a 48 week course is recommended for genotype 1 [172]. Although, the response of combination therapy against genotype 2 and 3 is better, still there are moderately high percentage of non-responders. The re-treatment response involving combination therapy in non-responders are still better in genotype 2 and 3 (50-60% SVR) compare to genotype 1 (14%) [173]. Genotype 4 presents advance liver disease in patients, and response to Interferon-Ribavirin combination therapy is moderate with ~60% SVR after 48 weeks treatment [174]. Similarly, among genotype 5 patients, the response rate achieved is more than 60% SVR, when treated with Interferon-Ribavirin combination therapy for 48 weeks [175]. HCV genotype 6 responds better to Interferon-Ribavirin combination therapy compare to genotype 1 with treatment duration of 48 weeks [176].

5. Hepatitis D virus

HDV was first discovered in 1977 among a group of patients infected with hepatitis B virus [177]. HDV depends on the HBV to provide hepatitis B surface antigen (HBsAg) for virion assembly and propagation [178]. There are approximately 350 million chronic HBV carriers of the virus, according to the available data 5% (15 million) of these HBV carriers are infected with HDV [179,180]. HDV is highly endemic in Mediterranean countries, Middle East, Central Africa, and northern parts of South America [181]. In contrast, in industrialized countries, its prevalence is low and its transmission is often associated with intravenous drug use [182]. HDV is transmitted through blood and body fluids, quite similar to that of HBV [183]. Hepatitis D symptoms are identical to other viral hepatitis diseases and include jaundice, fever, malaise, dark urine and nausea [183].

5.1. Disease severity

HDV propagates in human hepatocytes as its natural host but only in presence of hepatitis B virus, causing severe acute, fulminant or chronic hepatitis leading to liver cirrhosis [179, 184, 185]. HDV infection can occur either as a co-infection with HBV or as a superinfection in patients with chronic HBV infection [179]. The individuals with HBV-HDV co-infection resulted in more severe acute disease and a higher risk of fulminant hepatitis than HBV alone (1983). Only 2% of co-infected patients resulted in chronic infection [186]. Super infection with HDV in HBV chronic carriers leads to higher incidence of cirrhosis and hepatocellular carcinoma [187]. A factor that may influence the course of disease is the genetic heterogeneity of HDV prevalent in different geographical areas [188].

5.2. Genome organization

The HDV virion is a spherical particle of about 36-nm in diameter, which contains an envelope (HBsAg) and a nucleocapsid containing an RNA genome in complex with HDAg [189-191]. HDV particles consist of a negative sense, circular, single-strand RNA genome, approximately 1.7 kb in length. HDV anti-genome contains a unique open reading frame that encodes the small (sHD) and large hepatitis delta (LHD) proteins. The sHD and LHD correspond respectively to the small-p24 and the large-p27 hepatitis delta proteins [192]. The LHD amino acid sequence is identical to sHD except with the extension of 19 to 20 amino acids at carboxy-terminal end [192, 193]. sHD is required for viral replication and might promote RNA polymerase II elongation of nascent HDV RNA, while LHD inhibits HDV RNA replication and is required for HDV RNA packaging with the HBV envelope protein [194].

5.3. HDV genotypes and geographic distribution

To date researchers have identified 8 major clades or genotypes of hepatitis delta virus based on phylogenetic analysis and are labeled as HDV-1 to HDV-8 [195]. These genotypes are mostly defined based on the analysis of 357 nucleotide semi-conserved region of HDV genome [187,196,197] (Fig. 10).The sequence differences among these genotypes are significant; there is a divergence of 40% in nucleotide sequence and 35% in amino acid sequence of HDAg. Distribution of genotype 1 is ubiquitous which includes European, North American, African, and some Asian isolates [187,196-199]. Genotype 2 has been found in Japan, Taiwan and Yakoutia (Russia) [200]. Genotype 3 has been found exclusively in Central and South

America [187]. Genotype 4 was mostly prevalent in Japan and Taiwan [200,201]. Genotype 5-8 has been exclusively found in Africa [195] (Fig. 11).

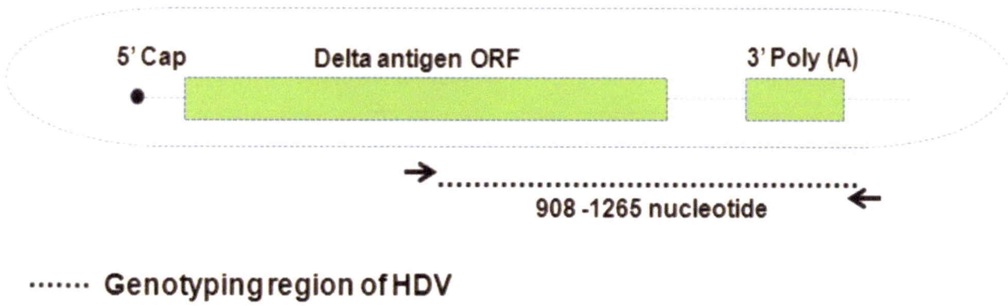

Figure 10. Genotyping region of HDV: The most widely used region for genotyping is spanning 908-1265 nucleotide, which encodes the second half of HDAg protein indicated by dotted line (...). (Adapted from: Ref. 190)

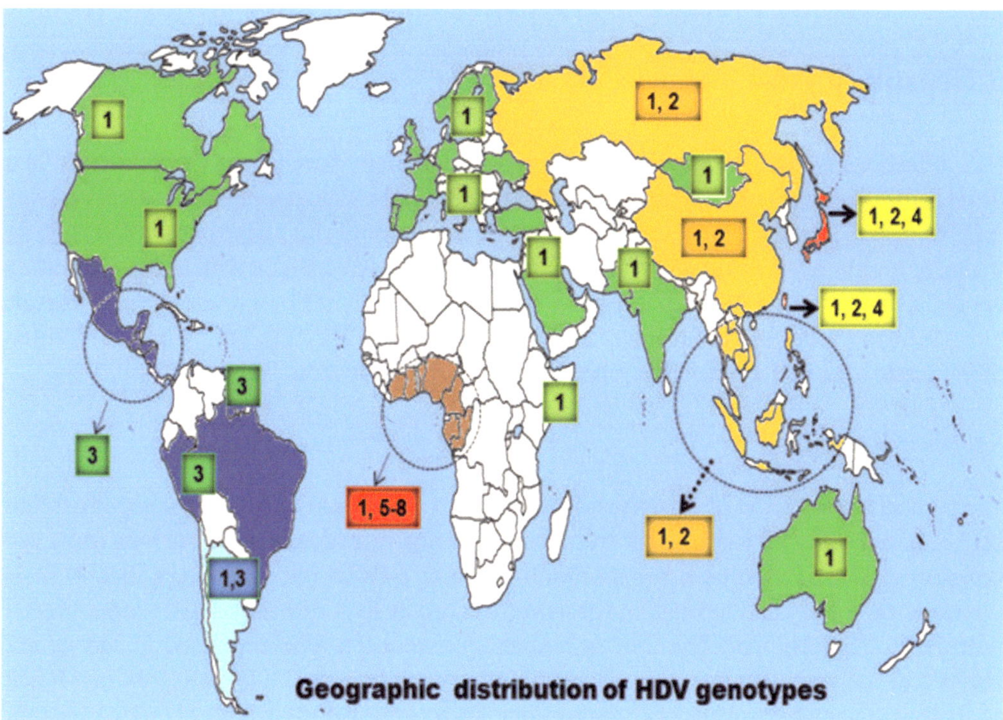

Figure 11. Worldwide geographic distribution of HDV. (Adapted from: Ref. 181 & 195)

5.4. Effect of genotype on disease severity

The genetic variant of hepatitis D virus along with geographical location and transmission route have been identified as important determinants of disease severity [202,203]. At one geographic location genotype 1 has been associated with fulminant hepatitis and hepatocellular carcinoma [196], while in other locality the same genotype have a mild clinical course [197,199]. The diversity observed among genotype HDV-2 has been associated with a less aggressive course, lower ALT values and HDV RNA levels than genotype HDV-1[196,204]. Genotype HDV-3 is endemic in northern South America and is associated with a severe clinical course [184]. Genotype HDV-4 (previously labeled HDV-IIb) also showed variable severity depending upon the geographic location [200,201,205]. Genotype HDV (5-8), mostly observed in African patients, most patients suffered from active chronic hepatitis or cirrhosis [181,195].

5.5. HDV Genotype and antiviral treatment response

There is no specific treatment for HDV infection. Treatment of chronic delta hepatitis is not very effective using long-term administration of high doses of interferon-alpha [206]. It is not known whether some HDV genotypes might be more susceptible to therapy than others. Although, there is no specific vaccine for HDV but vaccination of persons at high risk of acquiring HBV will prevent the acquisition of HDV infection.

6. Hepatitis E virus

HEV infection is a significant public health problem in many parts of the world, especially in developing countries [207-209]. It is estimated that about 2 billion people live in areas endemic for HEV [207,208]. HEV is transmitted via the fecal-oral route and target population includes young to middle aged adults [210]. Patients infected with HEV present with nausea, vomiting, anorexia, jaundice, abdominal pain, fever, and hepatomegaly [211]. It causes large outbreaks of acute hepatitis but usually resolves without any therapy [212-214]. The infected individual therefore develops antibodies that protect against future infection.

6.1. Disease severity

The clinical presentation of this disease ranges from subclinical to fulminant hepatic failure [215,216]. HEV is a major cause of fulminant hepatitis in endemic areas such as India and Bangladesh [216]. Hepatitis E has a mortality rate of 1-4% in the general population [211]. Increased morbidity and mortality is observed in chronic liver disease patients superinfected with HEV [215]. The endemic area is frequently associated with increased incidence and severity in pregnant women with around 15-20% mortality rate [217]. More than one-fourth of affected women have obstetric complications, such as premature rupture of membranes and intrauterine growth restriction [218,219]. It is unknown why HEV causes severe disease in pregnant women.

6.2. Genome organization

HEV is a spherical, non-enveloped virus of about 27–34 nm, classified currently as the sole member of the genus *Hepevirus* in the family *Hepeviridae* [210,220,221]. Its genome is a single stranded, positive-sense 5′capped RNA of approximately 7.2 kb in length [222,223]. It contains three overlapping open reading frames (ORF1, ORF2 and ORF3) flanked by short 5′ and 3′ untranslated regions (UTRs) [224,225] (Fig. 12). The ORF1 encodes a large non-structural protein with several putative functional motifs and domains such as methyltransferase, papain-like cysteine protease (PCP), RNA helicase and RNA dependent RNA polymerase (RdRp) [226]. The ORF2 encodes HEV capsid protein of 660 amino acids and encapsidate the viral RNA genome [227]. The ORF3 of HEV encodes a small protein of 123 amino acids that is essential for viral infectivity *in vivo*. Both the ORF2 and ORF3 proteins are translated from a single bicistronic subgenomic RNA [228].

6.3. HEV genotypes and geographic distribution

Four major genotypes (genotypes 1-4) of mammalian HEV have been identified on the basis of complete genome sequences [229,230]. Recently, partial sequence of HEV conserved region (i.e. ORF1 and ORF2) reflects nucleotide sequence heterogeneity and hence genotyping of HEV is possible without determining the entire genomic sequence [231,232] (Fig. 13). Regions within nucleotides 171–221, 280–310 and 6461–6495 were most conserved and represented the best targets for primer or probe design for genotyping and quantitation [232].

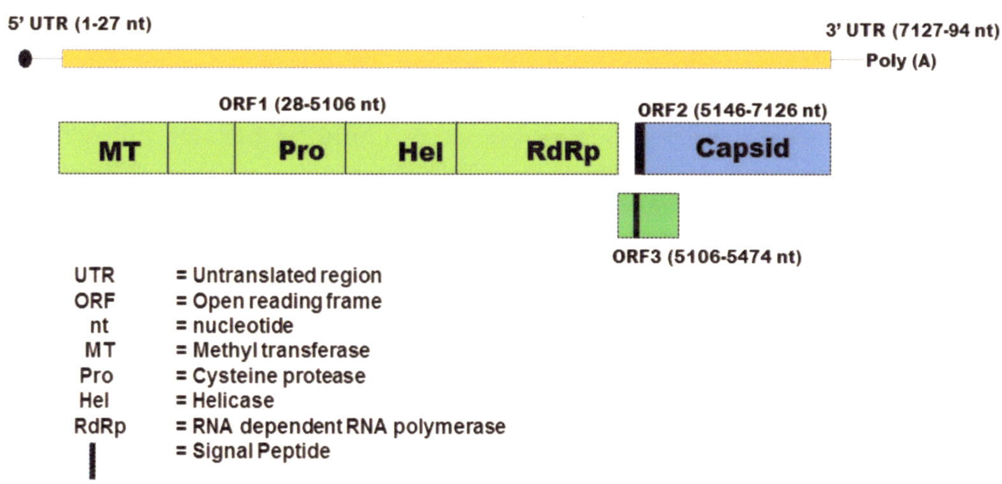

Figure 12. Genomic organization of HEV. HEV RNA is capped at the 5′ untranslated region (UTR) and polyadenylated at the 3′ UTR. ORF1 encodes the nonstructural polyprotein; methyltransferase (MeT), papain-like cysteine protease (PCP), RNA helicase (Hel) and RNA dependent RNA polymerase (RdRp). ORF2 encodes the viral capsid protein. ORF3 encodes a small regulatory phosphoprotein.(Adapted from: Ref. 222, 223 & 224)

Genotype 1 is mostly prevalent in Asia and Africa [230,233,234]. Genotype 2 is found in Central and South America as well in African countries (Fig. 14). Both genotype 1 and 2 outbreaks are the result of efficient human-to-human feco-oral transmission mostly in developing countries [231,234]. In industrialized countries, HEV genotype 1 infection is rare, therefore its presence there is treated as imported infectious disease [231]. Genotype 3 includes human and swine HEV strains from industrialized countries [235,236]. Finally, genotype 4 includes human and swine HEV strains from Asia, particularly China, Taiwan and Japan [234,237]. HEV strains of genotype 3 and 4 are maintained among animal species and occasionally infect humans probably due to inefficient cross-species transmission [235].

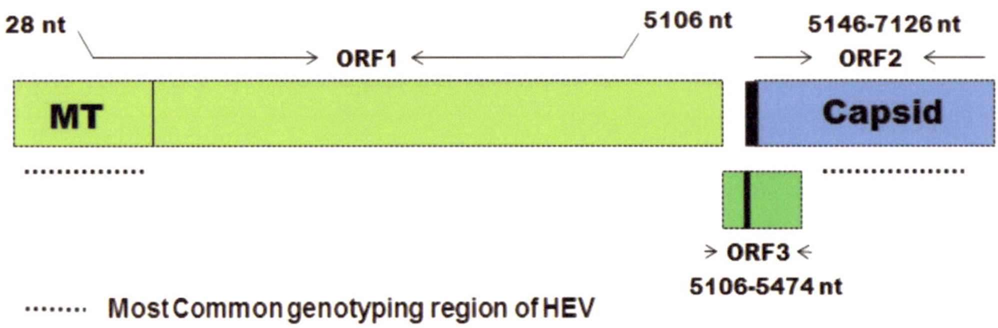

Figure 13. Genotyping region of HEV. The most widely used HEV genomic regions for genotyping are indicated by dotted line (...).

6.4. Genotype variations and disease severity

The severity of HEV associated acute hepatitis not only depends on the status of the host's immune system but also on viral factors such as genotypes. Hepatitis outbreaks in developing countries have been caused primarily by HEV genotype 1. Most of the patients suffering from hepatitis E caused by genotypes 1 are older children and young adults with mortality rate 1%[231,238]. A study from India reported that the viral load of genotype 1was significantly higher in pregnant patients than in non-pregnant patients, and high viral load might be a reason for severe liver disease in pregnant patients [239]. Genotype 2 is Mexican origin and mostly prevalent in central American and African countries, like genotype 1, it is mostly self-limiting. HEV genotype 3 is prevalent in industrialized nations and is rarely pathogenic. Recently, it has been reported that genotype 4 infected patients showed more severe form of the viral hepatitis than genotype 3 [240,241].

Most of the patients in this group belong to older age (~60 years) and the mortality rate is relatively high (6-10%) [231,242]. Japanese study suggested that the silent substitutions of U3148 and C5907 in the genotype 3 and 4 HEV strains are closely associated with the occurrence of fulminant and severe cases and found that C5907 is associated with high HEV load [243]. Thus, the genetic changes in hepatitis E virus genome may affect the effectiveness of virus transmission and hence the severity of HEV-associated hepatitis. Therefore, examination of HEV genotype is considered necessary in order to predict the clinical course and the outcome.

http://dx.doi.org/10.5772/55231

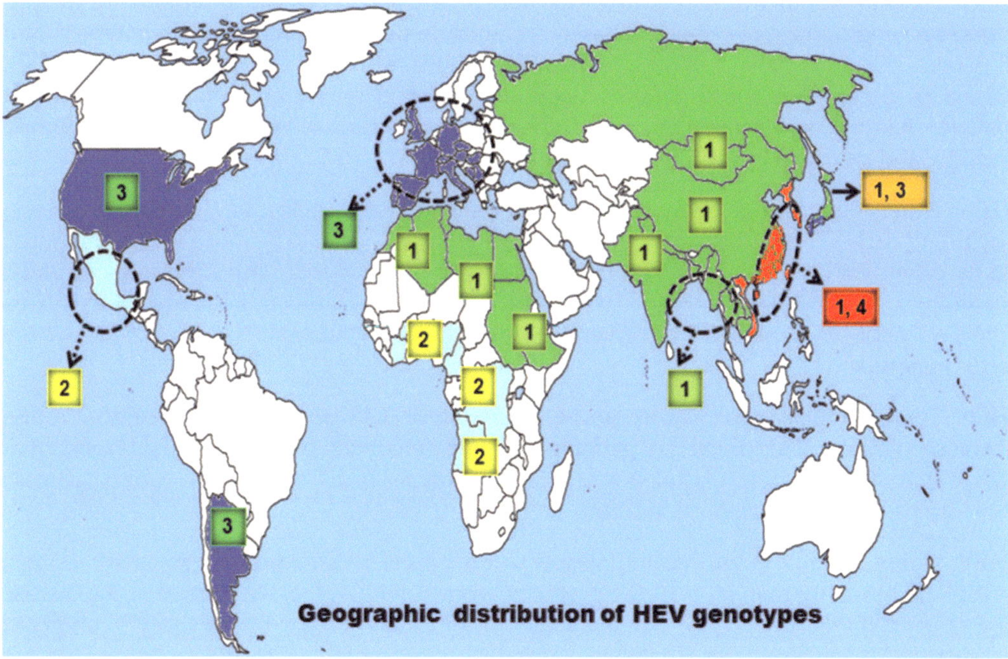

Figure 14. Worldwide geographic distribution of HEV: (Adapted from: Ref. 230,231,233,234 & 236)

6.5. HEV genotype and antiviral treatment response

Since most of the cases are self-limiting, acute HEV does not require antiviral therapy in immunocompetent patients related to any genotype. The immunosuppressed patients should be recommended ribavirin, so that these patients should not progressed to cirrhosis. Liver transplantation is the only treatment option for patients with fulminant hepatic failure due to HEV. All the four mammalian HEV strains belong to one serotype. Thus, only one hepatitis E vaccine is needed for broad protection. The first phase of the immunoprophylaxis of HEV is already tested for safety and immunogenicity [244]. The next phase is to make it available in the market, especially in developing countries so that it should be effectively controlled.

7. Conclusions

The analysis of genomic sequence heterogeneity among different isolates of hepatitis viruses (A-E) may provide an opportunity to decipher the course and pathogenesis of the virus. Although, lot of information are available in this area but still there are many contradictions and discrepancies.

HAV: There are contradictory findings regarding the role of nucleotide substitutions and genotypic variations in disease severity among patients contracted with hepatitis A in different geographical location.

HBV: There are conflicting report about the role of HBV genotypes and severity of the disease based on geographical distribution. Based on multiple studies, compared to genotype A and B patients, C and D patients have a higher risk of disease progression (i.e. cirrhosis & HCC). Similarly, genotype A and B patients responded better to interferon therapy than C and D patients. It is important to note that few studies find no association between genotypes, disease severity and response to treatment regimen.

HCV: Patients infected with any of the 6 HCV genotype can develop advanced liver disease, including cirrhosis and HCC. However, some genotypes appear to be more severe compared to the other. For example, genotype 1b is reported to be associated with a more severe and a more aggressive course compared to genotype 2. Presently, it is recommended all the patients irrespective of genotype should be given treatment, however treatment length depends on the virus genotype.

HDV: There are contradictory outcomes about the role of HDV genotypes and disease severity. At one geographical location HDV genotype 1 is associated with fulminant hepatitis and HCC while at another location it is not severe. Other genotypes of HDV also have variable disease severity based on geographical location.

HEV: Although HEV is self-limiting illness still it causes severe illness in pregnant women with high mortality rate. Most of the pregnant women with aggressive course of the disease are associated with genotype 1. There are lack of information regarding severity in pregnant women and other genotypes. There are contradictory report regarding the severity of disease and genotype 3 and 4, although a report from Japan suggests, silent substitutions of U3148 and C5907 in the genotype 3 and 4 with response to fulminant hepatitis.

Therefore, the genomic heterogeneity of hepatitis viruses is not the only critical factor that leads to disease progression, severity and final outcome. Hence, in combination with viral genomic heterogeneity other factors such as age, sex, geographical distribution, genetic polymorphism and host immune elements may play a vital role in deciding the clinical implications and final outcome of the infection.

Author details

Zahid Hussain*

Centre of Excellence in Biotechnology Research, King Saud University, Riyadh, Saudi Arabia

References

[1] Feinstone, S, Kapikian, M, Purcell, A, Z, & Hepatitis, R, H. A: detection by immune electron microscopy of a virus like antigen associated with acute illness. *Science*, 182, 1026

[2] World Health Organization(2000). Hepatitis A vaccines. *Wkly Epidemiol Rec* , 75, 38-44.

[3] Craig, A, & Schaffner, S. W. ((2004). Prevention of hepatitis A with the hepatitis A vaccine. *N Engl J Med350476481*

[4] Wasley, A, Fiore, A, Bell, B, & Hepatitis, P. A in the era of vaccination. *Epidemiol Rev. 28101111*

[5] Jacobsen, K, Wiersma, H, & Hepatitis, S, T. A virus seroprevalence by age and world region, 1990 and 2005. *Vaccine 2866536657*

[6] Feinstone, S.M. 1996 Hepatitis A Epidemiology and prevention. *Eur J Gastroenterol Hepatol* , 8, 300-5.

[7] Marinho, R, Valente, T, Ramalho, A, R, & De Moura, F,J. M, C. ((1997). The changing epidemiological pattern of hepatitis A in Lisbon, Portugal. *Eur J Gastroenterol Hepatol* , 9, 795-797.

[8] Hussain, Z, Das, B, Husain, C, Murthy, S, A, & Kar, N, S. Increasing trend of acute hepatitis A in north India: need for identification of high-risk population for vaccination. *J Gastroenterol Hepatol 21*, 689-693, 2006.

[9] Arankalle, V, Chadha, A, Chitambar, M, S, Walimbe, S, D, Chobe, A, M, & Gandhe, L, P. S, S. ((2001). Changing epidemiology of hepatitis A and E in urban and rural India (1982-1998). *J Viral Hepat 8293303*

[10] Hollinger, F. B, & Ticehurst, J.R. 1996 Hepatitis A Virus*Fields Virology*, 3rded.; Fields, B.N., Knipe, D.M., Howley, O.M., *et al.* Eds.; Lippincott Williams & Wilkins: Philadelphia, NY, USA, , 735-782.

[11] Debray, D, Cullufi, P, Devictor, D, Fabre, M, & Bernard, O. (1997). Liver failure in children with hepatitis A. *Hepatology* , 26, 1018-1022.

[12] Koff, R, Hepatitis, S, & , A. 351, 1643-1649.

[13] Grady, O, Schalm, J, G, & Williams, S,W. R. ((1993). Acute liver failure: redefining the syndromes. *Lancet, 273275*, 342

[14] Takashaki, Y, & Okuda, K. (1993). Fulminant and subfulminant hepatitis in Japan. *Indian J Gastroenterol121921*

[15] Acharya, S, Dasarathy, K, Kumer, S, et al. (1996). Fulminant hepatitis in a tropical population: clinical course, cause, and early predictors of outcome. *Hepatology, 23*, 1448-1455.

[16] Keeffe, E. B. ((1995). Is hepatitis A more severe in patients with chronic hepatitis B and other chronic liver disease? *Am J Gastroenterol* , 90, 201-205.

[17] Vento, S, Garofano, T, Rezzini, C, Cainelli, F, Casali, F, Ghirozi, G, Ferraro, T, & Concai, E. (1998). Fulminant hepatitis associated with hepatitis A virus superinfection in patients with chronic C. *N Engl J Med,* , 29, 286-290.

[18] Najarian, R, Caput, D, Gee, W, et al. (1985). Primary structure and gene organization of human hepatitis A virus. *Proc. Natl. Acad. Sci. USA8226272631*

[19] Borman, A, & Kean, M. K, M. (1997). Intact eukaryotic initiation factor 4G is required for hepatitis A virus internal initiation of translation. *Virology237129136*

[20] Totsuka, A, & Moritsugu, Y. (1999). Hepatitis A virus proteins. *Intervirology426368*

[21] Chang, K, Brown, H, & Lemon, E, A. S, M. ((1993). Cell type specific proteins which interact with the 5) non translated region of hepatitis A virus RNA. *J Virol* , 67, 6716-6725.

[22] Schultheiss, T, Kusov, Y, Gauss-muller, Y, & Proteinase, V. C of hepatitis A virus (HAV) cleaves the HAV polyprotein at all sites including VP1/2A and 2A/2B. *Virology198*, 275-281, 2-P3.

[23] Cohen, J. I, Ticehurst, J. R, Purcell, R. H, Buckler-white, A, & Baroudy, B. M. (1987). Complete nucleotide sequence of wild type hepatitis A virus: comparision with different strains of hepatitis A virus and other picornaviruses. *J Virol615059*

[24] Arauz-ruiz, P, Sundqvist, L, Garcia, Z, Taylor, L, Visona, K, Norder, H, & Magnius, L. O. (2001). Presumed common source outbreaks of hepatitis A in an endemic area confirmed by limited sequencing within the VP1 region. *J Med Virol 65449456*

[25] Costa-mattioli, M, Cristina, J, Romero, H, et al. (2002). Molecular evolution of hepatitis A virus: a new classification based on the complete VP1 protein. *J Virol7695169525*

[26] Khanna, B, Spelbring, J. E, Innis, B. L, & Robertson, B. H. (1992). Characterization of a genetic variant of human hepatitis A virus. *J Med Virol36118124*

[27] Robertson, B. H, Jansen, R. W, & Khanna, B. (1992). Genetic relatedness of hepatitis A virus strains recovered from different geographical regions. *J Gen Virol 7313651377*

[28] Ching, K. Z, Nakano, T, Chapman, L. E, Demby, A, & Robertson, B. H. (2002). Genetic characterization of wild-type genotype VII hepatitis A virus. *J Gen Virol 835360*

[29] Jansen, R. W, Siegl, G, & Lemon, S. M. (1990). Molecular epidemiology of human hepatitis A virus defined by an antigen-capture polymerase chain reaction method. *Proc. Natl. Acad. Sci. USA8728672871*

[30] Costa-mattioli, M. Di Napoli, A., Ferre, V., Billaudel, S., Perez-Bercoff, R., Cristina, J. (2003). Genetic variability of hepatitis A virus. *J Gen Virol 8431913201*

[31] Hussain, Z, Das, B. C, Husain, S. A, et al. (2005). Hepatitis A viral genotypes and clinical relevance: Clinical and molecular characterization of hepatitis A virus isolates from northern India. *Hepatol Res 321624*

[32] Fujiwara, K, Yokosuka, O, Ehata, T, et al. (2002). Association between severity of type A hepatitis and nucleotide variations in the 5′ non-translated region of hepatitis A virus RNA: strains from fulminant hepatitis have fewer nucleotide substitutions. *Gut 5*, 82-88.

[33] Kanda, T, Jeong, S. H, Imazeki, F, Fujiwara, K, & Yokosuka, O. (2010). Analysis of 5′ non-translated region of hepatitis A viral RNA genotype I from South Korea: comparison with disease severities. *PLoS One* 5, e15139

[34] Fujiwara, K, Yokosuka, O, Imazeki, F, et al. (2003). Analysis of the genotype determining region of hepatitis A viral RNA in relation to disease severities. *Hepatol Res* , 25, 124-134.

[35] Rezende, G, Roque-afonso, A. M, Samuel, D, et al. (2003). Viral and clinical factors associated with the fulminant course of hepatitis A infection. *Hepatology* , 38, 613-618.

[36] Normann, A, Jung, C, Vallbracht, A, & Flehmig, B. (2004). Time course of hepatitis A viremia and viral load in the blood of human hepatitis A patients. *J Med Virol* , 72, 10-16.

[37] Tjon, G. M, & Coutinho, R. A. van den Hoek A et al. ((2006). High and persistent excretion of hepatitis A virus in immunocompetent patients. *J Med Virol 78*, 1398-1405.

[38] Yoon, Y. K, Yeon, J. E, Kim, J. H, et al. (2011). Comparative analysis of disease severity between genotypes IA and IIIA of hepatitis A virus. *J Med Virol* , 83, 1308-1314.

[39] Coppola, N, Genovese, D, Pisaturo, M, et al. (2007). Acute hepatitis with severe cholestasis and prolonged clinical course due to hepatitis A virus Ia and Ib coinfection. *Clin Infect Dis* 44, ee77, 73.

[40] Tiollais, P, Pourcel, C, & Dejean, A. (1985). The hepatitis B virus. *Nature 317*, 489-495.

[41] Zuckerman, A. J. (1996). Hepatitis viruses. In Baron S, *et al.*. *Baron's Medical Microbiology* (4th ed.). University of Texas Medical Branch

[42] Tibbs, C. J, & Smith, H. M. (2001). Clinicians guide to viral hepatitis. 1st Edition. Arnold

[43] Kao, J. H, & Chen, D. S. (2002). Global control of hepatitis B virus infection. *Lancet Infect Dis 2*, 395-403.

[44] Hou, J, Liu, Z, & Gu, F. (2005). Epidemiology and Prevention of Hepatitis B Virus Infection. *International Journal of Medical Sciences* , 2, 50-57.

[45] Lee, W. M. (1997). Hepatitis B virus infection. *N Engl J Med* , 337, 1733-1745.

[46] Alter, M. J. (2003). Epidemiology and prevention of hepatitis B. *Semin liver Dis* , 23, 39-46.

[47] Gust, I, & Crowe, S. (1986). The global importance of viral hepatitis. Clin Trop Med Commun Dis , 1, 281-301.

[48] Custer, B, Sullivan, S. D, Hazlet, T. K, Iloeje, U, Veenstra, D. L, & Kowdley, K. V. (2004). Global epidemiology of hepatitis B virus. *J Clin Gastroenterol* 38, SS168, 158.

[49] Kidd-ljunggren, K, Myhre, E, & Bläckberg, J. (2004). Clinical and serological variation between patients infected with different Hepatitis B virus genotypes. *J Clin Microbiol* , 42, 5837-5841.

[50] Kao, J. H. (2003). Hepatitis B virus genotypes and hepatocellular carcinoma in Taiwan. *Intervirology 46*, 400-407.

[51] Fattovich, G, Stroffolini, T, Zagni, I, & Donato, F. (2004). Hepatocellular carcinoma in cirrhosis: incidence and risk factors. *Gastroenterology* 127, S, 35-50.

[52] Locarnini, S. A. (2002). Clinical relevance of viral dynamics and genotypes in hepatitis B virus. *Journal of Gastroenterology & Hepatology* 17, SS328, 322.

[53] Lavanchy, D. (2004). Hepatitis B virus epidemiology, disease burden, treatment, and current and emerging prevention and control measures. *Journal of Viral Hepatitis 11*, 97-107.

[54] Summers, J, & Mason, W. S. (1982). Replication of the genome of a hepatitis B-like virus by reverse transcription of an RNA intermediate. *Cell 29*, 403-415.

[55] Locarnini, S. (2004). Molecular virology of hepatitis B virus. *Semin Liver Dis* , 24, 3-10.

[56] Beck, J, & Nassal, M. (2007). Hepatitis B virus replication. *World J Gastroenterol* , 13, 48-64.

[57] Jilbert, A. R, Burrell, C. J, Triatni, M, & Kann, M. (2002). Hepatitis B virus replication. In *Hepatitis B Virus,* Edited by Lai C-L & Locarnini S. London: International Medical Press, 43-53.

[58] Seeger C & Mason WS(2000). Hepatitis B virus biology. *Microbiology & Molecular Biology Reviews* , 64, 51-68.

[59] Wu, H. L, Huang, L. R, Huang, C. C, et al. (2005). RNA interference-mediated control of hepatitis B virus and emergence of resistant mutant. *Gastroenterology* , 128, 708-716.

[60] Okamoto, H, Tsuda, F, Sakugawa, H, Sastrosoewignjo, R. I, Imai, M, Miyakawa, Y, & Mayumi, M. (1988). Typing hepatitis B virus by homology in nucleotide sequence: Comparison of surface antigen subtypes. *J Gen Virol* , 69, 2575-2583.

[61] Cao, G. W. (2009). Clinical relevance and public health significance of hepatitis B virus genomic variations. *World J Gastroenterol 15*, 5761-5769.

[62] Mcmahon, B. J. (2009). The influence of hepatitis B virus genotype and subgenotype on the natural history of chronic hepatitis B. *Hepatol Int 333442*

[63] Kurbanov, F, Tanaka, Y, & Mizokami, M. (2010). Geographical and genetic diversity of the human hepatitis B virus. *Hepatol Res 401430*

[64] Lin, C. L, & Kao, J. H. (2011). The clinical implications of hepatitis B virus genotype: Recent advances. *J Gastroenterol Hepatol* , 1, 123-30.

[65] Kao, J. H. (2002). Clinical relevance of hepatitis B viral genotypes: a case of deja vu? *Journal of Gastroenterology & Hepatology 17113115*

[66] Norder, H, Courouce, A. M, Coursaget, P, Echevarria, J. M, Lee, S. D, Mushahwar, I. K, & Robertson, B. H. Locarnini S & Magnius LO. ((2004). Genetic diversity of hepatitis B virus strains derived worldwide: genotypes, subgenotypes, and HBsAg subtypes. *Intervirology 47289309*

[67] Magnius LO & Norder H(1995). Subtypes, genotypes and molecular epidemiology of the hepatitis B virus as reflected by sequence variability of the S-gene. *Intervirology 382434*

[68] Mahtab, M. A, Rahman, S, Khan, M, & Karim, F. (2008). Hepatitis B virus genotypes: an overview. *Hepatobiliary Pancreat Dis Int* , 7, 457-464.

[69] Alvarado Mora MV, Romano CM, Gomes-Gouvea MS, Gutierrez MF, Botelho L, Carrilho FJ, Pinho JRR. ((2011). Molecular characterization of the Hepatitis B virus genotypes in Colombia: A Bayesian inferences on the genotype F. *Infection, genetics and Evolution* , 11, 103-108.

[70] Stuyver, L, De Gendt, S, Van Geyt, C, Zoulim, F, Fried, M, Schinazi, R. F, & Rossau, R. (2000). A new genotype of hepatitis B virus: completegenome and phylogenetic relatedness. *J Gen Virol 816774*

[71] Mizokamia, M, Nakanob, T, Oritob, E, Tanakab, Y, Sakugawac, H, Mukaided, M, Robertsone, H, & Hepatitis, B. B virus genotype assignment using restriction fragment length polymorphism patterns. *FEBS Letters 4506671*

[72] Grandjacques, C, Pradat, P, Stuyver, L, Chevallier, M, Chevallier, P, Pichoud, C, Maisonnas, M, Trepo, C, & Zoulim, F. (2000). Rapid detection of genotypes and mutations in the pre-core promoter and the pre-core region of hepatitis B virus genome: correlation with viral persistence and disease severity. *J Hepatol 33*, 430-439.

[73] Naito, H, Havashi, S, & Abe, K. (2001). Rapid and specific genotyping system for hepatitis B virus corresponding to six major genotypes by PCR using type-specific primers. *J Clin Microbiol 39*, 1686

[74] Chu, C. J, Keeffe, E. B, Han, S. H, Perrillo, R. P, Min, A. D, Soldevila-pico, C, et al. (2003). Hepatitis B virus genotypes in the United States: results of a nationwide study. *Gastroenterology* , 125, 444-451.

[75] Kumar, A, Kumar, S. I, Pandey, R, Naik, S, & Aggarwal, R. (2005). Hepatitis B virus genotype A is more often associated with severe liver disease in northern India than is genotype D. *Indian J Gastroenterol* , 24, 19-22.

[76] Sugauchi, F, Orito, E, Ichida, T, Kato, H, Sakugawa, H, Kakumu, S, Ishida, T, Chutaputti, A, Lai, C. L, Ueda, R, Miyakawa, Y, & Mizokami, M. (2002). Hepatitis B virus

of genotype B with or without recombination with genotype C over the precore region plus the core gene. *J Virol* , 76, 5985-5992.

[77] Lin, C. L, Chen, J. D, & Liu, C. J. (2007). Clinicopathological differences between hepatitis B viral genotype B- and C-related resectable hepatocellular carcinoma. *J Viral Hepat* 2007; , 14, 64-69.

[78] Zhang, H. W, Yin, J. H, & Li, Y. T. (2008). Risk factors for acute hepatitis B and its progression to chronic hepatitis in Shanghai, China. *Gut 5717131720*

[79] Matsuura, K, Tanaka, Y, & Hige, S. (2009). Distribution of hepatitis B virus genotypes among patients with chronic infection in Japan shifting toward an increase of genotype A. *J Clin Microbiol 4714761483*

[80] Arankalle, V. A, Murhekar, K. M, Gandhe, S. S, Murhekar, M. V, & Ramdasi, A. Y. Padbidri VS & Sehgal SC. ((2003). Hepatitis B virus: predominance of genotype D in primitive tribes of the Andaman and Nicobar islands, India (1989-1999). *J Gen Virol 8419151920*

[81] Chattopadhyay, S, Das, B. C, Hussain, Z, & Kar, P. (2006). Hepatitis B virus genotypes in acute and fulminant hepatitis patients from north India using two different molecular genotyping approaches. *Hepatol Res* , 35, 79-82.

[82] Abdo, A. A, Al-jarallah, B. M, Sanai, F. M, Hersi, A. S, Al-swat, K, Azzam, N. A, Al-dukhayil, M, Al-maarik, A, & Al-faleh, F. Z. (2006). Hepatitis B genotypes: relation to clinical outcome in patients with chronic hepatitis B in Saudi Arabia. *World J Gastroenterol 1270197024*

[83] Sanchez-tapias, J. M, Costa, J, & Mas, A. Bruguera M & Rodes J. ((2002). Influence of hepatitis B virus genotype on the long-term outcome of chronic hepatitis B in western patients. *Gastroenterology 12318481856*

[84] Pineiro YLFGMbayed VA and Campos RH. ((2003). Evolutionary history of hepatitis B virus genotype F: an in-depth analysis of argentine isolates. *Virus Genes 27103110*

[85] Suzuki, S, Sugauchi, F, Orito, E, Kato, H, Usuda, S, Siransy, L, Arita, I, Sakamoto, Y, Yoshihara, N, & Gohary, A. Ueda R & Mizokami M. ((2003). Distribution of hepatitis B virus (HBV) genotypes among HBV carriers in the Cote d'Ivoire: complete genome sequence and phylogenetic relatedness of HBV genotype E. *J Med Virol* , 69, 459-465.

[86] Arauz-Ruiz, Norder PH, Robertson BH, Magnius LO, Genotype H. ((2002). A new Amerindian genotype of hepatitis B virus revealed in Central America. *J Gen Virol 8320592073*

[87] Kato, H, Gish, R. G, Bzowej, N, Newsom, M, Sugauchi, F, Tanaka, Y, Kato, T, Orito, E, Usuda, S, & Ueda, R. Miyakawa Y& Mizokami M. ((2004). Eight genotypes (A-H) of hepatitis B virus infecting patients from San Francisco and their demographic, clinical, and virological characteristics. *J Med Virol 73516521*

[88] Devesa, M, Loureiro, C. L, Rivas, Y, Monsalve, F, Cardona, N, Duarte, M. C, Poblete, F, Gutierrez, M. F, Botto, C, & Pujol, F. H. (2008). Subgenotype diversity of hepatitis B virus American genotype F in Amerindians from Venezuela and the general population of Colombia. *J Med Virol* , 80, 20-26.

[89] Thuy, P. T, Alestig, E, Liem, N. T, Hannoun, C, & Lindh, M. C recombinant (putative genotype I) of hepatitis B virus is rare in Hanoi, Vietnam-genotypes B4 and C1 predominate. *J Med Virol* , 82, 1327-1333.

[90] Tatematsu, K, Tanaka, Y, & Kurbanov, F. (2009). A genetic variant of hepatitis B virus divergent from known human and ape genotypes isolated from a Japanese patient and provisionally assigned to new genotype J. *J Virol 831053847*

[91] Sumi, H, Yokosuka, O, Seki, N, Arai, M, Imazeki, F, Kurihara, T, et al. (2003). Influence of hepatitis B virus genotypes on the progression of chronic type B liver disease. *Hepatology* , 37, 19-26.

[92] Suzuki, Y, Kobayashi, M, & Ikeda, K. (2005). Persistence of acute infection with hepatitis B virus genotype A and treatment in Japan. *J MedVirol 76*, 33-39.

[93] Kao, J. H, Chen, P. J, Lai, M. Y, & Chen, D. S. (2000). Hepatitis B genotypes correlate with clinical outcomes in patients with chronic hepatitis B. *Gastroenterology* , 118, 554-559.

[94] Thakur, V, Guptan, R. C, Kazim, S. N, Malhotra, V, & Sarin, S. K. (2002). Profile, spectrum and significance of HBV genotypes in chronic liver disease patients in the Indian subcontinent. *J Gastroenterol Hepatol 17*, 165-70.

[95] Lindh, M, Hannoun, C, Dhillon, A. P, Norkrans, G, & Horal, P. (1999). Core promoter mutations and genotypes in relation to viral replication and liver damage in East Asian hepatitis B virus carriers. *J Infect Dis 179*, 775-782.

[96] Chan, H. L, Hui, A. Y, & Wong, M. L. (2004). Genotype C hepatitis B virus infection is associated with an increased risk of hepatocellular carcinoma. *Gut 53*, 1494-1498.

[97] Yuen, M. F, Sablon, E, Wong, D. K, Yuan, H. J, Wong, B. C, Chan, A. O, & Lai, C. L. (2003). Role of hepatitis B virus genotypes in chronic hepatitis B exacerbation. *Clin Infect Dis* , 37, 593-597.

[98] Orito, E, Ichida, T, Sakugawa, H, Sata, M, Horiike, N, Hino, K, Okita, K, Okanoue, T, Iino, S, Tanaka, E, Suzuki, K, Watanabe, H, Hige, S, & Mizokami, M. (2001). Geographic distribution of hepatitis B virus (HBV) genotype in patients with chronic HBV infection in Japan. *Hepatology 34*, 590-594.

[99] Chen, Y. C, Sheen, I. S, Chu, C. M, & Liaw, Y. F. (2002). Prognosis following spontaneous HBsAg seroclearance in chronic hepatitis B patients with or without concurrent infection. *Gastroenterology 12310841089*

[100] Hsu, Y. S, Chien, R. N, & Yeh, C. T. (2002). Long-term outcome after spontaneous HBeAg seroconversion in patients with chronic hepatitis B. *Hepatology 3515221527*

[101] Kao, J. H, Chen, P. J, Lai, M. Y, & Chen, D. S. (2004). Hepatitis B virus genotypes and spontaneous hepatitis B e antigen seroconversion in Taiwanese hepatitis B carriers. *J Med Virol 72*, 363-369.

[102] Wai, C. T, Fontana, R. J, & Polson, J. (2005). Clinical outcome and virological characteristics of hepatitis B-related acute liver failure in the United States. *J Viral Hepatol 12*, 192-198.

[103] Yuen, M. F, Wong, D. K, & Sablon, E. (2004). HBsAg seroclearance in chronic hepatitis B in the Chinese: virological, histological, and clinical aspects. *Hepatology 39*, 1694-1701.

[104] Imamura, T, Yokosuka, O, Kurihara, T, Kanda, T, Fukai, K, Imazeki, F, & Saisho, H. (2003). Distribution of hepatitis B viral genotypes and mutations in the core promoter and precore regions in acute forms of liver disease in patients from Chiba, Japan. *Gut* , 52, 1630-1637.

[105] Yuen, M. F, Tanaka, Y, & Mizokami, M. (2004). Role of hepatitis B virus genotypes Ba and C, core promoter and precore mutations on hepatocellular carcinoma: a case control study. *Carcinogenesis 25*, 1593-1598.

[106] Sharma, S, Sharma, B, & Singla, B. (2010). Clinical significance of genotypes and precore/basal core promoter mutations in HBV related chronic liver disease patients in North India. *Dig Dis Sci 55*, 794-802.

[107] Liu, S, Zhang, H, & Gu, C. (2009). Associations between hepatitis B virus mutations and the risk of hepatocellular carcinoma: a meta-analysis. *J Natl Cancer Inst 101*, 1066-82.

[108] Fan, Y. F, Lu, C. C, & Chen, W. C. (2001). Prevalence and significance of hepatitis B virus (HBV) pre-S mutants in serum and liver at different replicative stages of chronic HBV infection. *Hepatology 33*, 277-286.

[109] Sugauchi, F, Ohno, T, & Orito, E. (2003). Influence of hepatitis B virus genotypes on the development of pre-S deletions and advanced liver disease. *J Med Virol 70*, 537-544.

[110] Lin, C. L, Liu, C. H, & Wendy, C. (2007). Association of pre-S deletion mutant of hepatitis B virus with risk of hepatocellular carcinoma. *J Gastroenterol Hepatol 22*, 1098-1103.

[111] Liu, C. J, Kao, J. H, & Chen, D. S. (2005). Therapeutic implications of hepatitis B virus genotypes. *Liver Int* , 25, 1097-1107.

[112] Liu, C. J, & Kao, J. H. (2008). Genetic variability of hepatitis B virus and response to antiviral therapy. *Antivir Ther 13*, 613-624.

[113] Kao, J. H, Wu, N. H, Chen, P. J, Lai, M. Y, & Chen, D. S. (2000). Hepatitis B genotypes and the response to interferon therapy. *J Hepatol 339981002*

[114] Hou, J, & Schilling, R. Janssen HLA. ((2001). Molecular characteristics of hepatitis B virus genotype A confer a higher response to interferon treatment. *J Hepatol* 34, 15

[115] Wai, C. T, Chu, C. J, Hussain, M, & Lok, A. S. (2002). HBV genotype B is associated with better response to interferon therapy in HBeAg(+) chronic hepatitis than genotype C. *Hepatology 36*, 1425-1430.

[116] Erhardt, A, Blondin, D, & Hauck, K. (2005). Response to interferon alfa is hepatitis B virus genotype dependent: genotype A is more sensitive to interferon than genotype D. *Gut 54*, 1009-1013.

[117] Buti, M, Cotrina, M, Valdes, A, Jardi, R, Rodriguez-frias, F, & Esteban, R. (2002). Is hepatitis B virus subtype testing useful in predicting virological response and resistance to lamivudine? *J Hepatol* , 36, 445-446.

[118] Yuen, M. F, Wong, D. K, & Sablon, E. (2003). Hepatitis B virus genotypes B and C do not affect the antiviral response to lamivudine. *Antivir Ther* , 8, 531-534.

[119] Choo, Q. L, Kuo, G, Weiner, A. J, Overby, L. R, Bradley, D. W, & Houghton, M. (1989). Isolation of acDNA clone derived from a blood-borne non-A, non-B viral hepatitis genome. *Science* , 244, 359-362.

[120] Choo, Q. L, Richman, K. H, Han, J. H, et al. (1991). Genetic organization and diversity of the hepatitis C virus. *Proc Natl Acad Sci USA* , 88, 2451-2455.

[121] Van Der Poel, C. L, Reesink, H. W, Lelie, P. N, Leentvaar-kuypers, A, Choo, Q. L, Kuo, G, & Houghton, M. (1989). Anti-hepatitis C antibodies and non-A, non-B post-transfusion hepatitis in The Netherlands. *Lancet* , 2, 297-298.

[122] Saeed, A. A, Al-admawi, A. M, Al-rasheed, A, Fairclough, D, Bacchus, R, Ring, C, & Garson, J. (1991). Hepatitis C virus infection in Egyptian volunteer blood donors in Riyadh. *Lancet 338*, 459-460.

[123] MaheshwariA; Ray S; Thuluvath PJ. ((2008). Acute hepatitis C. *Lancet* , 372, 321-332.

[124] Rosen, H. R. (2011). Clinical practice. Chronic hepatitis C infection. *N Engl J Med* , 364, 2429-2438.

[125] Hoofnagle, J. H. (2002). Course and outcome of hepatitis C. *Hepatology 36,* SS29, 21.

[126] Alter, M. J, Margolis, H. S, Krawczynski, K, et al. (1992). The natural history of community-acquired hepatitis C in the United States. The Sentinel Counties chronic non-A, non-B Hepatitis Study Team. *N Engl J Med* , 327, 1899-1905.

[127] Fattovich, G, Giustina, G, Degos, F, et al. (1997). Effectiveness of interferon alfa on incidence of hepatocellular carcinoma and decompensation in cirrhosis type C. European Concerted Action on Viral Hepatitis (EUROHEP). *J Hepatol 27*, 201-205.

[128] Seeff LB & Hoofnagle JH(2003). Appendix: The National Institutes of Health Consensus Development Conference Management of Hepatitis C 2002. *Clinical Liver Disease* 7, 261-287.

[129] Poynard, T, & Yuen, M. F. Ratziu V & Lai CL. ((2003). Viral hepatitis C. *Lancet 362*, 2095-2100.

[130] Zoulim, F, & Chevallier, M. Maynard M & Trepo C. ((2003). Clinical consequences of hepatitis C virus infection. *Rev MedVirol 13*, 57-68.

[131] Takamizawa, A. C, Mori, I, & Fuke, S. (1991). Structure and organization of the hepatitis C virus genome isolated from human carriers. *J Virol* , 65, 1105-1113.

[132] Kato, N. (2000). Genome of human hepatitis C virus (HCV): gene organization, sequence diversity, and variation. *Microb Comp Genomics* , 5, 129-151.

[133] Houghton, M, Weiner, A, Han, J, Kuo, G, & Choo, Q. L. (1991). Molecular biology of the hepatitis C viruses: implications for diagnosis, development and control of viral disease. *Hepatology* , 14, 381-388.

[134] Weiner, A. J, Brauer, M. J, Rosenblatt, J, et al. (1991). Variable and hypervariable domains are found in the regions of HCV corresponding to the flavivirus envelope and NS1proteins and the pestivirus envelope glycoproteins. *Virology* , 180, 842-848.

[135] Tsukiyama-kohara, K, Iizuka, N, Kohara, M, & Nomoto, A. (1992). Internal ribosome entry site within hepatitis C virus RNA. *J Virol* , 66, 1476-1483.

[136] Ogata, N, Alter, H. J, Miller, R. H, & Purcell, R. H. (1991). Nucleotide sequence and mutation rate of the H strain of hepatitis C virus. *Proc Natl Acad Sci USA* , 88, 3392-3396.

[137] Simmonds, P, Holmes, E. C, Cha, T. A, et al. (1993). Classification of hepatitis C virus into six major genotypes and a series of subtypes by phylogenetic analysis of the NS-5 region. *J Gen Virol 74*, 2391-2399.

[138] Hoofnagle, J. H. (2002). Course and outcome of hepatitis C. *Hepatology* 36, SS29, 21.

[139] Franco, S, Gimenez-barcons, M, Puig-basagoiti, F, et al. (2003). Characterization and evolution of NS5A quasispecies of hepatitis C virus genotype 1b in patients with different stages of liver disease. *J Med Virol 71*, 195-204.

[140] Simmonds, P. (1995). Variability of hepatitis C virus. *Hepatology* , 21, 570-583.

[141] Robertson, B, Meyers, G, Howard, C, et al. (1998). Classification, nomenclature, and database development for hepatitis C virus (HCV) and related viruses: proposals for standardization. *Arch Virol 43*, 2493-503.

[142] Xavier, F, & Bukh, J. (1998). Methods for determining the hepatitis C genotype. *Viral Hepatitis Rev 4*, 1-19.

[143] Stuyver, L, Rossau, R, Wyseur, A, Duhamel, M, Vanderborght, B, Van Heuverswyn, H, & Maertens, G. (1993). Typing of hepatitis C virus isolates and characterization of new subtypes using a line probe assay. *J Gen Virol* , 74, 1093-1102.

[144] Okamoto, H, Sugiyama, Y, & Okada, S. et al. ((1992). Typing hepatitis C virus by polymerase chain reaction with type-specific primers: application to clinical surveys and tracing infectious sources. *J Gen Virol* , 73, 673-679.

[145] Zein, N. N, & Persing, D. H. (1996). Hepatitis C genotypes: current trends and future implications. *Mayo Clin Proc* , 71, 458-462.

[146] Zein, N. N. (2000). Clinical significance of hepatitis C virus genotypes. *Clinical Microbiology Reviews 13*, 223-235.

[147] Pawlotsky, J. M. (2003). Hepatitis C virus genetic variability: pathogenic and clinical implications. *Clinical Liver Disease 7*, 45-66.

[148] Nousbaum, J. B, Pol, S, Nalpas, B, Landais, P, Berthelot, P, & Bréchot, C. (1995). Hepatitis C virus type 1b (II) infection in France and Italy. Collaborative Study Group. *Ann Intern Med* , 122, 161-168.

[149] Takada, N, Takase, S, Takada, A, & Date, T. (1993). Differences in the hepatitis C virus genotypes in different countries. *J Hepatol* , 17, 277-283.

[150] Pawlotsky, J. M, Taskiris, L, Roudot-thoraval, F, Pellet, C, Stuyver, L, Duval, J, & Dhumeaux, D. (1995). Relationship between hepatitis C virus genotypes and sources of infection in patients with chronic hepatitis C. *J Infect Dis* , 171, 1607-1610.

[151] Chamberlain, R. W, Adams, N, Saeed, A. A, Simmonds, P, & Elliott, R. M. (1997). Complete nucleotide sequence of a type 4 hepatitis C virus variant, the predominant genotype in the Middle East. *J Gen Virol* , 78, 1341-1347.

[152] Agha, S, Tanaka, Y, Saudy, N, et al. (2004). Reliability of hepatitis C virus core antigen assay for detection of viremia in HCV genotypes 1, 2, 3, and 4 infected blood donors: A collaborative study between Japan, Egypt, and Uzbekistan. *J Med Virol 73*, 216-222.

[153] Cha, T. A, Beall, E, Irvine, B, Kolberg, J, Chien, D, Kuo, G, & Urdea, M. S. (1992). At least five related, but distinct, hepatitis C viral genotypes exist. *Proc Natl Acad Sci USA* , 89, 7144-7148.

[154] Blatt, L. M, Mutchnick, M. G, Tong, M. J, et al. (2000). Assessment of hepatitis C virus RNA and genotype from 6807 patients with chronic hepatitis C in United States. *J Viral Hepat* , 7, 196-202.

[155] Bruno, S, Silini, E, Crosignani, A, et al. (1997). Hepatitis C virus genotypes and risk of hepatocellular carcinoma in cirrhosis: a prospective study. *Hepatology* , 25, 754-758.

[156] Tassopoulos, N. C, Papatheodoridis, G. V, Katsoulidou, A, et al. (1998). Factors associated with severity and disease progression in chronic hepatitis C. *Hepatogastroenterology* , 45, 1678-1683.

[157] Lee, C. M, Hung, C. H, Lu, S. N, et al. (2006). Viral etiology of hepatocellular carcinoma and HCV genotypes in Taiwan. *Intervirology* , 49, 76-81.

[158] De Mitri, M. S, Poussin, K, Baccarini, P, et al. (1995). HCV-associated liver cancer without cirrhosis. *Lancet 345*, 413-415.

[159] Naoumov, N. V, Chokshi, S, Metivier, E, & Maertens, G. Johnson PJ & Williams R. ((1997). Hepatitis C virus infection in the development of hepatocellular carcinoma in cirrhosis. *J Hepatol 27*, 331-336.

[160] Reid, A. E, Koziel, M. J, Aiza, I, Jeffers, L, Reddy, R, Schiff, E, & Lau, J. Y. Dienstag JL & Liang TJ. ((1999). Hepatitis C virus genotypes and viremia and hepatocellular carcinoma in the United States. *Am J Gastroenterol 94*, 1619-1626.

[161] Charlton, M. Genotype b and severity of posttransplant recurrence of hepatitis C infection-unconvictable felon or wrongly accused? *Liver Transplantation 6*, 243-245.

[162] Serra, M. A, & Rodriguez, F. del Olmo JA, Escudero A &Rodrigo JM. ((2003). Influence of age and date of infection on distribution of hepatitis C virus genotypes and fibrosis stage. *J Viral Hepat 10*, 183-188.

[163] Hissar, S. S, Goyal, A, Kumar, M, et al. (2006). Hepatitis C virus genotype 3 predominates in North and Central India and is associated with significant histopathologic liver disease. *J Med Virol* , 78, 452-458.

[164] Adinolfi, L. E, Gambardella, M, Andreana, A, Tripodi, M. F, Utili, R, & Ruggiero, G. (2001). Steatosis accelerates the progression of liver damage of chronic hepatitis C patients and correlates with specific HCV genotype and visceral obesity. *Hepatology 33*, 1358-1364.

[165] Zekri, A. R, Bahnassy, A. A, Shaarawy, S. M, Mansour, O. A, Maduar, M. A, Khaled, H. M, & Ahmadi, O. (2000). Hepatitis C virus genotyping in relation to neu-oncoprotein overexpression and the development of hepatocellular carcinoma. *J Med Microbiol 49*, 89-95.

[166] Miller, F. D, & Abu-raddad, L. J. (2010). Evidence of intense ongoing endemic transmission of hepatitis C virus in Egypt. *Proc Natl Acad Sci USA* , 107, 14757-14762.

[167] Verbeeck, J, Peigue-lafeuille, H, Ross, R. S, et al. (2008). HCV genotype 5: epidemiology and spread of an uncommon genotype. *J Clin Virol* , 41, 170-171.

[168] Wong, D. A, Tong, L. K, & Lim, W. (1998). High prevalence of hepatitis C virus genotype 6 among certain risk groups in Hong Kong. *Eur J Epidemiol* , 14, 421-426.

[169] Saracco, G, Olivero, A, & Ciancio, A. Carenzi S & Rizzetto M. ((2003). Therapy of chronic hepatitis C: a critical review. *Current Drug Targets in Infectious Disorders 3,* 25-32.

[170] McHutchison JG & Fried MW(2003). Current therapy for hepatitis C: pegylated interferon and ribavirin. *Clin Liver Dis 7,* 149-161.

[171] Fried, M. W, Shiffman, M. L, Reddy, K. R, et al. (2002). Peginterferon alfa-2a plus ribavirin for chronic hepatitis C virus infection. *N Engl J Med* , 347, 975-982.

[172] Hadziyannis, S. J. Sette H Jr, Morgan TR et al. ((2004). Peginterferon-alpha2a and ribavirin combination therapy in chronic hepatitis C: A randomized study of treatment duration and ribavirin dose. *Ann Intern Med* , 140, 346-355.

[173] Shiffman, M. L. Di Bisceglie AM, Lindsay KL, et al. ((2004). Peginterferon alfa-2a and ribavirin in patients with chronic hepatitis C who have failed prior treatment. *Gastroenterology 126,* 1015-1023.

[174] Kamal, S. M, & Nasser, I. A. (2008). Hepatitis C genotype 4: What we know and what we don'tyet know. *Hepatology 47,* 1371-1383.

[175] Nguyen, M. H, & Keeffe, E. B. (2005). Prevalence and treatment of hepatitis C virus genotypes 4, 5, and 6. *Clin Gastroenterol Hepatol* 3, SS101, 97.

[176] Nguyen, M. H, Trinh, H. N, Garcia, R, Nguyen, G, Lam, K. D, & Keeffe, E. B. (2008). Higher rate of sustained virologic response in chronic hepatitis C genotype 6 treated with 48 weeks versus 24 weeks of peginterferon plus ribavirin. *Am J Gastroenterol* , 103, 1131-1135.

[177] Rizzetto, M, Canese, M, & Arico, S. (1977). Immunofluorescence detection of a new antigen antibody system (Delta/anti-Delta) associated to hepatitis B virus in liver and serum of HBs Ag carriers. *Gut 18,* 997-1003.

[178] Sureau, C, Guerra, B, & Lanford, R. E. (1993). Role of the large hepatitis B virus envelope protein in infectivity of the hepatitis delta virion. *J Virol* , 67, 366-372.

[179] Rizzetto, M, Ponzetto, A, & Forzani, I. (1991). Epidemiology of hepatitis delta virus: overview. *Prog Clin Biol Res* , 364, 1-20.

[180] Taylor, J. M. (2006). Hepatitis delta virus. *Virology* , 344, 71-76.

[181] Radjef, N, Gordien, E, Ivaniushina, V, et al. (2004). Molecular Phylogenetic Analyses Indicate a Wide and Ancient Radiation of African Hepatitis Delta Virus, Suggesting a Delta virus Genus of at Least Seven Major Clades. *J Virol* , 78, 2537-2544.

[182] Gaeta, G. B, Stroffolini, T, Chiaramonte, M, et al. (2000). Chronic hepatitis D: a vanishing disease? An Italian multicenter study. *Hepatology* , 32, 824-827.

[183] Polish, L. B, Gallagher, M, Fields, H. A, & Hadler, S. C. (1993). Delta hepatitis: molecular biology and clinical and epidemiological features. *Clin Microbiol Rev* , 6, 211-229.

[184] Hadler, S. C. Alcala de Monzon M, Rivero D, Perez M, Bracho A, Fields H. ((1992). Epidemiology and long-term consequences of hepatitis delta virus infection in the Yucpa Indians of Venezuela. *Am J Epidemiol 136,* 1507-1516.

[185] Casey, J. L. (1996). Hepatitis delta virus. Genetics and pathogenesis. *Clin Lab Med* , 16, 451-464.

[186] Rizzetto, M. (1983). The delta agent. *Hepatology* , 3, 729-737.

[187] Casey, J. L, Brown, T. L, Colan, E. J, Wignall, F. S, & Gerin, J. L. (1993). A genotype of hepatitis D virus that occurs in northern South America. *Proc Natl Acad Sci USA* , 90, 9016-9020.

[188] Wu, J. C, Choo, K. B, Chen, C. M, Chen, T. Z, Huo, T. I, & Lee, S. D. (1995). Genotyping of hepatitis D virus by restriction-fragment length polymorphism and relation to outcome of hepatitis D. *Lancet* , 346, 939-941.

[189] Bonino, F, Hoyer, B, Ford, E, Shih, J. W, Purcell, R. H, & Gerin, J. L. (1981). The delta agent: HBsAg particles with delta antigen and RNA in the serum of an HBV carrier. *Hepatology* , 1, 127-131.

[190] Wang, K. S, Choo, Q. L, Weiner, A. J, et al. (1986). Structure, sequence and expression of the hepatitis delta (δ) viral genome. *Nature* 323, 508-514 (Erratum, 328,456, 1987)

[191] Chao, M, Hsieh, S. Y, & Taylor, J. (1990). Role of two forms of hepatitis delta virusantigen: evidence for a mechanism of self-limiting genome replication. *J Virol* , 64, 5066-5069.

[192] Weiner, A. Q, Choo, L, Wang, K. S, et al. (1988). A single antigenomic open reading frame of the hepatitis delta virus encodes the epitope(s) of both hepatitis delta antigen polypeptides p27. *J Virol* 62, 594-599, 24and.

[193] Luo, G. X, Chao, M, Hsieh, S. Y, et al. (1990). A specific base transition occurs on replicating hepatitis delta virus RNA. *J Virol* , 64, 1021-1027.

[194] Yamaguchi, Y, Filipovska, J, Yano, K, et al. (2001). Stimulation of RNA polymerase II elongation by hepatitis delta antigen. *Science* , 293, 124-127.

[195] Le Gal FGault E, Ripault MP, Serpaggi J, Trinchet JC, Gordien E, Dény Eighth major clade for hepatitis delta virus. *Emerg Infect Dis* 12, 1447-1450, 2006.

[196] Wu, J. C, Chen, C. M, Sheen, I. J, Lee, S. D, Tzeng, H. M, & Choo, K. B. (1995). Evidence of transmission of hepatitis D virus to spouses from sequence analysis of the viral genome. *Hepatology 22,* 1656-1660.

[197] Shakil, A. O, Hadziyannis, S, & Hoofnagle, J. H. Di Bisceglie AM, Gerin JL, Casey JL. ((1997). Geographic distribution and genetic variability of hepatitis delta virus genotype I. *Virology* , 234, 160-167.

[198] Zhang, Y. Y, Tsega, E, & Hansson, B. G. (1996). Phylogenetic analysis of hepatitis D viruses indicating a new genotype I subgroup among African isolates. *J Clin Microbiol* , 34, 3023-3030.

[199] Niro, G. A, Smedile, A, Andriulli, A, Rizzetto, M, Gerin, J. L, & Casey, J. L. (1997). The predominance of hepatitis delta virus genotype I among chronically infected Italian patients. *Hepatology* , 25, 728-734.

[200] Wu, J. C, Chiang, T. Y, & Sheen, I. J. (1998). Characterization and phylogenetic analysis of a novel hepatitis D virus strain discovered by restriction fragment length polymorphism analysis. *J Gen Virol* , 79, 1105-1113.

[201] Watanabe, H, Nagayama, K, Enomoto, N, Chinzei, R, Yamashiro, T, Izumi, N, et al. (2003). Chronic hepatitis delta virus infection with genotype IIb variant is correlated with progressive liver disease. *J Gen Virol 84*, 3275-3289.

[202] Rizzetto, M, Hadziyannis, S, Hansson, B. G, Toukan, A, & Gust, I. (1992). Hepatitis delta virus infection in the world: epidemiological patterns and clinical. *Gastroenterol Internat* , 5, 18-32.

[203] Farci, P. (2001). Treatment of chronic hepatitis D. *Infections in Medicine.* , 18(10)

[204] Hsu, S. C, Syu, W. J, Sheen, I. J, Liu, H. T, Jeng, K. S, & Wu, J. C. (2002). Varied assembly and RNA editing efficiencies between genotypes I and II hepatitis D virus and their implications. *Hepatology* , 35, 665-672.

[205] Ma, S. P, Sakugawa, H, Makino, Y, Tadano, M, Kinjo, F, & Saito, A. (2003). The complete genomic sequence of hepatitis delta virus genotype IIb prevalent in Okinawa, Japan. *J Gen Virol* , 84, 461-464.

[206] Niro, G. A, Rosina, F, & Rizzetto, M. (2005). Treatment of hepatitis D. *J Viral Hepat 12*, 2-9.

[207] Panda, S. K, & Jameel, S. (1997). Hepatitis E virus: from epidemiology to molecular biology; *Vir Hep Rev 3*, 227-251.

[208] Jameel, S. (1999). Molecular biology and pathogenesis of hepatitis E virus; *Expert Rev Mol Med* , 1-16.

[209] Emerson, S. U, & Purcell, R. H. (2003). Hepatitis E Virus. *Rev Med Virol 13*, 145-154.

[210] Balayan, M. S, Andjaparidze, A. G, Savinskaya, S. S, et al. (1983). Evidence for a virus in non-A non-B hepatitis transmitted via fecal-oral route. *Intervirology* , 20, 23-31.

[211] Smith, J. L. (2001). A review of hepatitis E virus. *J Food Prot* , 64, 572-586.

[212] Suzuki, K, Aikawa, T, & Okamoto, H. (2002). Fulminant hepatitis E in Japan. *N Engl J Med* 347:1456

[213] Okamoto, H, Takahashi, M, & Nishizawa, T. (2003). Features of hepatitis E virus infection in Japan. *Intern Med 42*, 1065-1071.

[214] Dalton, H. R, Bendall, R, Ijaz, S, & Banks, M. (2008). Hepatitis E: an emerging infection in developed countries. *Lancet Infect Dis* , 8, 698-709.

[215] Hamid, S S, Atiq, M, Shehzad, F, Yasmeen, A, Nissa, T, Salam, A, Siddiqui, A, & Jafri, W. (2002). Hepatitis E virus superinfection in patients with chronic liver disease; *Hepatology 36*, 474-478.

[216] Sheikh, A, Sugitani, M, Kinukawa, N, et al. (2002). Hepatitis e virus infection in fulminant hepatitis patients and an apparently healthy population in Bangladesh. *Am J Trop Med Hyg* , 66, 721-724.

[217] Khuroo, M S, Teli, M R, Skidmore, S, Sofi, M. A, & Khuroo, M I. (1981). Incidence and severity of viral hepatitis in pregnancy. *Am J Med 70*, 252-255.

[218] Beniwal, M, Kumar, A, Kar, P, et al. (2003). Prevalence and severity of acute viral hepatitis and fulminant hepatitis during pregnancy: a prospective study from North India. *Indian J Med Microbiol* , 21, 184-185.

[219] Kumar, A, Beniwal, B, Kar, P, et al. (2004). Hepatitis E in pregnancy. Int J Gynaecol Obstet , 85, 240-244.

[220] Krawczynski, K, Aggarwal, R, & Kamili, S. (2000). Hepatitis E; *Infect Dis Clin North Am 14*, 669-687.

[221] ICTV Virus Taxonomy: (2009). release"Retrieved 2011-12-02

[222] Reyes, G. R, Purdy, M. A, Kim, J. P, Luk, K. C, Young, L. M, Fry, K. E, & Bradley, D. W. (1990). Isolation of a cDNA from the virus responsible for enterically transmitted non-A, non-B hepatitis. *Science* , 247, 1335-1339.

[223] Reyes, G. R, Huang, C. C, Tam, A. W, & Purdy, M. A. (1993). Molecular organization and replication of hepatitis E virus (HEV). *Arch Virol* , 7, 15-25.

[224] Tam, A. W, Smith, M. M, Guerra, M. E, Huang, C. C, Bradley, D. W, Fry, K. E, & Reyes, G. R. (1991). Hepatitis E virus (HEV): molecular cloning and sequencing of the full-length viral genome; *Virology 185*, 120-131.

[225] Tam, A. W, White, R, Reed, E, Short, M, Zhang, Y, Fuerst, T. R, & Lanford, R. E. (1996). In vitro propagation and production of hepatitis E virus from in vivo-infected primary macaque hepatocytes; *Virology 215*, 1-9.

[226] Ansari, I H, Nanda, S K, Durgapal, H, Agrawal, S, Mohanty, S K, Gupta, D, Jameel, S, & Panda, S. K. (2000). Cloning, sequencing, and expression of the hepatitis E virus (HEV) nonstructural open reading frame 1 (ORF1); *J Med Virol 60*, 275-283.

[227] Zafrullah, M, Ozdener, M H, Kumar, R, Panda, S K, & Jameel, S. (1999). Mutational analysis of glycosylation, membrane translocation, and cell surface expression of the hepatitis E virus ORF2 protein; *J Virol 73*, 4074-4082.

[228] Graff, J, Torian, U, Nguyen, H, & Emerson, S. U. (2006). A bicistronic subgenomic mRNA encodes both the ORF2 and ORF3 proteins of hepatitis E virus; *J Virol 80*, 5919-5926.

[229] Schlauder, G. G, & Mushahwar, I. K. (2001). Genetic heterogeneity of hepatitis E virus. *J Med Virol 65*, 282-292.

[230] Okamoto, H. (2007). Genetic variability and evolution of hepatitis E virus. *Virus Res* , 127, 216-228.

[231] Purcell, R. H, & Emerson, S. U. (2008). Hepatitis E: an emerging awareness of an old disease. *J Hepatol* , 48, 494-503.

[232] Lam, W. Y, Chan, R. C, Sung, J. J, & Chan, P. K. (2009). Genotype distribution and sequence variation of hepatitis E virus, Hong Kong. *Emerg Infect Dis* , 15, 792-794.

[233] Arankalle, V. A, Chobe, L. P, Joshi, M. V, Chadha, M. S, Kundu, B, & Walimbe, A. M. (2002). Human and swine hepatitis E virus from Western India belong to different genotypes. *J Hepatol* , 36, 417-425.

[234] Cooper, K, Huang, F. F, Batista, L, et al. (2003). Identification of genotype 3 hepatitis E virus (HEV) in serum and fecal samples from pigs in Thailand and Mexico, where genotype 1 and 2 HEV strains are prevalent in the respective human populations. *J Clin Microbiol* , 43, 1684-1688.

[235] Meng, X. J, Halbur, P. G, Shapiro, M. S, et al. (1998). Genetic and experimental evidence for cross-species infection by swine hepatitis E virus. *J Virol* , 72, 9714-9721.

[236] Ohnishi, S, Kang, J. H, Maekubo, H, et al. (2006). Comparison of clinical features of acute hepatitis caused by hepatitis E virus (HEV) genotypes 3 and 4 in Sapporo, Japan. *Hepatol Res* , 36, 301-307.

[237] Chobe, L. P, Lole, K. S, & Arankalle, V. A. (2006). Full genome sequence and analysis of Indian swine hepatitis E virus isolate of genotype 4. *Vet Microbiol 114*, 240-251.

[238] Viswanathan, R. (1957). Infectious hepatitis in Dehli (1955-56): a critical study; epidemiology. Indian J Med Res , 45, 1-30.

[239] Kar, P, Jilani, N, Husain, S. A, Pasha, S. T, Anand, R, Rai, A, & Das, B. C. (2008). Does hepatitis E viral load and genotypes influence the final outcome of acute liver failure during pregnancy? *Am J Gastroenterol* , 103, 2495-2501.

[240] Mizuo, H, Yazaki, Y, Sugawara, K, Tsuda, F, Takahashi, M, Nishizawa, T, & Okamoto, H. (2005). Possible risk factors for the transmission of hepatitis E virus and for the severe form of hepatitis E acquired locally in Hokkaido, Japan. *J Med Virol* , 76, 341-349.

[241] Abe, T, Aikawa, T, Akahane, Y, Arai, M, Asahina, Y, Atarashi, Y, et al. (2006). Demographic, epidemiological, and virological characteristics of hepatitis E virus infec-

tions in Japan based on 254 human cases collected nationwide [in Japanese]. Kanzo., 47, 384-91.

[242] Péron, J. M, Bureau, C, Poirson, H, et al. (2007). Fulminant liver failure from acute autochthonous hepatitis E in France: description of seven patients with acute hepatitis E and encephalopathy. *J Viral Hepat* , 14, 298-303.

[243] Inoue, J, Takahashi, M, Mizuo, H, Suzuki, K, Aikawa, T, Shimosegawa, T, & Okamoto, H. (2009). Nucleotide substitutions of hepatitis E virus genomes associated with fulminant hepatitis and disease severity. *Tohoku J Exp Med 218*, 279-284.

[244] Shrestha, M. P, Scott, R. M, & Joshi, D. M. Mammen MP Jr, Thapa GB, ThapaN, et al. ((2007). Safety and efficacy of a recombinant hepatitis E vaccine.*N Engl J Med* , 356, 895-903.

Chapter 3

Immunotherapy and Vaccine Development in Viral Hepatitis

Kazuto Tajiri and Yukihiro Shimizu

Additional information is available at the end of the chapter

http://dx.doi.org/10.5772/55525

1. Introduction

More than 300 million people and 170 million people are chronically infected with hepatitis B virus (HBV) and hepatitis C virus (HCV), respectively. To eradicate those viral infections, both prophylactic and therapeutic approaches are required. In HBV infection, there are global programs for prophylactic vaccination. However, some subjects, especially under immunocompromized state, are unable to acquire ant-HBs antibody (Ab) with conventional vaccination, and several attempts to improve the immunogenicity of HB vaccine have been made. On the other hand, development of effective prophylactic HCV vaccine has not been achieved mainly because of high rates of escape mutations within HCV envelope genes. We first focus on the recent development of prophylactic vaccine for HBV and HCV infections.

In the second half of the review, we summarized immunotherapeutic approach for both viral infections. Neither HBV nor HCV is cytopathic, and hepatitis is caused by the host immune response against virus-related peptides expressed on hepatocytes in conjunction with human leukocyte antigens (HLA). In acute self-limiting hepatitis, a broad immune response occurs that is strong enough to eradicate the virus or suppress viral replication [1], indicating that efficient induction of anti-viral immune response could have a potential to control viral infections. However, in chronic hepatitis, there are many mechanisms that hamper the antiviral immune response leading to persistent viral infection.

In chronic HBV infection, strong long-term viral suppression can now be achieved with various nucleoside and nucleotide analogs. However, there are some problems that must be solved in the near future. One of the problems in the treatment of nucleos(t)ide analogs is a low rate of HBe seroconversion even after long-term administration in $HBeAg^+$ patients. Moreover, reactivation rate of HBV replication is high in both $HBeAg^+$ and $HBeAg^-$ patients after cessation of the treatment, although drug-free viral controls would be better than long-term administration of the drugs in terms of control of medical costs and avoidance of adverse effects of these agents. Therefore, it would be beneficial to achieve long-term viral eradication even after cessation of nucleos(t)ide analogs in combination with efficient immunotherapy.

On the other hand, antiviral oral drugs, such as protease inhibitor or polymerase inhibitor showing potent antiviral ability [2], have been developed for chronic HCV infection. However, not all patients treated with these drugs could achieve sustained virological response and high medical cost for each patient is a global serious problem. Effective immunotherapy combined with these drugs may improve their antiviral effects and control medical costs also in hepatitis C.

2. Problems and recent advances in HBV vaccination

2.1. Non-responder for HBV vaccine (Table 1)

In HBV infection, HBV is transmitted at a high incidence rate by parenteral, percutaneous or sexual contact. Therefore, primary protection is very important and universal vaccination regardless of maternal HBsAg status is recommended. Most of countries have introduced HBV vaccination into their national immunization programs and more than 80% of infants have received HBV vaccine three times. In Taiwan, universal vaccination program of all newborns was introduced in 1986. After twenty years of the program, the rate of chronic HBV infection decreased from 9.8% to 1.2% and the risk of childhood HCC has been decreased by 70% [3, 4].

Host factors	
	Age > 40 years
	Obesity
	Smoking
	Genetics, certain HLA types
Other medical conditions	
	Diabetes
	Cirrhosis
	Renal failure
	Conditions requiring immunosuppressive therapy
Unrecognized chronic HBV infection	
Technical	
	Subcutaneous administration
	Freezing of vaccine

Table 1. Causes of non-responder to HBV vaccine

http://dx.doi.org/10.5772/55525

Non-responder for HBV vaccination and vaccine escape mutants are important problems to be focused in the future. The general recommendation for non-responders is to repeat a three-dose schedule; 50-75% is expected to respond to the second dose. Non-responders to the second dose should be evaluated for underlying chronic HBV infection. For hemodialysis patients, response may be improved by using double-dose vaccine [5]. Intradermal administration have been tried to improve the effectiveness of vaccination but is technically difficult [6] and long-term efficacy has not been demonstrated. Several trials to improve the effectiveness of HBV vaccination particularly in hemodialysis patients have been investigated (Table 2). Combined use of granulocyte macrophage-colony stimulating factor or levamisole as an adjuvant of HBV vaccination is a promising strategy [7-9]. New chemical adjuvant has also shown an excellent potential [10-12]. On the other hand, Interleukin (IL)-2 is not shown to be effective when used as an adjuvant [13,14]. Recently, a new HBV vaccine including preS lesion, which is known as an essential site for HBV-entry to hepatocyte, has been tried [15,16].

Materials	Mechanism	Effectiveness	ref
Adjuvant			
GM-CSF	dendritic cell activation	Meta-analysis: OR 4.63	[7]
Levamisole	interferon inducer	Meta-analysis: OR 2.43	[8]
	upregulation of defective immune function	Meta-analysis: OR 2.77	[9]
Interleukin-2	enhanced cellular immunity	RCT: no significant effect	[13, 14]
HB-AS04	upregulation of CD86, increased cytokine	RCT: Significant at month 3	[10]
(aluminium salt, monophosphoryl lipid (MPL))		RCT: Significant	[11]
HB-AS02	TLR4 agonist, improve antigen presentation	RCT: Significant	[12]
(MPL, QS21: extract from *Quillaja saponaria*)			
Pre-S			
Sci-B-Vac/BioHepB	block HBV-entry to hepatocyte?	preS1 antibody 50~60% positive	[15, 16]
(preS1/PreS2/preS)			

GM-CSF;granulocyte macrophage-colony stimulating factor, OR; Odds ratio, RCT; randomized controlled trial, TLR; toll-like receptor

Table 2. Human trials to improve the effectiveness of HBV vaccination

2.2. Escape mutant

Mutations in the small-S protein, commonly glycine to arginine substitution at codon 145 (G145R), have been found in some children born from mothers infected with hepatitis B [17]. Although these mutants have been found in many parts of the world, the prevalence appears to be low and decline in the efficacy of HBV vaccine has not been reported. However, a recent report showed that the mutant HBV was transmitted by sexual contact with a subject who had received universal HBV vaccination [18]. Application of HBV vaccine including preS protein to block infection of HBs mutant could be an effective strategy and should be investigated in the future.

3. Recent advances in HCV vaccine

In the analysis of secondary HCV infection after spontaneously clear primary infection, increased rate of spontaneous viral clearance and broader T-cell responses was found [19]. Actually, an animal study using chimpanzee showed that T-cell vaccine elicits effective immunity against HCV challenge thorough early $CD4^+$ and $CD8^+$ T-cell response [20]. These indicate the induction of protective memory responses against HCV during natural infection and also suggest a possibility for the development of effective prophylactic HCV vaccines.

B-cell response against HCV through the production of neutralizing antibodies has been analyzed for the development of HCV vaccine. In acute HCV infection, the detection of neutralizing antibodies and consequent rapid clearance of HCV had been reported [24]. On the other hand, delayed induction of these neutralizing antibodies has been shown in patients developing chronic HCV infection, [21]. These observations represent that the neutralizing antibodies could not control HCV infection and there are escape mechanisms of HCV from those antibodies. Actually, rapid evolution in the envelope glycoprotein sequences has been demonstrated as the mechanism of HCV evasion [22]. The HCV envelope glycoproteins, E1 and E2, have proven to be the essential region not only for viral attachment but also for viral endocytosis into hepatocytes [23]. Hypervariable region (HVR) is known to be located at the N-terminus of E2 region and is highly immunogenic and the region is necessary for binding to scavenger receptor class B type I (SR-BI), a lipoprotein receptor molecule involved in HCV entry [24,25]. Furthermore, conformational epitope within E2 is known to be conserved among various genotypes of HCV and is necessary for binding to CD81 [26,27]. While, E1 displays a relatively high degree of conservation within subtypes, also suggesting a high degree of intergenotypic cross-neutralization potential [28].

$CD4^+$ and $CD8^+$ T-cell are also important in viral clearance [29-31]. $CD4^+$ T-cells against conserved protein epitopes, such as HCV core, nonstructural (NS)3, NS4 and NS5, have been associated with self-limited infection of HCV. Trials for HCV prophylactic vaccines can be divided into two strategies to induce T-cell response or neutralizing antibodies, but both should be addressed together for an effective prophylaxis strategy. Since acute HCV infection is usually asymptomatic and is not associated with liver failure, prevention from acute to chronic HCV infection is another key goal of vaccine development.

Preclinical evaluation of prophylactic vaccine has been performed in chimpanzee, the only established model for the study of HCV infection in an immunocompetent host. These preclinical trials and the results are summarized in Table 3. Not only humoral responses but also cellular responses were elicited by vaccination, leading to viral clearance after HCV challenge [20,32-37]. Because many chimpanzees spontaneously resolve acute hepatitis C in unvaccinated control groups, definite conclusions for the efficacy of HCV vaccination should be analyzed in human studies. Most vaccine candidates were successful in inducing immune response and reducing viral load. However, protection of infection following challenge with heterologous strains was limited. Although these limited protection shows the difficulty in developing a vaccine against different isolates, these preclinical trials certainly provides information on potential and design of vaccine candidates. As phase I human clinical trial, E1/E2 vaccine adjuvanted with MF59 (an oil-in-water emulsion) was administered to healthy adults, and neutralizing antibodies could be induced without adverse events [38]. Furthermore, these antibodies showed the neutralizing capacities against heterologous virus strains [39]. Further trials should be made for the development of effective HCV vaccines.

Materials	Outocome	ref
E1/E2 protein	21 vaccinated/24 controls	[32]
	2/12 chronic infection after homologous challenge	
	1/9 chronic infection after heterologous challenge	
	Strong humoral immune response	
	15/24 chronic infection in controls	
DNA plasmid: E2	2 vaccinated/1 controls	[33]
	2/2: viral clearance	
	High anti-E2 antibodies in one vaccine	
	E2-specific CD4 T-cell response in the second	
DNA plasmid: Core-E1-E2, NS3-5	6 vaccinated/2 controls	[34]
	2/6: viral clearance	
	HCV-specific antibody and T-cell response	
	Reduced peak viral load in all animals 1 sterilizing immunity: high anti-E2 and strong cellular response	
	1/2 controls: viral clearance	
Adenovirus NS3-NS5B	5 vaccinated/5 controls	[20]
	4/5: viral clearance after 18 months	
	Peripheral and intrahepatic CD8 T-cell response	
	3/5 controls: viral clearance	
HCV like particle: Core E1-E2	4 vaccinated/4 controls	[35]
	4/4: viral clearance after 12 months	
	HCV specific CD4 and CD8 T-cell response	

Materials	Outocome	ref
	1/4 controls: viral clearance	
DNA plasmid: Core E1-E2 NS3	4 vaccinated/2 controls	[36]
	1/4: viral clearance	
	Reduction of HCV load in serum and liver	
	Strong HCV CD4 response	
	Anti-E1 and anti-E2 specific antibodies	
Vaccinia virus Core E1-E2-P7 -NS3-NS3	4 vaccinated/2 controls	[37]
	1/4: viral clearance after homologous	
	T-cell response: vigorous IFNγ production and moderate proliferation	

Table 3. Preclinical trials of HCV vaccines in chimpanzees

4. Immnunotherapy for viral hepatitis and vaccine development

To develop efficient immunotherapy, understanding of immune response for eradication or suppression of hepatitis virus during acute hepatitis is important. Moreover, the immunosuppressive mechanisms leading to persistent viral infection need to be analyzed.

4.1. Immune response in acute viral hepatitis

Immunological analysis has been extensively performed in transgenic and chimpanzee models of acute HBV infection. In one model, transgenic mice, in which infectious HBV virions replicate in the liver with expression of all HBV-related antigens, were injected with HBsAg-specific cytotoxic T lymphocytes (CTLs) that had been induced in nontransgenic mice. The transgenic mice produced interferon (IFN)-γ and tumor necrosis factor (TNF)-α, which purged viral RNA and DNA without destroying infected hepatocytes [40,41]. Importantly, this noncytolytic clearance of intracellular HBV is more efficient at controlling HBV replication than the killing of infected hepatocytes. This was confirmed in a chimpanzee infection model [42] and incubation phase of acute hepatitis B in humans [43].

The same is essentially true in acute HCV infection. Multispecific and vigorous CTL responses against HCV antigens are important for successful eradication of the virus. Moreover, a $CD4^+$ T cell response at an early stage of acute infection and persistence of the response are apparent in acute infection [44]. In contrast to acute HBV infection, the majority of patients with acute HCV infection progress to persistent infection, and the mechanisms underlying failure to eradicate the virus have been analyzed. The failure of $CD4^+$ T cell function is a key factor in HCV persistence and $CD4^+$ T cells from persistent infection do not produce Th1 cytokines, such as IFN-γ and IL-2, but produce IL-4 and IL-10, clearly distinct from those seen in patients with recovery [45]. Moreover, an early and strong Th1 response has been shown to play an important role in disease resolution.

The contributions of $CD4^+$ and $CD8^+$ T cells to the control of viral infection were analyzed in a chimpanzee model of acute hepatitis B and C by depleting either T cell population with monoclonal antibodies (Abs). The data showed that both $CD4^+$ and $CD8^+$ T cells are required for virus elimination [46,47].

4.2. Hierarchy of T cell response in viral hepatitis

The antigen-specificity of the T cell response to HBV in acute hepatitis has been analyzed, and it is clear that acute viral hepatitis involves a vigorous CTL response to multiple epitopes in the viral nucleocapsid, envelope, and polymerase proteins, while these are not seen in patients with chronic hepatitis [1]. Although multi-specificity of the CTL response is characteristic in acute hepatitis, there is known to be a hierarchy of epitope-specific $CD8^+$ T cell responses determined by cytokine production after peptide stimulation. In acute hepatitis B, $CD8^+$ T cell response to HBc18-27 (HLA-A2 restricted epitope) is dominant followed by the response to polymerase epitope (455 – 463), whereas envelope epitopes are always subdominant [48]. The hierarchy is clearly distinct from that observed in chronic hepatitis, in which the $CD8^+$ T cell response to envelope epitope (183 – 191) is always dominant. Interestingly, chronic hepatitis patients with lower HBV DNA levels in the serum show greater responses to HBc18-27 than those with high HBV DNA. These findings imply that the T cell response to HBcAg is important for viral control, which is important for designing peptide vaccines for the treatment of chronic HBV infection.

In acute HCV infection, the CTL responses were directed against multiple viral epitopes, in particular within the structural (core) and nonstructural (NS) regions of the virus (NS3, NS4, and NS5), and the CTL frequencies were higher in patients with acute infection [30,49]than in those who develop persistent infection. The hierarchy of HCV epitopes has not been analyzed extensively, but resolution of primary infection in the chimpanzee was shown to be associated with a dominant $CD4^+$ T cells response against epitopes including NS3 (GYKVLVLNPSV) [50].

4.3. Immune response in chronic viral hepatitis

In contrast to acute hepatitis, the T cell response to HBV is weak and is narrowly focused in chronically infected patients [51], suggesting that it may be a cause of persistent infection.

HBV-specific helper and CTLs are barely detectable in peripheral blood of patients with chronic hepatitis B (CHB) [52], possibly due to exhaustion by high viral load or tolerance to HBV.

In contrast to chronic HBV infection, CTL response against various HCV epitopes including core and envelope and NS regions can be detected in chronic HCV infection, especially in liver-infiltrating lymphocytes [53]. Although intrahepatic CTL response was shown associated with low viral load [54], the CTL response is not enough to terminate HCV infection possibly due to the presence of immunosuppressive mechanisms similar to chronic HBV infection.

4.4. Immunosuppressive mechanisms responsible for persistent hepatitis virus infection

4.4.1. Regulatory T cells (Tregs)

In HBV infection, significant accumulation of $CD4^+CD25^+FoxP3^+$ Treg cells in the liver was found in patients with chronic HBV infection. Moreover, patients with high viral load have a higher proportion of Tregs in the liver [55], suggesting that intrahepatic Tregs suppress antiviral immune responses in the liver in chronic hepatitis B virus infection. In HCV infection, several groups have also shown a higher frequency of $CD4^+CD25^+$ regulatory T cells in the blood of chronically HCV-infected patients versus recovered or healthy individuals [56,57] and the presence of $CD4^+FoxP3^+$ T cells in the liver of chronically HCV-infected patients [58].

4.4.2. Programmed Death-1 (PD-1)

PD-1 is a surface receptor critical for the regulation of T cell function [59,60]. Binding to PD-1 by its ligands PD-L1 and PD-L2 results in the antigen-specific inhibition of T cell proliferation, cytokine production, and cytolytic function, leading to exhaustion of T cells.

Intrahepatic HBV-specific $CD8^+$ T cells express higher levels of PD-1, and upregulation of intrahepatic PD-1/PD-L1 is associated with liver inflammation and ALT elevation [64]. PD-1/PD-L1 blockade increased $CD8^+$ T cell proliferation and enhanced IFN-γ and IL-2 production by intrahepatic lymphocytes [61].

In chronic HCV infection, circulating and intrahepatic HCV-specific $CD8^+$ T cells were found to express high levels of PD-1 [62], and PD-1 expression level in the liver is higher than that in peripheral blood. Increased expression of PD-1 is associated with $CD8^+$ T cell dysfunction, and functional restoration is achieved by blocking the signal from PD-1 [63]. Interestingly, HCV core protein induces PD-1 and PD-L1 on T cells from healthy donors [64], indicating that immunosuppressive ability of HCV core protein is mediated by the upregulation of inhibitory molecules on T cells. Increased PD-1 expression on HCV-specific CTLs was reported to be significantly associated with poor response to antiviral therapy [65].

4.4.3. IL-10

IL-10 is an important cytokine with anti-inflammatory properties, and is produced by activated monocytes/macrophages and T cell subsets, including Treg and Th1 cells [66]. In chronic HBV infection, HBcAg stimulates the production of IL-10, which negatively regulates HBcAg-specific Th17 cell responses in CHB patients [67].

In HCV infection, HCV proteins have been shown to induce IL-10 from monocytes in patients with chronic HCV infection, leading to suppression of antiviral immune response [68].

4.4.4. T-cell immunoglobulin and mucin domain-containing molecule-3 (Tim-3)

Recently, an inhibitory molecule, Tim-3, has been reported. A high frequency of Tim3-expressing $CD4^+$ and $CD8^+$ T cells are found in chronic HBV infection, and the frequency of

Tim-3[+] T cells was positively correlated with the severity of liver inflammation, and negatively correlated with plasma IFN-γ levels [69]. Tim-3 was also highly expressed on CD4[+] and CD8[+] T cells in HCV infection, with the highest levels seen on HCV-specific CTLs. Tim-3 expression is associated with reduced Th1/Tc1 cytokine production, and blocking the Tim-3 – Tim-3 ligand interaction could enhance CD4[+] and CD8[+] T cell proliferation in response to HCV-specific antigens [70].

4.4.5. Dysfunction of Dendritic Cells (DCs)

In patients with CHB, maturation of DCs from peripheral blood of patients after incubation with cytokines is lower than that of normal subjects with lower expression of HLA-DR and costimulatory molecules in the former population [71], leading to low allostimulatory function of DCs from CHB patients. Interestingly, impaired function of monocyte-derived DCs from patients with CHB could be reversed by inhibiting viral replication with nucleoside analogs such as lamivudine [72]. Type 2 precursor plasmacytoid dendritic cells (pDCs), which are the most important cells in antiviral innate immunity, were also reported to have quantitative and qualitative impairment in patients with chronic HBV infection [73]. Recently, HBV itself was shown to inhibit the functions of pDCs [74].

In chronic hepatitis C, DCs from patients also show impaired immunostimulatory function, which could be induced by HCV [75] or NS4 protein [76]. Monocyte-derived DCs from HCV patients were shown to induce proliferation of CD4[+]CD25[+]FoxP3[+] regulatory T cells, which limit proliferation of HCV-specific T lymphocytes [77]. DCs in HCV patients thus inhibit T cell responses via a variety of mechanisms.

5. Immunotherapeutic trials for viral hepatitis

Previous basic analyses and human trials in HBV infection are listed in Tables 4 and 5, respectively, and those in HCV infection are summarized in Tables 6 and 7.

Animal model	Immunotherapy	Results	Ref
Peptide vaccination			
HBV transgenic mice	A synthesized fusion peptide, consisting HBcAg18-27 and HIV Tat49-57 adjuvanted with CpG ODN	Decreased in serum HBV DNA levels and the expression levels of HBsAg and HBcAg in the liver	[79]
Protein vaccination			
HBV transgenic mice	HBsAg vaccine	Most of the mice showed reduction of HBV DNA levels and disappearance of HBeAg and HBsAg	[83]

Animal model	Immunotherapy	Results	Ref
Woodchuck hepatitis Virus infection	Combination of vaccine of HBV large surface protein and clevudine	Restored T-cell response to Pre-S and S region.	[85]
Mice	Chimeric HBsAg-preS1 protein	Primed both HBcAg-specific T cells and antibodies to preS1.	[86]
Balb/c and HBV transgenic mice	Chimeric HBsAg-preS1 protein	Induced strong anti-HBc and moderate anti-preS1 immune response, and reduced HBsAg and HBV DNA in HBV-Tg mice.	[96]
Balb/c mice	Chimeric protein with HBcAg and carboxy terminus of the Hsp65	Induced moderate anti-HBc immune response and strong HBcAg-specific T cells response.	[97]
Balb/c and HBV transgenic mice	HBsAg, HBcAg and heat shock protein gp96	Decreased serum HBsAg and HBcAg expression in hepatocytes by 45% and 90%, respectively. Decreased serum HBV DNA to below or close to the detection limit.	[98]
Balb/c and HBV transgenic mice	Fusion protein with protein transduction domains from HIV-1-Tat and HBcAg	Induced HBcAg-specific CTLs and enhanced production of IFN-γ, IL-2, IL-4 and IL-10. Reduced HBV DNA and HBsAg in the serum and HBsAg expression in liver tissue of HBV transgenic mice.	[99]
DNA immunization			
Woodchuck	DNA vaccine expressing WHsAg was administered by electroporation	Induced dose-dependent antibody and T cell responses to WHsAg more efficiently than conventional hypodermic needle injection.	[104]
Acute DHBV infection	DNA vaccine expressing DHBc and Pre-S/S and entecavir Boosted with fowl poxvirus vectors expressing DHBc and Pre-S/S	Cleared DHBV infection at a rate of 100%.	[105]
Chronic DHBV infection	DNA vaccine encoding the HBV large envelope and/or core protein with or without lamivudine	Reduced viremia and liver DHBV cccDNA in 33% of ducks. Seroconversion to anti-pre S in 67% of ducks showing cccDNA clearance.	[106]
HBV transgenic mice	DNA vaccine expressing HBcAg fused to extracellular	Reduced serum HBV DNA and HBcAg in the liver. Clearance of serum HBsAg was also observed.	[107]

Animal model	Immunotherapy	Results	Ref
	domain of CTLA-4. Mice were challenged by pAAVNBV1.2		
HBV transgenic mice	DNA vaccine expressing HBsAg fused to extracellular domain of CTLA-4.	Serum levels of HBsAg and HBV DNA were decreased by induction of anti-HBs Ab and HBsAg-specific CD8+ T cell response.	[108]
DC immunization			
HBV transgenic mice	Activated bone marrow-derived DCs	Broke CTL tolerance to HBsAg.	[121]
HBV transgenic mice	HBV-specific peptide-pulsed DCs	Reduced in the serum HBsAg and HBV DNA.	[122]
HBV transgenic mice	Anti-CD40 agonistic monoclonal Ab	Induced noncytopathic inhibition of HBV replication mediated by antiviral cytokines (IL-12 and TNF-α) produced by activated intrahepatic APCs.	[123]
Cytokines and adjuvants			
HBV transgenic mice	Recombinant IL-12	Markedly inhibited HBV replication in the liver.	[132]
HBV transgenic mice	α-galactosylceramide that can activate NKT cells	Induced complete inhibition of HBV replication.	[133]
HBV transgenic mice	Recombinant IL-18	Inhibited HBV replication noncytopathically, mediated by activation of resident intrahepatic NK cells and NKT cells.	[134]
Gene therapy			
HBsAg transgenic mice	Lentivectors expressing HBsAg and IgFc fusion Ag	Induced seroconversion to anti-HBs.	[100]
Adjuvant			
HBV transgenic mice	Cationic lipid DNA complexes and HBsAg	Suppressed HBV DNA in hepatocytes non-cytopathically.	[101]
Woodchuck	Cationic liposomes and non-coding DNA was administered with WHsAg intramuscularly	Induced rapid and high Ab and T cell response to WHsAg.	[102]

CpG ODN; CpG oligodeoxynucleotide, WHV; woodchuck hepatitis virus, DHBV; duck hepatitis B virus, cccDNA; covalently closed circular DNA, DC; dendritic cells, CTL; cytotoxic T lymphocytes, APC; Antigen-presenting cells, NKT; natural killer T, Ig; immunoglobulin

Table 4. Immunotherapeutic approaches for animal models of HBV infection

Immunotherapy	Results	Ref
Peptide vaccination		
A vaccine with HBc18-27 peptide comprised of a T-helper cell epitope and two palmitic acid residues	Low levels of CTL activity were induced but no significant changes in liver biochemistry or viral serology were observed.	[80]
Protein vaccination		
PreS2/S (GenHevac B) or S (Recombivax).	HBe/anti-HBe seroconversion was observed in 13% and HBV DNA negativity was in 16% of the treated patients.	[84]
Oral administration of HBV envelope proteins (HBsAg+preS1+preS2)	Induced histological improvement in 30%, HBeAg negativity in 26.3% and HBsAg-specific T cell proliferation in 78% of the treated patients.	[87]
Combination of lamivudine and HBsAg vaccine	Induced sustained negativity of HBV DNA in 1/4 of the patients.	[88]
The combination with lamivudune and HBsAg vaccine in HBeAg^{+} cases	No improvement of HBe seroconversion rate was observed in comparison with lamivudine therapy alone.	[89]
Combination of lamivudine and HBsAg vaccine	HBV DNA became undetectable in 64% of the patients, and was decreased in the remaining patients.	[90]
Intradermal HBsAg vaccine and laimvudine in combination with IL-2	Induced significant HBV DNA loss in the serum in two of five of the treated patients.	[91]
IFN-α-2b monotherapy (9 months) or IFN-α-2b plus pre-S2/S vaccine	Induced greater reduction in HBV DNA in patients with combination HBV therapy than those who received IFN-α-2b monotherapy.	[92]
Complexes composed of yeast-derived hepatitis B surface antigen (HBsAg) and antibodies	HBeAg seroconversion rate was 21,6% and was correlated with decrease of HBsAg and HBV DNA.	[93]
HB preS/S vaccine (GenHevac B)	Caused no effect on HBV DNA and seroconversion of HBeAg to HBeAg in the immunotolerant phase of children with chronic HBV infection.	[94,95]
DNA immunization		
DNA vaccine encoding HBV envelope protein	Induced an increase in HBV-specific IFN-γ-secreting T cells in nonresponders to conventional therapies, and HBV DNA levels were transiently decreased in 50% of vaccinated patients.	[109]
DNA vaccine encoding PreS and S in patients with lamivudine breakthrough	Induced IFN-γ-producing T cells specific for preS or S antigen. Two of 10 patients showed seroconversion to anti-HBe.	[110]
DNA vaccine encoding HBsAg followed by recombinant modified vaccinia virus Ankara expressing HBsAg	Failed in decrease in AST or ALT and did not reduce HBV viremias.	[111]
DC immunization		

Immunotherapy	Results	Ref
Activated DCs from PBL pulsed with HBsAg	Induced anti-HBs and HBsAg-specific cellular immnunity in some patients.	[124]
PBL-derived DCs from chronic hepatitis B incubated with a cocktail of cytokines: IL1-β, PGE2, IL-6 and TNF-α, and pulsed with HBsAg or HBcAg	Induced autologous T cell proliferation and Ag-specific IFN-γ production.	[125]
Peripheral blood-derived DCs, activated with GM-CSF and IL-4 pulsed with HBsAg.	Both patients with normal and elevated ALT responded equally to DC vaccine and 53% of the patients showed induction of HBeAg negativity.	[126]
Activated DCs from PBL with GM-CSF and IL-4, pulsed with two peptides, HBc18-27 and PreS2 44-53.	Undetectable HBV DNA was achieved in 46.3% and 3.13% of $HBeAg^-$ and $HBeAg^+$ patients, respectively. ALT normalization was observed in 69% and 30.5% of $HBeAg^-$ and $HBeAg^+$ patients, respectively.	[127]
Cytokines		
GM-CSF	Safe and tolerable up to 1.0mg/kg body weight, and induced HBV DNA negativity in 4/8 patients.	[135]
Combination therapy with GM-CSF and HBsAg vaccine in HBV carrier children	Significantly reduced serum HBV DNA.	[136]
High dose of IL-12 (0.5μg/kg)	HBV DNA clearance was observed in 25% of the patients.	[137]
Combination of IL-12 and lamivudine	Stimulated T cell response to HBV with IFN-γ production. However, IL-12 was unable to suppress re-elevation of HBV DNA after cessation of lamivudine.	[138]
Combination of IL-12 and IL-18	Stimulated IFN-γ production by CD4+ T cells isolated from peripheral blood in response to HBcAg, and the effect was greater than those observed with either cytokine alone.	[139]
Thymosin-α 1(Talpha1)		
Combination of Talpha1 and IFN-α	No significant differences was observed as compared with IFN-α monotherapy with respect to HBeAg seroconversion, changes in histology, normalization of ALT or loss of HBV DNA.	[140]
Talpha1 alone	At 12 months after cessation of therapy, 36.4% of patients treated with 1.6mg of Talpha1 achieved ALT normalization, 15% achieved HBV DNA clearance by transcription-mediated amplification, and 22.8% achieved clearance of HBeAg.	[141]
Comparative effect of Talpha1 and IFN-α	Talpha1 treatment was more effective in achieving ALT normalization and HBV DNA negativity at the end of the follow-up period than IFN-α.	[142]

Immunotherapy	Results	Ref
Combination of Talpha1 and lamivudine	No any additional antiviral effect compared with lamivudine monotherapy as assessed by HBe seroconversion and the emergence of viral breakthrough.	[143]
Combination therapy with lamivudine and Talpha1	Induced significantly higher rates of ALT normalization, virological response, and HBeAg seroconversion than lamivudine monotherapy.	[145]
CTL; cytotoxic T lymphocytes, GM-CSF; granulocyte macrophage-colony stimulating factor		

Table 5. Immunotherapeutic trials for chronic HBV infection in humans

Animal model	Vaccine	Results	Ref.
Protein vaccination			
Chimpanzee	Recombinant HCV-like particles containing core, E1 and E2 proteins	Increased in peripheral and intrahepatic T cell proliferative responses against the HCV proteins.	[35]
DNA immunization			
HCV transgenic mouse model	The combination of DNA vaccination encoding HCV core and mouse IL-2	Broke tolerance against HCV and activates previously tolerant T cells.	[112]
Mice expressing HCV antigens in the liver	HCV NS3/NS4 DNA vaccine	Induced HCV-specific CD8+ T cells expressing IFN-γ and CCR5 and cleared HCV NS3 expressing hepatocytes.	[113]
Mice	Murine DCs with CFm40L transfected with adenovirus encoding HCV NS3	Induced CD4+ and CD8+ T cell response against HCV NS3.	[114]
Mice	DCs transfected with adenovirus encoding HCV NS3	Induced multiepitopic CD4+ (Th1) and D8+ T cell response and down-regulated the expression of HCV RNA in the liver.	[115]
Balb/c and HLA-A2.1 trangenic mice	DCs transfected with adenovirus encoding HCV NS3	Induced NS3-specific cell mediated and humoral immune response.	[116]
Chimpanzee with HCV-challenge	Recombinant adenoviral vectors encoding the HCV NS3-5B (genotype 1b) and with NS3-5B–encoding plasmid DNA in a combined modality regimen	HCV NS3-NS5, HCV-specific T cells appeared earlier, maintained better functionality, and persisted at higher frequencies. The T cells controlled HCV-challenge.	[117]
DC immunization			

Animal model	Vaccine	Results	Ref.
HCV transgenic mouse model	DCs treated with peptide inhibitors of IL-10	Induced strong anti-HCV T cell responses	[128]
Gene therapy			
C57BL/6 and BALB/c mice	Adenovirus-besed HCV vaccine by fusing HCV NS3 to MHC class II chaperone protein invariant chain	Induced CD8+ T cells expressing IFN-γ, TNF-α, IL-2, CD27 and CD127. The CD8+ T cells protected mice from infection with recombinant vaccinia virus expressing HCV NS3 of heterologous 1b strains	[129]

Table 6. Immunotherapeutic approaches for animal models of HCV infection

Immunotherapy	Results	Ref.
Peptide vaccination		
A vaccine, IC41, containing 7 relevant HCV T cell epitopes and the Th1 adjuvant poly-L-arginine	Induced HCV-specific Th1/Tc1 responses in a subset of HCV patients not responding to or relapsing from standard therapy. However, only a minimal decrease in HCV viremia was induced by the vaccination.	[81]
Vaccination with a peptide derived from HCV core protein	Induced both cellular and humoral responses in nearly all HCV patients with different HLA class I-A alleles, and reduced serum ALT and AFP levels in 29% and 50% of patients, respectively.	[82]
DNA vaccination		
A new vaccine, CIGB0230, consisting of a mixture of plasmid expressing HCV structural antigens and HCV recombinant core protein	Induced specific T cell proliferation and IFN-γ production in 73%. More than 40% of the vaccines showed improvement of liver histology, despite persistent detection of HCV RNA.	[99]
DC vaccination		
Human DCs from HCV-infected patienst with CFh40L transfected with adenovirus encoding HCV NS3	Induced CD4+ and CD8+ T cell response against HCV NS3 in HCV-infected patients	[114]
Monocyte-derived DCs loaded with lipopeptides consisting of HCV-specific HLA-A2.1-restricted CTL epitopes	Induced HCV-specific CD8+ T cell responses with IFN-γ production in PBL in HCV patients in whom conventional IFN-based therapy has failed. However, ALT levels were not elevated and viral load was not decreased.	[118]
Human DCs infected with adenoviral vectors harboring HCV core and NS3	Induced CD4+ and CD8+ T cell response against HCV core and NS3 in healthy subjects	[130]
Human DCs infected with adenoviral vectors harboring HCV NS genes	DCs transfected with adenovirus NS3/NS4 efficiently induced HCV-specific immunity in healthy subjects	[131]

Immunotherapy	Results	Ref.
Cytokine		
Talpha1	Patients with chronic HCV infection who had been nonresponders to prior IFN-α and ribavirin were treated with Talpha1, PEG-IFN α-2a, and ribavirin for 48 weeks. Twenty-four percent of the treated patients with genotype 1 achieved a sustained virological response.	[144]
Blockade of inhibitory signals		
Blocking PD-1, CTLA-4 and IL-10 combined with therapeutic vaccination	Synergistically enhanced functional CD8+ T cell response and improve viral control in chronically infected mice. Moreover, addition of stimulatory signals, such as IL-2, could further increase the efficacy of the therapy in chronic viral infection	[146]
Combined blockade of CTLA-4 and PD-1	Combined blockade of CTLA-4 and PD-1, but not blocking of either molecule, can reverse CD8+ T cell exhaustion in HCV infected patients	[147]
Blocking Tim-3/Tim-3 ligand	Blocking Tim-3/Tim-3 ligand induced intrahepatic T cell proliferation and IFN-γ production in response to HCV antigens in HCV-infected patients	[70]
Blockade of Tim-3 on human HCV-specific CTLs	Blockade of Tim-3 on human HCV-specific CTLs fron HCV-infected patients increased cytotoxicity against an HCVAg-expressing hepatocyte cell line that expresses HCV epitopes	[149]
Gene transfection		
Human T cells transduced with HCV TCR specific for HCV NS3 1071-1081 (HLA A2-restricted epitope)	T cells recognized the peptide and produced IFN-γ, IL-2 and TNF-α in healthy subjects	[119]
Two adenoviral vectors expressing NS3, 4 and 5 proteins from HCV genotype 1B	Induced HCV-specific CD4+ and CD8+ T cells subsets secreting IL-2, IFN-γ, and TNF-α and could be sustained for at least a year after boosting.	[120]
Recombinant virus		
Recombinant poxvirus vaccine, TG4040, that expresses the hepatitis C virus (HCV) proteins NS3, NS4, and NS5B.	It was safe and well-tolerated. It induced HCV-specific immune response and a transient decrease in HCV viremia (>1log) in 33% of HCV-infected patients.	[103]

CTLA-4; cytotoxic T lymphocyte antigen-4, PD-1; programmed death-1, Tim-3; T cell Immunoglobulin and Mucin domain containing-3

Table 7. Immunotherapeutic approach for chronic HCV infection in humans

5.1. Suppression of viral replication

High viral load has been shown to suppress $CD4^+$ and $CD8^+$ T cells in addition to induction of Tregs, which could be reversed by antiviral therapy [78]. Therefore, immunotherapy followed by restoration of virus-specific T cell response with antiviral therapy could be more efficient.

5.2. Induction of immune response to hepatitis virus

5.2.1. Peptide immunization

A fusion peptide consisting of HBc18-27 and HIV Tat49-57 was synthesized, and the vaccination induced significant anti-viral effect in HBV transgenic mice [79]. However, in humans, peptide vaccine containing highly immunogenic HBc18-27 administered to CHB patients, showed disappointing results [80], because there was no induction of a significant antiviral T cell response.

In HCV infection, a vaccine, IC41, containing 7 HCV T cell epitopes and the Th1 adjuvant induced HCV-specific Th1/Tc1 responses in chronic HCV patients, but anti-viral effects were minimal [81]. Another HCV vaccine with a peptide derived from HCV core protein induced both cellular and humoral responses in HCV patients and reduced serum alanine aminotransferase (ALT) and alpha-fetoprotein (AFP) in some patients [82].

5.2.2. Protein immunization

In a model of HBV in transgenic mice, HBsAg vaccine in complete Freund's adjuvant once a month for 12 months induced reduction in HBV DNA, and the disappearance of HBeAg and HBsAg in most mice treated [83]. Interestingly, some mice developed anti-HBs in the sera. However, several human trials with HBsAg vaccine showed limited efficacy if used as monotherapy.

Recently, HB vaccine containing not only S protein but also preS has been used with increased immunogenicity [84-88], or has been combined with lamivudine [89,90], IL-2 [91] or IFN-α [92] leading to potential improvement of clinical efficacy [93-95]. Moreover, vaccines containing HBcAg have been developed, and some showed significant anti-viral effect in HBV transgenic mice [96-99]. Because T cell response to HBcAg is important for viral control, these vaccines may have a promising immunothepapeutic potential also in humans. Recently, some trials to enhance the immunogenicity of HBV vaccine in combination with adjuvant or by using viral vectors have been made [100-102].

In HCV infection, a recombinant poxvirus vaccine expressing HCV NS3, NS4 and NS5B, TG4040, has been recently developed [103] and administered to HCV patients. The vaccine was safe and induced HCV-specific cellular immune response and reduction in viremia. These data are encouraging, and further large scale clinical trials need to be done.

5.2.3. DNA immunization

Injection of plasmid DNA has been shown to strongly elicit both cellular and humoral immune responses. DNA vaccine is now shown to be safe and well-tolerated, and has been tried in humans with some encouraging anti-viral effects both in mice and humans [104].

In a model of duck hepatitis B virus infection, DNA vaccine encoding HBV large envelope and/or core protein was shown to induce reduction in not only viremia [105] but also cccDNA in the liver in one third of ducks receiving DNA monotherapy or combination treatment along with lamivudine [106]. This finding is encouraging because clearance of cccDNA from the liver is the goal of treatment for HBV infection, but is difficult to achieve using IFN-α or nucleoside analogs. More recently, DNA vaccine expressing HBcAg or HBsAg in combination with extracellular domain of CTLA-4 have been developed and showed significant anti-viral effects in HBV transgenic mice [107,108]. In humans, safety and therapeutic potential of DNA vaccines have been already explored in chronic HBV carriers [109-111].

In HCV infection, DNA vaccine encoding HCV core and IL-2 breaks tolerance and activates previously tolerant T cells in HCV transgenic mice [112]. NS3-specific T cells were induced by DNA immunization in mice models [113-116]. In chimpanzee models, NS3-specific T cells were also induced and HCV-challenge could be controlled [117]. In HCV patients, a new DNA vaccine, CIGB0230, consisting of a mixture of plasmid expressing HCV structural antigens induced HCV-specific T cell response and improved liver histology [118]. Furthermore, trials to elicit HCV-specific T cells response by transduction of HCV-specific T cell receptor or by new type vaccines have been made [119,120].

5.2.4. DC immunization

DCs are specialized antigen-presenting cells that can induce strong immune responses in T and B cell. We have previously shown that activated bone marrow-derived DCs can break CTL tolerance to HBsAg in HBV transgenic mice [121]. Thereafter, several immunotherapies with activated DCs have been applied in both animals and humans. In a recent study performed in HBV transgenic mice, peptide-pulsed DCs were shown to significantly reduce the concentrations of serum HBsAg and HBV DNA [122], indicating therapeutic potential in chronic HBV infection. Moreover, when intrahepatic antigen-presenting cells, including DCs, were activated by injection of anti-CD40 agonistic Ab, HBV replication was inhibited by a noncytopathic mechanism possibly through production of antiviral cytokines such as TNF-α and IL-12 [123]. Although no CTL response against HBV antigens was reported in this study, the in vivo activation of DCs could be an alternative way for inducing antiviral immune responses including possible activation of CTLs against HBV. In humans, injection of activated DCs loaded with HBV peptide or protein achieved the induction of HBV-specific immunity [124,125] and a reduction in HBV DNA level in some patients [126,127]. HBeAg negativity was achieved in more than half of the treated patients in one study [126].

In HCV infection, DCs treated with peptide inhibitors of IL-10 were shown to induce strong anti-HCV T cells response in HCV transgenic mice [128], suggesting a strategy to augment the immunogenic function of DCs. Recently, murine DCs infected with adenovirus encoding HCV NS3 were used as vaccines, and showed induction of NS3-specific T cell response and antiviral effect [129]. In humans, DCs infected with adenovirus vectors harboring HCV core or NS genes, especially NS3, were administered in healthy subjects [130,131] and HCV patients [114,118], and those DCs induced $CD4^+$ and $CD8^+$ T cell response in both populations. Although preparation of activated and mature DCs incurs financial costs and requires experienced researchers, immunotherapy with DCs is a promising method.

5.2.5. Cytokines and Thymosin-α1 (Talpha1)

Cytokines, such as IL-12 [132] and IL-18 [133], and the activation of NKT cells [134] were shown to inhibit HBV replication noncytopathically in HBV transgenic mice. In humans, GM-CSF [135,136] and IL-12 [137-139] have been used for treatment with some antiviral effects. They have been used as monotherapy or in combination with HBsAg vaccine or lamivudine.

Talpha1, a synthetic 28-amino acid peptide, is able to enhance the Thl immune response and also exerts a direct antiviral mechanism of action. It has been used for the treatment of chronic HBV [140-143] and HCV [144] infection in humans, and showed antiviral effect with some efficacy. Although antiviral effect by the addition of Talpha1 to lamivudine or IFN-α therapy was controversial, a meta analysis demonstrated that the combination therapy with lamivudine and Talpha1 showed significantly higher rates of ALT normalization, virological response, and HBeAg seroconversion as compared with lamivudine monotherapy [145]. It is of note that HBeAg seroconversion rate was 45% in the combination group, which was significantly higher than that with lamivudine monotherapy (15%).

5.2.6. Blockade of inhibitory signals

There have been several basic attempts to improve the efficacy of immunotherapy. Among these reports, augmentation or restoration of T cell response by blocking the inhibitory signals have been extensively analyzed in vitro. It has been demonstrated that exhausted T cells

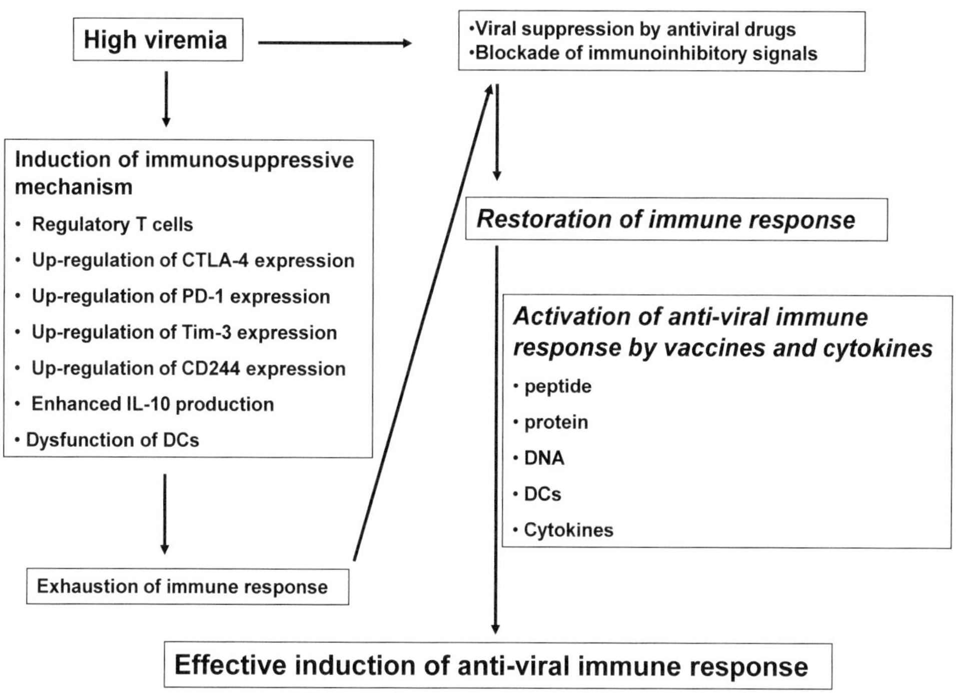

Figure 1.

express not only PD-1, but also CTLA-4 [146,147], CD244 [148] or Tim-3 [70,149], and blocking of these molecules in combination could be better than blocking any single molecule to achieve full activation of the exhausted T cells.

6. Conclusion

There have been several advances in immunotherapy and vaccine development both for prophylactic and therapeutic purposes in HBV and HCV infections and some of the data are promising. For therapeutic purposes, viral suppression, stimulation of antiviral immune response with vaccines with peptides, proteins, plasmid or DC, blockade of immunoinhibitory signals must be combined to achieve desirable antiviral effects (Fig.1). Further studies are required to explore the best protocols and their most efficient combinations to become a promising and practical treatment.

Author details

Kazuto Tajiri[1] and Yukihiro Shimizu[2]

1 The Third Department of Internal Medicine, University of Toyama, Toyama, Japan

2 Gastoenterology Unit, Takaoka City Hospital, Toyama, Japan

References

[1] Rehermann, B. Immunopathogenesis of viral hepatitis. Bailliere's clinical gastroenterology (1996). , 10, 483-500.

[2] Gane, E. J, Roberts, S. K, Stedman, C. A, et al. Oral combination therapy with a nucleoside polymerase inhibitor (RG7128) and danoprevir for chronic hepatitis C genotype 1 infection (INFORM-1): a randomised, double-blind, placebo-controlled, dose-escalation trial. Lancet (2010). , 376, 1467-1475.

[3] Ni, Y. H, Huang, L. M, Chang, M. H, et al. Two decades of universal hepatitis B vaccination in taiwan: impact and implication for future strategies. Gastroenterology (2007). , 132, 1287-1293.

[4] Chang, M. H, You, S. L, Chen, C. J, et al. Decreased incidence of hepatocellular carcinoma in hepatitis B vaccinees: a 20-year follow-up study. Journal of the National Cancer Institute (2009). , 101, 1348-1355.

[5] Rangel, M. C, Coronado, V. G, Euler, G. L, & Strikas, R. A. Vaccine recommendations for patients on chronic dialysis. The Advisory Committee on Immunization Practices and the American Academy of Pediatrics. Seminars in dialysis (2000). , 13, 101-107.

[6] Fabrizi, F, Andrulli, S, Bacchini, G, Corti, M, & Locatelli, F. Intradermal versus intramuscular hepatitis b re-vaccination in non-responsive chronic dialysis patients: a prospective randomized study with cost-effectiveness evaluation. Nephrol Dial Transplant (1997). , 12, 1204-1211.

[7] Fabrizi, F, Ganeshan, S. V, Dixit, V, & Martin, P. Meta-analysis: the adjuvant role of granulocyte macrophage-colony stimulating factor on immunological response to hepatitis B virus vaccine in end-stage renal disease. Alimentary pharmacology & therapeutics (2006). , 24, 789-796.

[8] Fabrizi, F, Dixit, V, Messa, P, & Martin, P. Meta-analysis: levamisole improves the immune response to hepatitis B vaccine in dialysis patients. Alimentary pharmacology & therapeutics (2011). , 32, 756-762.

[9] Alavian, S. M, & Tabatabaei, S. V. Effects of oral levamisole as an adjuvant to hepatitis B vaccine in adults with end-stage renal disease: a meta-analysis of controlled clinical trials. Clinical therapeutics (2010). , 32, 1-10.

[10] Tong, N. K, Beran, J, Kee, S. A, et al. Immunogenicity and safety of an adjuvanted hepatitis B vaccine in pre-hemodialysis and hemodialysis patients. Kidney international (2005). , 68, 2298-2303.

[11] Kong, N. C, Beran, J, Kee, S. A, et al. A new adjuvant improves the immune response to hepatitis B vaccine in hemodialysis patients. Kidney international (2008). , 73, 856-862.

[12] Tielemans, C. L, Vlasak, J, Kosa, D, et al. Immunogenicity and safety of an investigational AS02(v)-adjuvanted hepatitis B vaccine in patients with renal insufficiency who failed to respond or to maintain antibody levels after prior vaccination: results of two open, randomized, comparative trials. Vaccine (2011). , 29, 1159-1166.

[13] Jungers, P, Devillier, P, Salomon, H, Cerisier, J. E, & Courouce, A. M. Randomised placebo-controlled trial of recombinant interleukin-2 in chronic uraemic patients who are non-responders to hepatitis B vaccine. Lancet (1994). , 344, 856-857.

[14] Mauri, J. M, & Valles, M. Effects of recombinant interleukin-2 and revaccination for hepatitis B in previously vaccinated, non-responder, chronic uraemic patients. Collaborative Group of Girona. Nephrol Dial Transplant (1997). , 12, 729-732.

[15] Hellstrom, UB, Madalinski, K, Sylvan, SP, & Pre, . 1 epitope recognition in newborns after vaccination with the third-generation Sci-B-Vac vaccine and their relation to the antibody response to hepatitis B surface antigen. Virology journal 2009;6:7

[16] Sylvan, S. P, Madalinski, K, & Hellstrom, U. B. Anti-preS responses influence the anti-HBs response in newborns after vaccination with the third generation Sci-B-Vac vaccine. Vaccine (2009). , 28, 446-451.

[17] Carman, W. F, Zanetti, A. R, Karayiannis, P, et al. Vaccine-induced escape mutant of hepatitis B virus. Lancet (1990). , 336, 325-329.

[18] Stramer, S. L, Wend, U, Candotti, D, et al. Nucleic acid testing to detect HBV infection in blood donors. The New England journal of medicine (2011). , 364, 236-247.

[19] Osburn, W. O, Fisher, B. E, Dowd, K. A, et al. Spontaneous control of primary hepatitis C virus infection and immunity against persistent reinfection. Gastroenterology (2010). , 138, 315-324.

[20] Folgori, A, Capone, S, Ruggeri, L, et al. A T-cell HCV vaccine eliciting effective immunity against heterologous virus challenge in chimpanzees. Nature medicine (2006). , 12, 190-197.

[21] Pestka, J. M, Zeisel, M. B, Blaser, E, et al. Rapid induction of virus-neutralizing antibodies and viral clearance in a single-source outbreak of hepatitis C. Proceedings of the National Academy of Sciences of the United States of America (2007). , 104, 6025-6030.

[22] Von Hahn, T, Yoon, J. C, Alter, H, et al. Hepatitis C virus continuously escapes from neutralizing antibody and T-cell responses during chronic infection in vivo. Gastroenterology (2007). , 132, 667-678.

[23] Bartosch, B, Dubuisson, J, & Cosset, F. L. Infectious hepatitis C virus pseudo-particles containing functional E1-E2 envelope protein complexes. The Journal of experimental medicine (2003). , 197, 633-642.

[24] Scarselli, E, Ansuini, H, Cerino, R, et al. The human scavenger receptor class B type I is a novel candidate receptor for the hepatitis C virus. The EMBO journal (2002). , 21, 5017-5025.

[25] Bartosch, B, Vitelli, A, Granier, C, et al. Cell entry of hepatitis C virus requires a set of co-receptors that include the CD81 tetraspanin and the SR-B1 scavenger receptor. The Journal of biological chemistry (2003). , 278, 41624-41630.

[26] Owsianka, A. M, Timms, J. M, Tarr, A. W, et al. Identification of conserved residues in the E2 envelope glycoprotein of the hepatitis C virus that are critical for CD81 binding. Journal of virology (2006). , 80, 8695-8704.

[27] Perotti, M, Mancini, N, Diotti, R. A, et al. Identification of a broadly cross-reacting and neutralizing human monoclonal antibody directed against the hepatitis C virus E2 protein. Journal of virology (2008). , 82, 1047-1052.

[28] Leroux-roels, G, Batens, A. H, Desombere, I, et al. Immunogenicity and tolerability of intradermal administration of an HCV E1-based vaccine candidate in healthy volun-

teers and patients with resolved or ongoing chronic HCV infection. Human vaccines (2005). , 1, 61-65.

[29] Cooper, S, Erickson, A. L, Adams, E. J, et al. Analysis of a successful immune response against hepatitis C virus. Immunity (1999). , 10, 439-449.

[30] Lechner, F, Wong, D. K, Dunbar, P. R, et al. Analysis of successful immune responses in persons infected with hepatitis C virus. The Journal of experimental medicine (2000). , 191, 1499-1512.

[31] Grakoui, A, Shoukry, N. H, Woollard, D. J, et al. HCV persistence and immune evasion in the absence of memory T cell help. Science (New York, NY (2003). , 302, 659-662.

[32] Choo, Q. L, Kuo, G, Ralston, R, et al. Vaccination of chimpanzees against infection by the hepatitis C virus. Proceedings of the National Academy of Sciences of the United States of America (1994). , 91, 1294-1298.

[33] Forns, X, Payette, P. J, Ma, X, et al. Vaccination of chimpanzees with plasmid DNA encoding the hepatitis C virus (HCV) envelope E2 protein modified the infection after challenge with homologous monoclonal HCV. Hepatology (Baltimore, Md (2000). , 32, 618-625.

[34] Youn, J. W, Park, S. H, Lavillette, D, et al. Sustained E2 antibody response correlates with reduced peak viremia after hepatitis C virus infection in the chimpanzee. Hepatology (Baltimore, Md (2005). , 42, 1429-1436.

[35] Elmowalid, G. A, Qiao, M, Jeong, S. H, et al. Immunization with hepatitis C virus-like particles results in control of hepatitis C virus infection in chimpanzees. Proceedings of the National Academy of Sciences of the United States of America (2007). , 104, 8427-8432.

[36] Rollier, C. S, Paranhos-baccala, G, Verschoor, E. J, et al. Vaccine-induced early control of hepatitis C virus infection in chimpanzees fails to impact on hepatic PD-1 and chronicity. Hepatology (Baltimore, Md (2007). , 45, 602-613.

[37] Youn, J. W, Hu, Y. W, Tricoche, N, et al. Evidence for protection against chronic hepatitis C virus infection in chimpanzees by immunization with replicating recombinant vaccinia virus. Journal of virology (2008). , 82, 10896-10905.

[38] Frey, S. E, Houghton, M, Coates, S, et al. Safety and immunogenicity of HCV E1E2 vaccine adjuvanted with MF59 administered to healthy adults. Vaccine (2010). , 28, 6367-6373.

[39] Stamataki, Z, Coates, S, Abrignani, S, Houghton, M, & Mckeating, J. A. Immunization of human volunteers with hepatitis C virus envelope glycoproteins elicits antibodies that cross-neutralize heterologous virus strains. The Journal of infectious diseases (2011). , 204, 811-813.

[40] Guidotti, L. G, Ishikawa, T, Hobbs, M. V, et al. Intracellular inactivation of the hepatitis B virus by cytotoxic T lymphocytes. Immunity (1996). , 4, 25-36.

[41] Guidotti, L. G, & Chisari, F. V. Noncytolytic control of viral infections by the innate and adaptive immune response. Annual review of immunology (2001). , 19, 65-91.

[42] Guidotti, L. G, Rochford, R, Chung, J, et al. Viral clearance without destruction of infected cells during acute HBV infection. Science (New York, NY (1999). , 284, 825-829.

[43] Webster, G. J, Reignat, S, Maini, M. K, et al. Incubation phase of acute hepatitis B in man: dynamic of cellular immune mechanisms. Hepatology (Baltimore, Md (2000). , 32, 1117-1124.

[44] Semmo, N, & Klenerman, P. CD4+ T cell responses in hepatitis C virus infection. World J Gastroenterol (2007). , 13, 4831-4838.

[45] Tsai, S. L, Liaw, Y. F, Chen, M. H, Huang, C. Y, & Kuo, G. C. Detection of type 2-like T-helper cells in hepatitis C virus infection: implications for hepatitis C virus chronicity. Hepatology (Baltimore, Md (1997). , 25, 449-458.

[46] Thimme, R, Wieland, S, Steiger, C, et al. CD8(+) T cells mediate viral clearance and disease pathogenesis during acute hepatitis B virus infection. Journal of virology (2003). , 77, 68-76.

[47] Bassett, S. E, Guerra, B, Brasky, K, et al. Protective immune response to hepatitis C virus in chimpanzees rechallenged following clearance of primary infection. Hepatology (Baltimore, Md (2001). , 33, 1479-1487.

[48] Webster, G, & Bertoletti, A. Quantity and quality of virus-specific CD8 cell response: relevance to the design of a therapeutic vaccine for chronic HBV infection. Molecular immunology (2001). , 38, 467-473.

[49] Cucchiarini, M, Kammer, A. R, Grabscheid, B, et al. Vigorous peripheral blood cytotoxic T cell response during the acute phase of hepatitis C virus infection. Cellular immunology (2000). , 203, 111-123.

[50] Shoukry, N. H, Sidney, J, Sette, A, & Walker, C. M. Conserved hierarchy of helper T cell responses in a chimpanzee during primary and secondary hepatitis C virus infections. J Immunol (2004). , 172, 483-492.

[51] Chisari, F. V, & Ferrari, C. Hepatitis B virus immunopathology. Springer seminars in immunopathology (1995). , 17, 261-281.

[52] Ferrari, C, Penna, A, Bertoletti, A, et al. Cellular immune response to hepatitis B virus-encoded antigens in acute and chronic hepatitis B virus infection. J Immunol (1990). , 145, 3442-3449.

[53] Koziel, M. J, Dudley, D, Afdhal, N, et al. HLA class I-restricted cytotoxic T lymphocytes specific for hepatitis C virus. Identification of multiple epitopes and characteri-

zation of patterns of cytokine release. The Journal of clinical investigation (1995). , 96, 2311-2321.

[54] Freeman, A. J, Pan, Y, Harvey, C. E, et al. The presence of an intrahepatic cytotoxic T lymphocyte response is associated with low viral load in patients with chronic hepatitis C virus infection. Journal of hepatology (2003). , 38, 349-356.

[55] Stoop, J. N, Claassen, M. A, Woltman, A. M, et al. Intrahepatic regulatory T cells are phenotypically distinct from their peripheral counterparts in chronic HBV patients. Clinical immunology (Orlando, Fla (2008). , 129, 419-427.

[56] Cabrera, R, Tu, Z, Xu, Y, et al. An immunomodulatory role for CD4(+)CD25(+) regulatory T lymphocytes in hepatitis C virus infection. Hepatology (Baltimore, Md (2004). , 40, 1062-1071.

[57] Boettler, T, Spangenberg, H. C, Neumann-haefelin, C, et al. T cells with a CD4+CD25+ regulatory phenotype suppress in vitro proliferation of virus-specific CD8+ T cells during chronic hepatitis C virus infection. Journal of virology (2005). , 79, 7860-7867.

[58] Sturm, N, Thelu, M. A, Camous, X, et al. Characterization and role of intra-hepatic regulatory T cells in chronic hepatitis C pathogenesis. Journal of hepatology (2010). , 53, 25-35.

[59] Francisco, L. M, Sage, P. T, Sharpe, A. H, & The, P. D. pathway in tolerance and autoimmunity. Immunological reviews (2010). , 236, 219-242.

[60] Fife, B. T, & Pauken, K. E. The role of the PD-1 pathway in autoimmunity and peripheral tolerance. Annals of the New York Academy of Sciences (2011). , 1217, 45-59.

[61] Fisicaro, P, Valdatta, C, Massari, M, et al. Antiviral intrahepatic T-cell responses can be restored by blocking programmed death-1 pathway in chronic hepatitis B. Gastroenterology (2010). e681-684, 138, 682-693.

[62] Golden-mason, L, Palmer, B, Klarquist, J, et al. Upregulation of PD-1 expression on circulating and intrahepatic hepatitis C virus-specific CD8+ T cells associated with reversible immune dysfunction. Journal of virology (2007). , 81, 9249-9258.

[63] Penna, A, Pilli, M, Zerbini, A, et al. Dysfunction and functional restoration of HCV-specific CD8 responses in chronic hepatitis C virus infection. Hepatology (Baltimore, Md (2007). , 45, 588-601.

[64] Yao, Z. Q, King, E, Prayther, D, Yin, D, & Moorman, J. T cell dysfunction by hepatitis C virus core protein involves PD-1/PDL-1 signaling. Viral immunology (2007). , 20, 276-287.

[65] Golden-mason, L, Klarquist, J, Wahed, A. S, & Rosen, H. R. Cutting edge: programmed death-1 expression is increased on immunocytes in chronic hepatitis C virus

and predicts failure of response to antiviral therapy: race-dependent differences. J Immunol (2008). , 180, 3637-3641.

[66] Sabat, R, Grutz, G, Warszawska, K, et al. Biology of interleukin-10. Cytokine & growth factor reviews (2010). , 21, 331-344.

[67] Li, J, Wu, W, Peng, G, et al. HBcAg induces interleukin-10 production, inhibiting HBcAg-specific Th17 responses in chronic hepatitis B patients. Immunology and cell biology (2010). , 88, 834-841.

[68] Barrett, L, Gallant, M, Howley, C, et al. Enhanced IL-10 production in response to hepatitis C virus proteins by peripheral blood mononuclear cells from human immunodeficiency virus-monoinfected individuals. BMC immunology (2008).

[69] Ju, Y, Hou, N, Zhang, X. N, et al. Blockade of Tim-3 pathway ameliorates interferon-gamma production from hepatic CD8+ T cells in a mouse model of hepatitis B virus infection. Cellular & molecular immunology (2009). , 6, 35-43.

[70] Golden-mason, L, Palmer, B. E, Kassam, N, et al. Negative immune regulator Tim-3 is overexpressed on T cells in hepatitis C virus infection and its blockade rescues dysfunctional CD4+ and CD8+ T cells. Journal of virology (2009). , 83, 9122-9130.

[71] Wang, F. S, Xing, L. H, Liu, M. X, et al. Dysfunction of peripheral blood dendritic cells from patients with chronic hepatitis B virus infection. World J Gastroenterol (2001). , 7, 537-541.

[72] Beckebaum, S, Cicinnati, V. R, Zhang, X, et al. Hepatitis B virus-induced defect of monocyte-derived dendritic cells leads to impaired T helper type 1 response in vitro: mechanisms for viral immune escape. Immunology (2003). , 109, 487-495.

[73] Duan, X. Z, Wang, M, Li, H. W, et al. Decreased frequency and function of circulating plasmocytoid dendritic cells (pDC) in hepatitis B virus infected humans. Journal of clinical immunology (2004). , 24, 637-646.

[74] Woltman, A. M. Ter Borg MJ, Binda RS, et al. Alpha-galactosylceramide in chronic hepatitis B infection: results from a randomized placebo-controlled Phase I/II trial. Antiviral therapy (2009). , 14, 809-818.

[75] Eksioglu, E. A, Bess, J. R, Zhu, H, et al. Hepatitis C virus modulates human monocyte-derived dendritic cells. Journal of viral hepatitis (2010).,, 17, 757-769.

[76] Takaki, A, Tatsukawa, M, Iwasaki, Y, et al. Hepatitis C virus NS4 protein impairs the Th1 polarization of immature dendritic cells. Journal of viral hepatitis (2010). , 17, 555-562.

[77] Dolganiuc, A, Paek, E, Kodys, K, Thomas, J, & Szabo, G. Myeloid dendritic cells of patients with chronic HCV infection induce proliferation of regulatory T lymphocytes. Gastroenterology (2008). , 135, 2119-2127.

[78] Boni, C, Penna, A, Ogg, G. S, et al. Lamivudine treatment can overcome cytotoxic T-cell hyporesponsiveness in chronic hepatitis B: new perspectives for immune therapy. Hepatology (Baltimore, Md (2001). , 33, 963-971.

[79] Wang, S, Han, Q, Zhang, N, et al. HBcAg18-27 epitope fused to HIV-Tat 49-57 adjuvanted with CpG ODN induces immunotherapeutic effects in transgenic mice. Immunology letters (2010). , 127, 143-149.

[80] Heathcote, J, Mchutchison, J, Lee, S, et al. A pilot study of the CY-1899 T-cell vaccine in subjects chronically infected with hepatitis B virus. The CY1899 T Cell Vaccine Study Group. Hepatology (Baltimore, Md (1999). , 30, 531-536.

[81] Klade, C. S, Wedemeyer, H, Berg, T, et al. Therapeutic vaccination of chronic hepatitis C nonresponder patients with the peptide vaccine IC41. Gastroenterology (2008). , 134, 1385-1395.

[82] Yutani, S, Komatsu, N, Shichijo, S, et al. Phase I clinical study of a peptide vaccination for hepatitis C virus-infected patients with different human leukocyte antigen-class I-A alleles. Cancer science (2009). , 100, 1935-1942.

[83] Akbar, S. M, Kajino, K, Tanimoto, K, et al. Placebo-controlled trial of vaccination with hepatitis B virus surface antigen in hepatitis B virus transgenic mice. Journal of hepatology (1997). , 26, 131-137.

[84] Pol, S, Nalpas, B, Driss, F, et al. Efficacy and limitations of a specific immunotherapy in chronic hepatitis B. Journal of hepatology (2001). , 34, 917-921.

[85] Menne, S, Tennant, B. C, Gerin, J. L, & Cote, P. J. Chemoimmunotherapy of chronic hepatitis B virus infection in the woodchuck model overcomes immunologic tolerance and restores T-cell responses to pre-S and S regions of the viral envelope protein. Journal of virology (2007). , 81, 10614-10624.

[86] Malik, I. R, Chen, A, Brass, A, et al. A bi-functional hepatitis B virus core antigen (HBcAg) chimera activates HBcAg-specific T cells and preS1-specific antibodies. Scandinavian journal of infectious diseases (2012). , 44, 55-59.

[87] Safadi, R, Israeli, E, Papo, O, et al. Treatment of chronic hepatitis B virus infection via oral immune regulation toward hepatitis B virus proteins. The American journal of gastroenterology (2003). , 98, 2505-2515.

[88] Senturk, H, Tabak, F, Ozaras, R, et al. Efficacy of pre-S-containing HBV vaccine combined with lamivudine in the treatment of chronic HBV infection. Digestive diseases and sciences (2009). , 54, 2026-2030.

[89] Vandepapeliere, P, Lau, G. K, Leroux-roels, G, et al. Therapeutic vaccination of chronic hepatitis B patients with virus suppression by antiviral therapy: a randomized, controlled study of co-administration of HBsAg/AS02 candidate vaccine and lamivudine. Vaccine (2007). , 25, 8585-8597.

[90] Al-mahtab, M, Rahman, S, Akbar, S. M, et al. Combination therapy with antiviral drugs and hepatitis B vaccine in incidentally-detected and asymptomatic chronic hepatitis virus B carriers at Bangladesh. Viral immunology (2010). , 23, 335-338.

[91] Dahmen, A, Herzog-hauff, S, Bocher, W. O, Galle, P. R, & Lohr, H. F. Clinical and immunological efficacy of intradermal vaccine plus lamivudine with or without interleukin-2 in patients with chronic hepatitis B. Journal of medical virology (2002). , 66, 452-460.

[92] Helvaci, M, Kizilgunesler, A, Kasirga, E, et al. Efficacy of hepatitis B vaccination and interferon-alpha-2b combination therapy versus interferon-alpha-2b monotherapy in children with chronic hepatitis B. Journal of gastroenterology and hepatology (2004). , 19, 785-791.

[93] Wang, X. Y, Zhang, X. X, Yao, X, et al. Serum HBeAg sero-conversion correlated with decrease of HBsAg and HBV DNA in chronic hepatitis B patients treated with a therapeutic vaccine. Vaccine (2010). , 28, 8169-8174.

[94] Dikici, B, Bosnak, M, Ucmak, H, et al. Failure of therapeutic vaccination using hepatitis B surface antigen vaccine in the immunotolerant phase of children with chronic hepatitis B infection. Journal of gastroenterology and hepatology (2003). , 18, 218-222.

[95] Yalcin, K, Danis, R, Degertekin, H, et al. The lack of effect of therapeutic vaccination with a pre-S2/S HBV vaccine in the immune tolerant phase of chronic HBV infection. Journal of clinical gastroenterology (2003). , 37, 330-335.

[96] Chen, X, Li, M, Le, X, Ma, W, & Zhou, B. Recombinant hepatitis B core antigen carrying preS1 epitopes induce immune response against chronic HBV infection. Vaccine (2004). , 22, 439-446.

[97] Yang, B. F, Zhao, H. L, Xue, C, et al. Recombinant heat shock protein 65 carrying hepatitis B core antigen induces HBcAg-specific CTL response. Vaccine (2007). , 25, 4478-4486.

[98] Wang, S, Qiu, L, Liu, G, et al. Heat shock protein gp96 enhances humoral and T cell responses, decreases Treg frequency and potentiates the anti-HBV activity in BALB/c and transgenic mice. Vaccine (2011). , 29, 6342-6351.

[99] Chen, X, Lai, J, Pan, Q, et al. The delivery of HBcAg via Tat-PTD enhances specific immune response and inhibits Hepatitis B virus replication in transgenic mice. Vaccine (2010). , 28, 3913-3919.

[100] Hong, Y, Peng, Y, Mi, M, et al. Lentivector expressing HBsAg and immunoglobulin Fc fusion antigen induces potent immune responses and results in seroconversion in HBsAg transgenic mice. Vaccine (2011). , 29, 3909-3916.

[101] Morrey, J. D, Motter, N. E, Chang, S, Fairman, J, & Breaking, B. and T cell tolerance using cationic lipid--DNA complexes (CLDC) as a vaccine adjuvant with hepatitis B

virus (HBV) surface antigen in transgenic mice expressing HBV. Antiviral research (2011). , 90, 227-230.

[102] Cote, P. J, Butler, S. D, George, A. L, et al. Rapid immunity to vaccination with woodchuck hepatitis virus surface antigen using cationic liposome-DNA complexes as adjuvant. Journal of medical virology (2009). , 81, 1760-1772.

[103] Habersetzer, F, Honnet, G, Bain, C, et al. A poxvirus vaccine is safe, induces T-cell responses, and decreases viral load in patients with chronic hepatitis C. Gastroenterology (2011). e891-894, 141, 890-899.

[104] Liu, K. H, Ascenzi, M. A, Bellezza, C. A, et al. Electroporation enhances immunogenicity of a DNA vaccine expressing woodchuck hepatitis virus surface antigen in woodchucks. Journal of virology (2011). , 85, 4853-4862.

[105] Miller, D. S, Boyle, D, Feng, F, et al. Antiviral therapy with entecavir combined with post-exposure "prime-boost" vaccination eliminates duck hepatitis B virus-infected hepatocytes and prevents the development of persistent infection. Virology (2008). , 373, 329-341.

[106] Thermet, A, Buronfosse, T, Werle-lapostolle, B, et al. DNA vaccination in combination or not with lamivudine treatment breaks humoral immune tolerance and enhances cccDNA clearance in the duck model of chronic hepatitis B virus infection. The Journal of general virology (2008). , 89, 1192-1201.

[107] Yin, Y, Wu, C, Song, J, et al. DNA immunization with fusion of CTLA-4 to hepatitis B virus (HBV) core protein enhanced Th2 type responses and cleared HBV with an accelerated kinetic. PloS one (2011). e22524

[108] Zhou, C, Peng, G, Jin, X, Tang, J, & Chen, Z. Vaccination with a fusion DNA vaccine encoding hepatitis B surface antigen fused to the extracellular domain of CTLA4 enhances HBV-specific immune responses in mice: implication of its potential use as a therapeutic vaccine. Clinical immunology (Orlando, Fla (2010). , 137, 190-198.

[109] Mancini-bourgine, M, Fontaine, H, Scott-algara, D, et al. Induction or expansion of T-cell responses by a hepatitis B DNA vaccine administered to chronic HBV carriers. Hepatology (Baltimore, Md (2004). , 40, 874-882.

[110] Mancini-bourgine, M, Fontaine, H, Brechot, C, Pol, S, & Michel, M. L. Immunogenicity of a hepatitis B DNA vaccine administered to chronic HBV carriers. Vaccine (2006). , 24, 4482-4489.

[111] Cavenaugh, J. S, Awi, D, Mendy, M, et al. Partially randomized, non-blinded trial of DNA and MVA therapeutic vaccines based on hepatitis B virus surface protein for chronic HBV infection. PloS one (2011). e14626

[112] Encke, J, Geissler, M, Stremmel, W, & Wands, J. R. DNA-based immunization breaks tolerance in a hepatitis C virus transgenic mouse model. Human vaccines (2006). , 2, 78-83.

[113] Lang Kuhs KAToporovski R, Ginsberg AA, et al. Peripheral immunization induces functional intrahepatic hepatitis C specific immunity following selective retention of vaccine-specific CD8 T cells by the liver. Human vaccines (2011). , 7, 1326-1335.

[114] Echeverria, I, Pereboev, A, Silva, L, et al. Enhanced T cell responses against hepatitis C virus by ex vivo targeting of adenoviral particles to dendritic cells. Hepatology (Baltimore, Md (2011). , 54, 28-37.

[115] Zabaleta, A, Llopiz, D, Arribillaga, L, et al. Vaccination against hepatitis C virus with dendritic cells transduced with an adenovirus encoding NS3 protein. Mol Ther (2008). , 16, 210-217.

[116] Xiang, M, Eisenbach, C, Lupu, C. M, et al. Induction of antigen-specific immune responses in vivo after vaccination with dendritic cells transduced with adenoviral vectors encoding hepatitis C virus NS3. Viral immunology (2006). , 19, 210-219.

[117] Zubkova, I, Choi, Y. H, Chang, E, et al. T-cell vaccines that elicit effective immune responses against HCV in chimpanzees may create greater immune pressure for viral mutation. Vaccine (2009). , 27, 2594-2602.

[118] Gowans, E. J, Roberts, S, Jones, K, et al. A phase I clinical trial of dendritic cell immunotherapy in HCV-infected individuals. Journal of hepatology (2010). , 53, 599-607.

[119] Zhang, Y, Liu, Y, Moxley, K. M, et al. Transduction of human T cells with a novel T-cell receptor confers anti-HCV reactivity. PLoS pathogens (2010). e1001018

[120] Barnes, E, Folgori, A, Capone, S, et al. Novel adenovirus-based vaccines induce broad and sustained T cell responses to HCV in man. Science translational medicine (2012). ra111

[121] Shimizu, Y, Guidotti, L. G, Fowler, P, & Chisari, F. V. Dendritic cell immunization breaks cytotoxic T lymphocyte tolerance in hepatitis B virus transgenic mice. J Immunol (1998). , 161, 4520-4529.

[122] Jiang, W. Z, Fan, Y, Liu, X, et al. Therapeutic potential of dendritic cell-based immunization against HBV in transgenic mice. Antiviral research (2008). , 77, 50-55.

[123] Kimura, K, Kakimi, K, Wieland, S, Guidotti, L. G, & Chisari, F. V. Activated intrahepatic antigen-presenting cells inhibit hepatitis B virus replication in the liver of transgenic mice. J Immunol (2002). , 169, 5188-5195.

[124] Akbar, S. M, Furukawa, S, Horiike, N, et al. Safety and immunogenicity of hepatitis B surface antigen-pulsed dendritic cells in patients with chronic hepatitis B. Journal of viral hepatitis (2011). , 18, 408-414.

[125] Duan, X. Z, He, H. X, & Zhuang, H. Restoration in vitro of impaired T-cell responses in patients with chronic hepatitis B by autologous dendritic cells loaded with hepatitis B virus proteins (R2). Journal of gastroenterology and hepatology (2006). , 21, 970-976.

[126] Chen, M, Li, Y. G, Zhang, D. Z, et al. Therapeutic effect of autologous dendritic cell vaccine on patients with chronic hepatitis B: a clinical study. World J Gastroenterol (2005). , 11, 1806-1808.

[127] Luo, J, Li, J, Chen, R. L, et al. Autologus dendritic cell vaccine for chronic hepatitis B carriers: a pilot, open label, clinical trial in human volunteers. Vaccine (2010). , 28, 2497-2504.

[128] Diaz-valdes, N, Manterola, L, Belsue, V, et al. Improved dendritic cell-based immunization against hepatitis C virus using peptide inhibitors of interleukin 10. Hepatology (Baltimore, Md (2011). , 53, 23-31.

[129] Mikkelsen, M, Holst, P. J, Bukh, J, Thomsen, A. R, & Christensen, J. P. Enhanced and sustained CD8+ T cell responses with an adenoviral vector-based hepatitis C virus vaccine encoding NS3 linked to the MHC class II chaperone protein invariant chain. J Immunol (2011). , 186, 2355-2364.

[130] Li, W, Krishnadas, D. K, Li, J, Tyrrell, D. L, & Agrawal, B. Induction of primary human T cell responses against hepatitis C virus-derived antigens NS3 or core by autologous dendritic cells expressing hepatitis C virus antigens: potential for vaccine and immunotherapy. J Immunol (2006). , 176, 6065-6075.

[131] Tian, Y, Zhang, H. H, Wei, L, et al. The functional evaluation of dendritic cell vaccines based on different hepatitis C virus nonstructural genes. Viral immunology (2007). , 20, 553-561.

[132] Cavanaugh, V. J, Guidotti, L. G, & Chisari, F. V. Interleukin-12 inhibits hepatitis B virus replication in transgenic mice. Journal of virology (1997). , 71, 3236-3243.

[133] Kimura, K, Kakimi, K, Wieland, S, Guidotti, L. G, & Chisari, F. V. Interleukin-18 inhibits hepatitis B virus replication in the livers of transgenic mice. Journal of virology (2002). , 76, 10702-10707.

[134] Kakimi, K, Guidotti, L. G, Koezuka, Y, & Chisari, F. V. Natural killer T cell activation inhibits hepatitis B virus replication in vivo. The Journal of experimental medicine (2000). , 192, 921-930.

[135] Martin, J, Bosch, O, Moraleda, G, et al. Pilot study of recombinant human granulocyte-macrophage colony-stimulating factor in the treatment of chronic hepatitis B. Hepatology (Baltimore, Md (1993). , 18, 775-780.

[136] Wang, J, Zhu, Q, Zhang, T, & Yu, H. A pilot study on the combined therapy of granulocyte-macrophage colony-stimulating factor and hepatitis B vaccine on chronic hepatitis B virus carrier children. Chinese medical journal (2002). , 115, 1824-1828.

[137] Zeuzem, S, & Carreno, V. Interleukin-12 in the treatment of chronic hepatitis B and C. Antiviral research (2001). , 52, 181-188.

[138] Rigopoulou, E. I, Suri, D, Chokshi, S, et al. Lamivudine plus interleukin-12 combination therapy in chronic hepatitis B: antiviral and immunological activity. Hepatology (Baltimore, Md (2005). , 42, 1028-1036.

[139] Szkaradkiewicz, A, Jopek, A, & Wysocki, J. Effects of IL-12 and IL-18 on HBcAg-specific cytokine production by CD4 T lymphocytes of children with chronic hepatitis B infection. Antiviral research (2005). , 66, 23-27.

[140] Arase, Y, Tsubota, A, Suzuki, Y, et al. A pilot study of thymosin alpha1 therapy for chronic hepatitis B patients. Internal medicine (Tokyo, Japan) (2003). , 42, 941-946.

[141] Iino, S, Toyota, J, Kumada, H, et al. The efficacy and safety of thymosin alpha-1 in Japanese patients with chronic hepatitis B; results from a randomized clinical trial. Journal of viral hepatitis (2005). , 12, 300-306.

[142] You, J, Zhuang, L, Cheng, H. Y, et al. Efficacy of thymosin alpha-1 and interferon alpha in treatment of chronic viral hepatitis B: a randomized controlled study. World J Gastroenterol (2006). , 12, 6715-6721.

[143] Lee, H. W, Lee, J. I, Um, S. H, et al. Combination therapy of thymosin alpha-1 and lamivudine for HBeAg positive chronic hepatitis B: A prospective randomized, comparative pilot study. Journal of gastroenterology and hepatology (2008). , 23, 729-735.

[144] Poo, J. L. Sanchez Avila F, Kershenobich D, et al. Efficacy of triple therapy with thymalfasin, peginterferon alpha-2a, and ribavirin for the treatment of hispanic chronic HCV nonresponders. Annals of hepatology (2008). , 7, 369-375.

[145] Zhang, Y. Y, Chen, E. Q, Yang, J, Duan, Y. R, & Tang, H. Treatment with lamivudine versus lamivudine and thymosin alpha-1 for e antigen-positive chronic hepatitis B patients: a meta-analysis. Virology journal (2009).

[146] Ha, S. J, West, E. E, Araki, K, Smith, K. A, & Ahmed, R. Manipulating both the inhibitory and stimulatory immune system towards the success of therapeutic vaccination against chronic viral infections. Immunological reviews (2008). , 223, 317-333.

[147] Nakamoto, N, Cho, H, Shaked, A, et al. Synergistic reversal of intrahepatic HCV-specific CD8 T cell exhaustion by combined PD-1/CTLA-4 blockade. PLoS pathogens (2009). e1000313

[148] Raziorrouh, B, Schraut, W, Gerlach, T, et al. The immunoregulatory role of CD244 in chronic hepatitis B infection and its inhibitory potential on virus-specific CD8+ T-cell function. Hepatology (Baltimore, Md (2010). , 52, 1934-1947.

[149] Mcmahan, R. H, Golden-mason, L, Nishimura, M. I, et al. Tim-3 expression on PD-1+ HCV-specific human CTLs is associated with viral persistence, and its blockade restores hepatocyte-directed in vitro cytotoxicity. The Journal of clinical investigation (2010). , 120, 4546-4557.

Section 2

Management of Chronic Viral Hepatitis

Chapter 4

Clinical Application of Non-Invasive Markers of Liver Fibrosis

Hadi Parsian, Maryam Alizadeh and
Yousef Yahyapour

Additional information is available at the end of the chapter

http://dx.doi.org/10.5772/55422

1. Introduction

Liver is one of the most important organs in our body and any damage on this vital organ may be life threatening. Various factors such as toxins, heavy metals, drugs and infection with hepatitis viruses are able to influence on the function of this organ. One of the most important effects of these factors on liver is gradual necrosis of active liver cells and if this disturbance remained untreated, can lead to liver fibrosis, cirrhosis and finally death. Therefore, it is necessary to diagnose the liver fibrosis. Nowadays physicians rely on liver biopsy to evaluate liver fibrosis. This method was named as 'gold standard' for many years, but it seems researchers prefer to say "The best, not the gold standard". Because of liver biopsy limitations (inter-observer variation amongst pathologists, fibrosis staging systems and sampling errors), patients and also physicians like to estimate the liver fibrosis stages and inflammation grades noninvasively. Therefore we had to find non invasive markers for estimation of liver fibrosis stage.

There are various serum based biomarkers, individually or in an algorithm model for estimation of liver fibrosis stage. The list of serum marker algorithms for assessment of liver fibrosis is increasing. [1-6]. In the last decade, the list of liver fibrosis noninvasive tools is increased rapidly. Some of them (such as transient ultrasound elastography [FibroScan], acoustic radiation force impulse [ARFI], magnetic resonance imaging [MRI], doppler analysis, computed tomography [CT], real-time elastography, tissue strain imaging, supersonic shear imaging, diffusion-weighted MRI, magnetic resonance spectroscopy, positron emission tomography [PET] and single photon emission computed tomography [SPECT] [5-8]) are beyond the scope of this chapter. In this chapter, we will focus on serum noninvasive algorithm-based scores surrogate of liver biopsy.

2. List of serum noninvasive algorithm-based scores

There are some serum-based noninvasive markers individually or in an algorithm-based score that proposed instead of liver biopsy. These markers are usable in clinic, because the physicians are able to request analysis of them frequently, during the treatment and for assessing the treatment efficacy, too.

The lists of individual markers are long. The most common of them that are introduced from the past are: aspartate aminotransferase (AST), alanine aminotransferase (ALT), bilirubin, alkaline phosphatase, albumin, prothrombin time and gamma glutamyl transferase [2-6]. Now it is proposed that some of these simple tests are not able to predict liver injury accurately. For example Seto showed that an elevation of serum ALT levels is not able to predict liver injury [9].

There are some markers that newly introduced and most well-known of them are: α-2-macroglobulin, apolipoprotein A1, collagen markers such as procollagen I carboxyl terminal peptide (PICP), procollagen III amino terminal peptide (PIIINP), procollagen IV C peptide, procollagen IV N peptide (7-S collagen) and collagen IV, collagenases (metalloproteinase) and their inhibitors (tissue inhibitors of metalloproteinase), glycoproteins such as human cartilage glycoprotein (YKL-40), fibronectin, laminin, osteonectin, tenascin, glycosaminoglycans such as perlecan, hyaluronic acid, decorin, aggrecan, lumican, fibromodulin and the others [2-4, 10-12]. Some of these parameters increased in various diseases such as cancer; therefore before the using of these parameters for estimation of liver fibrosis, we had to exclude the other diseases [13].

It seems that these serum individual markers are useful for establishing the presence, but not absence of the fibrosis. For overcome on this problem, researchers combined the results of panels of markers and proposed various algorithms. Interestingly, in some algorithms improve in diagnostic accuracy of these noninvasive markers were observed. Again the lists of these markers are long. Some of the most well-known of them are:

AST to platelet ratio index, Age-platelet index, PGA index, Forns, Bonacini, De Ritis, PATEL, Leroy, FibroSpect, European Liver Fibrosis score, Fibrometer, Hepascore, SHASTA Index, FIB-4, SteatoTest, NAFLD Fibrosis Score, Cirrhosis discriminate score, BARD score, Hui model, FibroMeter NAFLD, Fibrosis Probability Index, Lok index, Fibro Q and the others.

The aim of this chapter is describing the formula, usability and diagnostic accuracy of some of the most common and available serum noninvasive algorithm-based scores in various liver diseases in a simple manner.

3. Age-Platelet (AP) index

Age and platelet counts are major constituents of this index. This index is calculated according to the following instruction:

Platelets counts $(10^9/l)$: 225 = 0; 200-224 = 1; 175-199 = 2; 150-174 = 3; 125-149 = 4; <125 = 5

Age (years) <30 = 0; 30-39 = 1; 40-49 = 2; 50-59 = 3; 60-69 = 4; 70 = 5

Sum of age and platelets counts scores are AP index [14]. Various studies proposed that this index is a good index for estimating liver fibrosis stage. For example in a study that carried out by Lackner [15] on HCV patients, area under the ROC curve (AUROC) was 0.740 for prediction of significant fibrosis and for prediction of cirrhosis, AUROC was 0.910 (according to Ishak score). In another study on 62 hepatitis patients, Parsian et al reported an AUROC of 0.818 for discrimination of patients with liver fibrosis vs. control group and an AUROC of 0.518 for discrimination of patients with mild from those with significant fibrosis [16]. There are other studies that discussed diagnostic accuracy of this simple index [17].

4. AST to Platelet Ratio Index (APRI)

APRI score was initially described by Wai et al [18]. This index is dependent to two routine tests, i.e. aspartate aminotransferase and platelet count and simply calculated by this formula:

$$\text{APRI} = \left[(\text{AST, upper limit of normal}) / \text{platelet count } \left(10^9 / \text{L}\right)\right] \times 100$$

Several studies have suggested that the APRI may be a useful noninvasive marker of hepatic fibrosis. Shin et al showed that in chronic hepatitis B patients, the predictive power of detecting significant fibrosis based on the AUROC is 0.850–0.950 and concluded that this index is a useful indirect marker for estimating significant fibrosis [19].

The AUROC of APRI in HCV patients was reported better in female (0.871) than in male (0.753). Among female cases, an APRI value >1.4 was 91% sensitive and 75% specific in detecting a staging score >2. The corresponding values among male cases were 60% and 77%, respectively [8].

5. AAR index (Deritis index)

There is another simple index that used for evaluation of liver fibrosis and researchers named it AAR index. By dividing the levels of two routine enzymes, i.e. AST and ALT, we are able to calculate it [20].

In a study that carried out on 111 NAFLD patients, researchers found an AUC of 0.61 with an AST/ALT ratio of 0.8 for the prediction of advanced fibrosis [21]. Park et al reported that AST/ALT > or = 1 is highly specific but not diagnostic for the presence of cirrhosis in patients with chronic HCV infection and concluded that the ratio reflects the grade of fibrosis in these patients [22].

6. Fibro Q

Fibro Q is a index that is more complicated than previous indices and is dependent to age (years), AST level, platelet count and also PT International Normalized Ratio (INR). PT INR measures the extrinsic pathway of coagulation. We are able to calculate this index by the following formula [23].

Fibro Q = [(10 × age (years) × AST × PT INR)/ (PLT × ALT)].

In 2012, Hsieh et al showed that FibroQ is a simple and useful test for predicting significant fibrosis in patients with chronic hepatitis C [24]. In our previous study, we found that this index had a reasonable AUROC for discrimination of patients with liver fibrosis vs. control and not for discrimination of patients with severe liver fibrosis vs. mild liver fibrosis [11].

7. FIB4

Other simple index that related to age (years), AST and ALT levels (U/L) and platelet count, is FIB-4 [25]. By the following formula, one can calculate its value:

$$\text{FIB-4} = [\text{age (year)} \times \text{AST (U/L)}] / [\text{PLT} (10^9/\text{L}) \times \text{ALT (U/L)})^{1/2}].$$

Yang et al reported that FIB-4 index had a significant power for differentiation between patients with mild and significant fibrosis in nonalcoholic fatty liver disease (0.24 ± 0.12 vs. 0.31 ± 0.21, P = 0.010) and the AUROC of FIB4 was 0.810. They reported that FIB4 might be useful as a noninvasive hepatic fibrosis scores for predicting hepatic fibrosis in patients with NAFLD [6]. Shah et al [8] in a study on 541 NAFLD adults found that among various serum based algorithms, FIB4 had better diagnostic accuracy for estimation of liver fibrosis.

8. BARD score

In 2008, Harrison et al proposed an index and named it BARD score. The constituents of this score are body-mass index (BMI), AST/ALT ratio (AAR), and presence of type 2 diabetes mellitus (DMt2). They combined these three simple variables to propose a score for predicting advanced fibrosis. Calculating of this score is simple:

BMI ≥ 28 kg/m^2 = 1 point, BMI <28 kg/m^2 = 0 point; AST/ALT ratio ≥ 0.8 = 2 points, AST/ALT ratio < 0.8 = 0 points; freshly recognized or preexisting DMt2 = 1 point.

A total of 2-4 points (sum of the score of BMI, AST/ALT ratio and presence or absence of DMt2) indicate significant fibrosis [26]. In a study that carried out by Wyszomirska in 2010, validation of this score on nonalcoholic fatty liver disease (NAFLD) evaluated. They reported that this scoring system has value for diagnosis of advanced fibrosis in NAFLD patients and if it is possible using of this system in clinic, most patients don’t need to undergo liver biopsy [27]. As another try to determine the validation of this score, Ruffillo et al, evaluated the diagnostic accuracy of this score in NAFLD patients and concluded that this score is useful in identifying patients without severe fibrosis [28].

9. Enhanced Liver Fibrosis (ELF)

This liver fibrosis score is derived from markers that are not available in routine clinical laboratories [29-30]. It was shown that this score has good diagnostic accuracy for the detection of moderate and severe fibrosis [31].

ELF panel constituents are matrix metalloproteinase 1 inhibitor, hyaluronic acid, and amino-terminal peptide of pro-collagen III.

ELF score can calculate by this formula [32]:

Discriminant score = - 7.412 + [ln (HA) × 0.681) + ln (PIIINP) × 0.775) + ln (TIMP1) × 0.494] + 10

In a study that carried out by Nobili et al on 112 NAFLD subjects, concluded that the ELF test is able to accurately discriminate patients with liver fibrosis and can be used for assessing the level of liver fibrosis in pediatric patients [30].

10. Cirrhosis Discriminate Score (CDS) Bonacini

This simple score is proposed by Bonacini [33] and its constituents are AST/ALT, PT-INR and platelet count in a simple manner as described in table 1 [34]. According to this score, different points are given to ingredients of this index and ultimately they added together.

Parametes/Score	0	1	2	3	4	5	6
INR	<1.1	1.1-1.4	>1.4				
ALT/AST ratio	>1.7	1.7-1.2	1.19-0.6	<0.6			
PLT ×1 000 /mm^3	>340	340-280	279-220	219-160	159-100	99-40	<40

Table 1. Determinants of Bonacini score.

There are various studies that analyzed the accuracy of this index for assessing liver fibrosis. For example in a study by Colli et al [34] on 176 patients with chronic HCV infection, they observed that this score was able to identify 67% of patients with a high (>75%) or low (<10%) probability of cirrhosis, and ultimately 33% of the HCV patients need liver biopsy for assessing their liver fibrosis score. Against the above study, there are some studies that found this score was not able to detect severe fibrosis and observed this score has low power of discrimination [35].

11. Fibrotest (FT)

Fibrotest is consisting of a panel of five biomarkers that proposed for evaluation of liver fibrosis stage. Constituents of this index are alpha2-macroglobulin, haptoglobin, apolipoprotein A1, gamma glutamyl transpeptidase and total bilirubin [36] and the formula of this index is:

Fibrotest=4467 × log [alpha2-macroglobulin (gr/l)] – 1357 × log [haptoglobin (gr/l)] + 0.0821 × [age (years)] +1737 × log [bilirubin (μmol/l)] - 1184 × [apolipoprotein A1 (gr/l)] + 0.301 × sex (male=1, female=0) – 5.054

FT is the most studied test and now there are various studies that proposed this test has considerable ability for discrimination of liver fibrosis without significant divergence among liver diseases. For example its ability on hepatitis C, hepatitis B, alcoholic and nonalcoholic fatty liver disease was shown [37-40].

In a study that carried out by Sebastiani et al [41] the ability of several noninvasive markers including FT on 110 CHB patients were assessed. They found that the Fibrotest and APRI had the highest diagnostic accuracy for discrimination of patients with severe stage of liver fibrosis. In another study on 221 chronic alcoholic liver disease patients, Naveau et al [42] reported that in heavy alcohol drinkers, this test is able to estimate the liver fibrosis stage and by this test is possible to decrease the need for liver biopsy.

12. Fibrometer

Fibrometer is a regression algorithm that proposed for evaluation of liver fibrosis stage in liver diseases. Glucose, AST, ferritin, platelet, ALT, body weight and age are the variables that this score is derived from them. First time, this score proposed by Cales et al [43]. Calculation of this score is simple by the following formula:

Fibrometer= 0.4184 glucose (mmol/l) + 0.0701 AST (IU/l) + 0.0008 ferritin (μg/l) - 0.0102 platelet (G/l) - 0.0260 ALT (UI/l) + 0.0459 body weight (kg) + 0.0842 age (yr) + 11.6226.

Various groups of researchers determined the diagnostic accuracy of this index versus liver biopsy in liver disease. For example Cale et al [44] analyzed the accuracy of this index on 235 NAFLD patients. They observed that this score, in comparison with the other scores such as APRI, had higher accuracy rate for significant fibrosis and had lower misclassification rate. Finally, they concluded that Fibrometer had a reasonable performance.

13. Fibrosis Probability Index (FPI) or sud index

This index is depended on: any history of alcohol use, patient age, cholesterol level, AST activity and HOMA-IR index (Homeostasis model assessment: insulin resistance) [45]. First time Sud et al proposed this index and published the results of their study in hepatology journal [46]. They considered and analyzed thirty-five variables in 176 HCV patients and proposed a fibrosis probability index (FPI) for estimation of the liver fibrosis stages by some of these parameters. In addition, they tested the accuracy of this index in another study consists of 126 patients.

Fibrosis probability index (FPI) = 10.929 + (1.827 × Ln AST) +(0.081 × age) + (0.768 × past alcohol use) + (0.385 × HOMA-IR) – (0.447 × cholesterol).

It seems, this index that proposed by this research team can be used as a noninvasive tools for estimation of liver fibrosis and this confirmed by others [47].

14. Forns score

Another score for assessing the liver fibrosis score is Forn score [48]. Constituents of this score are age, platelet count, GGT, and cholesterol. One can calculate this index by this equation:

Forns index: $[7.811 - 3.131 \times \ln(\text{platelet count}) + 0.781 \times \ln(\text{GGT}) + 3.467 \times \ln(\text{age}) - 0.014 \times \text{cholesterol}]$

In their study on 476 CHC patients, Forn et al reported the AUROC of this score was 0.86 for the estimation group and 0.81 for the validation group. Yang et al [6] evaluated the accuracy of Forn score in 77 NAFLD children and according to the severity of their necroinflmmatory injuries, divided the patients to two groups: mild fibrosis (stage 0-1) vs. significant fibrosis (stage 2-4). They analyzed diagnostic accuracy of some simple algorhitms such as AAR, APARI and FIB-4, in addition to Forn score. They observed that among these algorithms, only APRI and FIB4 had a significant difference between patients with mild and significant fibrosis.

15. Hepascore

Hepascore is a more complicated score for estimation of liver fibrosis stage. Age, gender, bilirubin, GGT, hyaluronic acid and alpha2-macroglobulin are constituents of this score [49]. In this score that was proposed by Adams et al for the first time, they added a single direct biomarker of hepatic fibrosis i.e. hyaluronic acid in their algorithm.

By this formula, we can calculate this score:

$$\text{Hepascore} = y/(1 + y), \text{ where } y = \exp(-4.185818 - 0.0249 \times \text{age} + 0.7464 \times \text{gender (male = 1, female = 0)} + 1.0039 \times \alpha2\text{-macroglobulin} + 0.0302 \times \text{hyaluronic acid} + 0.0691 \times \text{bilirubin} - 0.0012 \times \text{GGT}.$$

In their study, Adams et al on 221 HCV patients reported AUROCs of 0.82, 0.90 and 0.89 for the diagnosis of significant fibrosis, extensive fibrosis and cirrhosis, respectively.

In another study on patients with chronic hepatitis C virus, Becker et al [50] reported that Hepascore is able to predict liver fibrosis and maybe by this score a need for liver biopsy is decrease. Bourliere et al reported that the accuracy of Hepascore for excluding the cirrhosis was excellent [51].

16. HUI model

Hui et al performed a retrospective study on 235 CHB patients and by univariate analysis and multivariate logistic regression generated this predictive model. They concluded that this model is able to predict absence of significant fibrosis, accurately. Body mass index (BMI), platelet count, serum albumin, and total bilirubin levels are the constituents of this model [52]. Calculation of this model is very simple and we can calculate this model score by this following formula.

Hui score = 3.148 + 0.167× BMI + 0.088×bilirubin - 0.151× albumin - 0.019 × platelet

In a study that carried out by Sebastiani on 110 CHB patients, some indices such as, APRI, Forns' index, Hui's model and Fibrotest were determined. They reported that performance of these methods for discrimination of patients with significant fibrosis as positive predictive values (PPV) was excellent, i.e. 100% for Forns and greater than 92% for APRI, GUCI, Fibrotest and Hui model [41].

17. Leroy score or MP3 model

Leroy et al used extracellular matrix component i.e. procollagen III amino terminal peptide (PIIINP) and matrix metalloproteinases-1 (MMP-1) for proposing this model. They determined serum levels of hyaluronate (HA), PIIINP, MMP-1, MMP-2, MMP-9 and their tissue inhibitors of metalloproteinases (TIMP-1 and TIMP-2) in 194 chronic hepatitis C patients and 194 healthy people. They found that six markers (MMP-2, TIMP-1, HA, PIIINP, MMP-1 and MMP-9) were significantly correlated with liver fibrosis and by using regression model they proposed their index according to the following formula:

MP3= 0.5903 × log PIIINP (ng/mL) - 0.1749 × log MMP-1 (ng/mL)

They showed that their scoring system is able to differentiate between mild and significant fibrosis and pointed that maybe this score can provide a useful tool for evaluating liver fibrosis [53].

18. Lok index

Another simple scoring system for estimation of liver fibrosis stage that proposed by Lok et al is Lok index [54]. This index is based on serum AST and ALT levels, platelet count and PT-INR. One can calculate this index according to a simple formula:

Lok index = - 5.56 - 0.0089 × platelet $(10^3 mm^3)$ + 1.26 × AST/ALT ratio + 5.27 × INR

For this scoring system two cut points introduced: 0.2 to rule out cirrhosis and 0.5 to confirm cirrhosis. All values that are between these cut points are considered indeterminate. Lok et al in their cohort study on 1,141 patients with CHC, introduced this score and reported an AUROC of 0.78-0.81 to detect cirrhosis.

There are various studies that used this score for estimation of liver fibrosis stage. Castera et al reported that this index has a reasonable performance [55]. Masuzaki studied 386 CHC patients for determining the diagnostic accuracy of this index in comparison with the other noninvasive indices such as APRI. They reported that Lok index and APRI were correlated with histological fibrosis stages (rho=0.581, and 0.460, respectively) and reported an AUROC (95% CI) of Lok index and APRI of 0.787 (0.741-0.832) and 0.692(0.639-0.745), respectively [56].

19. FIBROSpect or PATEL index

Patel et al [57] by combing the serum levels of hyaluronic acid (HA), tissue inhibitors of metalloproteinase 1 (TIMP-1) and alpha2-macroglobulin (A2M), introduced this index that is also has another name, FibroSpect. Against the much scores that are based on the routine and simple laboratory tests, this score is based on the specific and non routine laboratory test. In a study that carried out by their research team on 696 HCV patients, they introduced this scoring system and reported an AUROC of 0.830 for the diagnosis of significant fibrosis.

There are some studies that confirmed the diagnostic accuracy of this scoring system and reported the excellency of this scoring system for estimation of liver fibrosis [58].

20. PGA index

PGA index can be calculated by the sum of three tests, i.e., P, prothrombin time; G, gamma-glutamyl transpeptidase and A, apoliprotein AI and is ranged from 0 to 12 [59].

There are various studies that showed the accuracy of this index in patients with various chronic liver diseases [60-61]. These studies reported that this score has highest accuracy for detecting cirrhosis in patients with alcoholic liver disease.

Against the above mentioned studies, Yang et al didn't find similar results [6]. In their study on 77 NAFLD children, diagnostic accuracy of PGA index (AUROC=0.45) in addition to the other tests such as AAR (0.53), APRI (0.70), Forns index (0.73) and FIB-4 (0.81) were compared. They concluded that among these indices, APRI and FIB4 had the highest performance for discrimination of patients with mild from significant fibrosis.

21. SHASTA index

This index first time introduced by Kelleher et al [62]. They studied 95 patients that had HIV/HCV co-infection and determined the serum levels or activity of ALT, AST, APRI, albumin, total bilirubin, hyaluronic acid (HA) and YKL-40. They observed that among these tests, only serum HA, albumin and AST were useful for discrimination of mild from advanced fibrosis. Finally they constructed a predictive model by these factors (HA, albumin and AST) and named it SHASTA Index. This index can be calculated by the following formula:

Risk score = -3.84 +1.70 (1 if HA 41–85 ng/ml, 0 otherwise) +3.28 (1 if HA>85 ng/ml, 0 otherwise) +1.58 (albumin <3.5 g/dl, 0 otherwise) +1.78 (1 if AST >60 IU/l, 0 otherwise).

A cut off of 0.8 of this index showed specificity and positive predictive value of 100%. A cutoff of <0.30 was associated with a sensitivity and negative predictive value of 88% and 94%, respectively.

22. STEATO test panel

This index is an index that proposed by researchers for estimation of liver steatosis in alcoholic, NAFLD, hepatitis C and B patients. By combining the simple parameters such as age, sex, and BMI with AST, ALT, bilirubin, GGT, alpha2-macroglobulin, apolipoprotein AI, haptoglobin, glucose, cholesterol, and triglyceride this index proposed. First time, Poynard et al proposed this index by the above mentioned variables. They found that steatoTest is able to predict liver steatosis and can decrease the need for liver biopsy [63].

In a study that carried out by Lassailly, diagnostic accuracy of this panel confirmed on two hundred and eighty-eight patients with morbid obesity and concluded that this panel is able to reduce the need for biopsy [64].

23. NAFLD fibrosis score

Components of this score that proposed by Angulo et al are age (years), body mass index, impaired fasting glucose (IFG) or presence the diabetes, AST, ALT, platelet count, and serum albumin levels [65]. They proposed this index as a predictive model for estimation of liver fibrosis. By using the following formula, we are able to calculate this scoring system.

$$\text{NAFLD fibrosis score} = -1.675 + 0.037\times \text{age (years)} + 0.094 \times \text{BMI} \left(\text{kg/m}^2\right) + 1.13 \times \text{IFG/diabetes (yes = 1, no = 0)} + 0.99 \times \text{AST/ALT ratio} - 0.013 \times \text{platelets} \left(10^9/\text{l}\right) - 0.66\times \text{albumin (gr/dl)}$$

A score value < -1.455 (lowest cut point) is able to exclude advanced liver fibrosis and a value > 0.676 (high cutoff) is able to predict advanced liver. Values between these two values are considered as indeterminate liver fibrosis and maybe patients with this result had to undergo liver biopsy.

Shah et al studied diagnostic accuracy of this scoring model in 541 adults with NAFLD for estimation of liver fibrosis and found an AUROC (95% confidence interval [CI]) of 0.768; (0.720 – 0.816) for this model [8]. In another study that carried out by Ruffillo et al on 138 NAFLD patients, they concluded that this scoring model is useful for identifying patients without severe fibrosis, but it has some indeterminate results [28]. In another study that carried out by Yang et al on 77 NAFLD children, AUROC of NAFLD fibrosis score was determined 0.58 for discrimination of mild from significant liver fibrosis [65].

24. Göteborg University Cirrhosis Index (GUCI index)

First time, this index proposed by Kandemir et al [66].They analyzed blood samples from 68 CHC patients for aspartate aminotransferase, prothrombin INR, and platelet count and found a strong association between the fibrosis stage and their proposed index. The GUCI index can be calculate by this formula:

$$\text{GUCI} = \text{Normalized AST} \times \text{prothrombin-INR} \times 100 / \text{Platelet count} \left(\times 10^9/\text{L}\right)$$

They concluded that this index can discriminate patients with severe fibrosis (stage 3-4) from those without severe fibrosis (stage 0-2).

25. King score

This score introduced by Cross et al and is a simple index that derived from age, AST activity INR and platelet count, as follow for the estimation of liver fibrosis.

$$\text{King's Score} = [\text{age (years)} \times \text{AST (IU/l)} \times \text{INR}] / \text{platelets}(10^9/\text{L})$$

Cross et al in their study on 923 CHC patients introduced this scoring model. They reported AUROCs for predicting of cirrhosis and significant fibrosis of 0.91 and 0.79 (respectively) and the results was confirmed in a validation study. They concluded that this scoring is an applicable index for predicting of cirrhosis in chronic hepatitis C patients [67].

Diagnostic accuracy of this scoring model determined in another study. Cross et al performed another study on 187 CHC patients and evaluated the diagnostic accuracy of King score (KS) model and Fibroscan (FS). For diagnosis of significant fibrosis, AUROCs for FS, KS and FS + KS were 0.83, 0.82 and 0.85 (respectively) and for the diagnosis of cirrhosis these values were 0.96, 0.89 and 0.93, respectively [68].

26. Predicted Liver Fibrosis score (PLF score)

Bota et al in their study on 212 CHC patients proposed a scoring system for estimation of liver fibrosis and named it predicted liver fibrosis score [69]. Constituents of their score are transient elastography (TE), APRI score, Forns score, FIB-4 score and King score. Their scoring formula is:

$$\text{Predicted liver fibrosis score (PLF score)} = 0.956 + 0.084 \times \text{TE} - 0.004 \times \text{King Score} + 0.124 \times \text{Forns score} + 0.202 \times \text{APRI score.}$$

They found a good correlation (r = 0.68) for their score with liver fibrosis and concluded that this complex formula that derived from the other algorithms, is able to predict sever fibrosis and its performance is better than TE.

The cut off values, AUROC, positive and negative predictive values of the above mentioned algorithms for estimation of liver fibrosis severity in chronic viral hepatitis and/or NAFLD/NASH is summarized in the table 2.

Noninvasive Test	Variables	Disease	Cut off	AUROC	PPV	NPV	Explanations
AAR	AST and ALT	HCV	≥1	NA	73.7	88.1	
AP	Age and platelets counts	HCV	≥6	t=0.76 v=0.69	96	NA	
APRI	AST and platelets counts	HCV	≥1.5 ≤0.5	t=0.80 v=0.88	91	90	≈Ishak 3-6 ≈Ishak 0-2
BARD score	BMI, AST, ALT and type 2 diabetes mellitus	NAFLD/ NASH	2-4 2	NA	43 27-81	96 45-95	Advanced liver fibrosis (F3-4)
CDS	PT-INR, AST, ALT and platelets counts	HCV	>8	NA	92.6	NA	≈Knodell 3-4
ELF	Matrix metalloproteinase 1 inhibitor, hyaluronic acid, and aminoterminal peptide of pro-collagen III	HBV HCV NAFLD	>0.102 <0.102	0.8	35	92	≈ Scheuer 3-4 ≈ Scheuer 0-2
FIB4	Age, AST, ALT and platelet count	HCV	<1.45 >3.25	0.76	65	90	≈Ishak <4-6 ≈Ishak ≥4-6
Fibro Q	Age, AST, platelet count and PT-INR	HBV HCV	1.6 2.6	F2-4= 0.783 F4=0.791	93 11.3	41 100	
Fibrometer	Glucose, AST, ferritin, platelet, ALT, body weight and age	NAFLD	NA	NA	88	92	
FIBROSpect	Hyaluronic acid, tissue inhibitors of metalloproteinase 1 and alpha2-macroglobulin	HCV	0.82-0.97	NA	90	58	For stage ≥F2
FORNS SCORE	Age, platelet count, GGT, and cholesterol	HCV	≥6.9 <4.2	t=0.86 v=0.81	66	96	≈ Scheuer 2-4 ≈ Scheuer 0-1
FPI	Alcohol use, age, cholesterol, AST and HOMA-IR index	HCV	<0.2 ≥0.8	t=0.84 v=0.77	87	77.4	≈F0-F1 ≈F2-F4
FT	Alpha2-macroglobulin, haptoglobin, apolipoprotein A1, gamma glutamyl transpeptidase and bilirubin	HCV HBV	0.75-1.00 ≈F4 0.73-0.74≈F3-F4 0.59-0.72≈F3 0.49-0.58≈F2 0.32-0.48≈F1-F2 0.28-0.31≈F1 0.22-0.27≈F0-F1 0.00-0.21≈F0	t=0.83 v=0.87	78 76 76 67 61	- - - - 85 91 92 94	

Noninvasive Test	Variables	Disease	Cut off	AUROC	PPV	NPV	Explanations
Göteborg University Cirrhosis Index (GUCI index)	AST,PT-INR, and platelet count	HCV	NA	F4=0.85	F4=31	F4=97	
Hepascore	Age, gender, bilirubin, GGT, hyaluronic acid and alpha2-macroglobulin	HCV	≥0.5 <0.5	t=0.85 v=0.82	88	98	≈F2-F4 ≈F0-F1
HUI model	BMI, platelet count, albumin and bilirubin	HBV	<0.15	t=0.803 v=0.765 entire cohort=0.791	NA	NA	
King Score	Age, AST, INR and platelet count	HCV	≥12.3 ≥16.7	F3-6=0.79 F5-6=0.91	81 56	77 96	
Leroy score or MP3 model	Procollagen III amino terminal peptide and matrix metalloproteinases-1	HCV	NA	≥F2, 0.82	≥F2=89	≥F2=84	
Lok index	AST, ALT, platelet count and PT-INR	HCV	NA	F4=0.78-.0.81	F4=32-75	F4= 84-91	
NAFLD fibrosis score	Age, BMI, impaired fasting glucose (IFG) or presence the diabetes, AST, ALT, platelet count, and serum albumin levels	NAFLD/ NASH	-1.455 0.676	NA	30-56 82-90	88-93 85-86	
PLF score	Transient elastography, APRI score, Forns score, FIB-4 score and King score	HCV	F ≥ 1= 1.77 F ≥ 2= 2.88 F ≥ 3=2.47 F=4, = 2.98	0.76 0.78 0.86 0.97	99.5 96.4 85.1 70.7	18.1 21.4 78.6 99.4	
SHASTA index	ALT, AST, APRI, albumin, total bilirubin, hyaluronic acid and YKL-40	HCV	>.08 <0.3	0.87	100	94 21.4	Ishak ≥3 Ishak ≤2
STEATO test panel	ALT, α2-macroglobulin , apolipoprotein A-I, haptoglobin, total bilirubin, GGT, cholesterol, triglycerides, glucose, age, gender and BMI	NAFLD	0.3 0.5 0.7	NA	22 29 33	100 95 92	For predicting liver steatosis greater than 5%.

Table 2. An alphabetical order of various noninvasive serum indices to detect liver fibrosis in patients with chronic viral hepatitis and/or NAFLD/NASH.

Abbreviations

AUROC, area under receiver operating characteristic curve; NA, Not available; PPV, positive predictive value; NPV, negative predictive value; ALT, alanine aminotransferase; AST, aspartate aminotransferase; MMP, metalloproteinases TIMP, tissue inhibitors of matrix metalloproteinases; HOMA-IR, homeostasis model assessment of insulin resistance; INR, international normalized ratio for prothrombie; t, training group; v, validation group [3, 15, 22,23, 52, 63, 67, 69, 71].

27. Conclusion

Liver biopsy still has an important role in the estimation of liver fibrosis stage, but it is not very far that this invasive method will completely replace with the other noninvasive methods such as serum based biomarkers [70]. Therefore development of non-invasive methods is still needed and we should work harder for finding an appropriate method. Maybe with finding some appropriate biomarkers, we can completely obsolete the liver biopsy.

Acknowledgements

The authors greatly thanks from all patients that permitted to the researchers to analyze their serum or tissue for research purposes.

Author details

Hadi Parsian[1,2], Maryam Alizadeh[2] and Yousef Yahyapour[1,3]

*Address all correspondence to: hadiparsian@yahoo.com

1 Cellular and Molecular Biology Research Center, Babol University of Medical Sciences, Babol, Iran

2 Department of Biochemistry and Biophysics, Babol University of Medical Sciences, Babol, Iran

3 Department of Microbiology and Immunology, Babol University of Medical Sciences, Babol, Iran

References

[1] Bedossa P, Carrat F. Liver biopsy: The best, not the gold standard. Journal of Hepatology 2009; 50: 1–3.

[2] Stella M. Martınez, Gonzalo Crespo, Miquel Navasa, and Xavier Forns. Noninvasive Assessment of Liver Fibrosis. Hepatology 2011; 53: 325-35.

[3] Papastergiou V, Tsochatzis E, Burroughs AK. Non-invasive assessment of liver fibrosis. Annals of Gastroenterology 2012; 25: 1-14.

[4] Rossi E, Adams LA, Bulsara M, Jeffrey GP. Assessing Liver Fibrosis with Serum Marker Models. Clin Biochem Rev 2007; 28: 1-10.

[5] Baranova A, La P, Birerdinc A and Younossi ZM. Non-Invasive markers for hepatic fibrosis. BMC Gastroenterology 2011; 11: 91.

[6] Yang H R, Kim H R, Kim M J, Ko J S, and Seo J K. Noninvasive Parameters and hepatic fibrosis scores in children with nonalcoholic fatty liver disease. World J Gastroenterol. 2012 7; 18(13): 1525–30.

[7] Diarmuid S, Manning Nezam, H. Afdhal. Diagnosis and Quantitation of Fibrosis. Gastroenterology 2008; 134: 1670–81.

[8] Shah AG, Lydecker A, Murray K, Tetri BN, Contos MJ, Sanyal AJ; Nash Clinical Research Network. Comparison of noninvasive markers of fibrosis in patients with nonalcoholic fatty liver disease. Clin Gastroenterol Hepatol. 2009 Oct; 7(10): 1104-12. Epub 2009 Jun 10.

[9] Seto W-K, Lai C-L, Ip PPC, Fung J, Wong DK-H, et al. A Large Population Histology Study Showing the Lack of Association between ALT Elevation and Significant Fibrosis in Chronic Hepatitis B. PLoS ONE 2012; 7(2): e32622. doi:10.1371/journal.pone.0032622.

[10] Mato JM, Lu SC. Where are we in the search for noninvasive nonalcoholic steatohepatitis biomarkers? Hepatology 2011 Oct; 54(4): 1115-7. doi: 10.1002/hep.24642.

[11] Parsian H, Nouri M, Rahimipour A, Somi MH, Qujeq D. Comparison of five liver fibrosis indexes with serum levels of laminin and N terminal peptide of procollagen type III in chronic hepatitis patients. Liver Biopsy. Rijeka, Croatia: InTech. 2011.

[12] Parsian H, Rahimipour A, Nouri M, Somi M Hand Qujeq D. Assessment of liver fibrosis development in chronic hepatitis b patients by serum hyaluronic acid and laminin levels. Acta Clin Croat 2010; 49: 257-65.

[13] Aghcheli K, Parsian H,, Qujeq D, Talebi M, Mosapour A, Khalilipour E, Islami F, Semnani S, Malekzadeh R. Serum hyaluronic acid and laminin as potential tumor markers for upper gastrointestinal cancers. European Journal of Internal Medicine 2012; 23: 58–64.

[14] Poynard T, Bedossa P. Age and platelet count: a simple index for predicting the presence of histological lesions in patients with antibodies to hepatitis C virus. METAVIR and CLINIVIR Cooperative Study Groups. J Viral Hepatol 1997; 4: 199-208.

[15] Lackner C, Struber G, Liegl B, Leibl S, Ofner P, Bankuti C, Bauer B, Stauber RE. Comparison and Validation of Simple Noninvasive Tests for Prediction of Fibrosis in Chronic Hepatitis C. Hepatology 2005; 41(6): 1376-82.

[16] Parsian H. Is the aspartate transaminase to platelet ratio adequate for the assessment of liver fibrosis in patients with chronic liver disease? Hepat Mon. 2011; 11(5): 380-81.

[17] Yilmaz Y, Yonal O, Kurt R, Bayrak M, Aktas B, Ozdogan O. Noninvasive assessment of liver fibrosis with the aspartate transaminaseto platelet ratio index (APRI): Usefulness in patients with chronic liver disease. Hepat Mon 2011; 11(2): 103-7.

[18] Wai CT, Greenson JK, Fontana RJ, Kalbfleisch JD, Marrero JA, Conje evaram HS, et al. A simple noninvasive index can predict both significant fibrosis and cirrhosis in patients with chronic hepatitis C. Hepatology 2003; 38(2): 518-26.

[19] Shin WG, Park SH, Jang MK, Hahn TH, Kim JB, Lee MD, Kim DJ,. Jun SY, Park CK. Aspartate aminotransferase to platelet ratio index (APRI) can predict liver fibrosis in chronic hepatitis B. Digestive and Liver Disease 2008; 40: 267–74.

[20] Williams AL, Hoofnagle JH. Ratio of serum aspartate to alanine aminotransferase in chronic hepatitis Relationship to cirrhosis. Gastroenterology 1988; 95: 734-9.

[21] Kruger FC, Daniels CR, Kidd M, Swart G, Brundyn K, Rensburg KV, Kotze M. APRI: A simple bedside marker for advanced fibrosis that can avoid liver biopsy in patients with NAFLD/NASH. S Afr Med J 2011; 101: 477-80.

[22] Park GJ, Lin BP, Ngu MC, Jones DB, Katelaris PH. Aspartate aminotransferase: alanine aminotransferase ratio in chronic hepatitis C infection: is it a useful predictor of cirrhosis?J Gastroenterol Hepatol 2000 Apr; 15(4): 386-90.

[23] Hsieh YY, Tung SY, Lee IL, Lee K, Shen CH, Wei KL, Chang TC, Chuang CS, Wu CS, Lin YH. FibroQ: An Easy and Useful Noninvasive Test for Predicting Liver Fibrosis in Patients with Chronic Viral Hepatitis. Chang Gung Med J 2009; 32(6): 614-22.

[24] Hsieh YY, Tung SY, Lee K, Wu CS, Wei KL, Shen CH, Chang TS and Lin YH. Routine blood tests to predict liver fibrosis in chronic hepatitis C. World J Gastroenterol 2012; 18(8): 746-53.

[25] Sterling RK, Lissen E, Clumeck N, Sola R, Correa MC, Montaner J, et al. Development of a simple noninvasive index to predict significant fibrosis in patients with HIV/HCV coinfection. Hepatology 2006; 43: 1317-25.

[26] Harrison SA, Oliver D, Arnold HL, Gogia S, Neuschwander-Tetri BA. Development and validation of a simple NAFLD clinical scoring system for identifying patients without advanced disease. Gut. 2008 Oct; 57(10): 1441-7. Epub 2008 Apr 4.

[27] Raszeja-Wyszomirska J, Szymanik B, Ławniczak M, Kajor M, Chwist A, Milkiewicz P, Hartleb M. Validation of the BARD scoring system in Polish patients with nonalcoholic fatty liver disease (NAFLD). BMC Gastroenterol 2010 Jun; 28(10): 67.

[28] Ruffillo G, Fassio E, Alvarez E, Landeira G, Longo C, Domínguez N, Gualano G. Comparison of NAFLD fibrosis score and BARD score in predicting fibrosis in nonalcoholic fatty liver disease. J Hepatol 2011 Jan; 54(1): 160-3. Epub 2010 Aug 22.

[29] Rosenberg WM, Voelker M, Thiel R, et al. Serum markers detect the presence of liver fibrosis: a cohort study. Gastroenterology 2004; 127: 1704–13.

[30] Nobili V, Parkes J, Bottazzo G, Marcellini M, Cross R, Newman D, Vizzutti F, Pinzani M, Rosenberg WM. Performance of ELF serum markers in predicting fibrosis stage in pediatric non-alcoholic fatty liver disease. Gastroenterology. 2009 Jan; 136(1): 160-7. Epub 2008 Sep 20.

[31] Parkes J, Guha IN, Roderick P, Harris S, Cross R, Manos MM, Irving W, Zaitoun A, Wheatley M, Ryder S, Rosenberg W. Enhanced Liver Fibrosis (ELF) test accurately identifies liver fibrosis in patients with chronic hepatitis C. J Viral Hepat. 2011 Jan; 18(1): 23-31. doi: 10.1111/j.1365-2893.2009.01263.x.

[32] Parkes J, Bialek SR, Bell BP, et al. ELF serum markers accurately distinguish fibrosis severity in chronic hepatitis C: an external validation study. Hepatology 2006; 44(Suppl 1): 321.

[33] Bonacini M, Hadi G, Govindarajan S, Lindsay KL. Utility of a discriminant score for diagnosing advanced fibrosis or cirrhosis in patients with chronic hepatitis C virus infection. Am J Gastroenterol 1997; 92: 1302-4.

[34] Agostino Colli, Alice Colucci, Silvia Paggi, Mirella Fraquelli, Sara Massironi, Marco Andreoletti, Vittorio Michela, Dario Conte. Accuracy of a predictive model for severe hepatic fibrosis or cirrhosis in chronic hepatitis C. World J Gastroenterol 2005; 11(46): 7318-22.

[35] Saadeh S, Cammell G, Carey WD, Younossi Z, Barnes D, Easley K. The role of liver biopsy in chronic hepatitis C. Hepatology 2001; 33: 196-200.

[36] Contreras RH, Callewaert NLM. Serum marker for measuring liver fibrosis. U.S. patent 7244619; 2007.

[37] Poynard T, Imbert-Bismut F, Munteanu M, Messous D, Myers RP, Thabut D, et al. Overview of the diagnostic value of biochemical markers of liver fibrosis (FibroTest, HCVFibrosure) and necrosis (ActiTest) in patients with chronic hepatitis C. Comp Hepatol 2004; 3: 8.

[38] Poynard T, Imbert, Bismut F, Munteanu M, Ratziu V. FibroTest-FibroSURE: Towards a universal biomarker of liver fibrosis. Expert Rev Mol Diagn 2005; 5: 15–21.

[39] Morra R, Munteanu M, Imbert Bismut F, Messous D, Ratziu V, Poynard T. FibroMAX: Towards a new universal biomarker of liver disease. Expert Rev Mol Diagn 2007; 7: 481–90.

[40] Poynard T, Morra R, Halfon P, Castera L, Ratziu V, Imbert,Bismut F, et al. Meta-analyses of Fibrotest diagnostic value in chronic liver disease. BMC Gastroenterol 2007; 7: 40.

[41] Sebastiani G, Vario A, Guido M, Alberti A. Sequential algorithms combining non-invasive markers and biopsy for the assessment of liver fibrosis in chronic hepatitis B. World J Gastroenterol 2007; 13: 525-31.

[42] Naveau S, Raynard B, Ratziu V, Abella A, Imbert-Bismut F, Messous D, Beuzen F, Capron F, Thabut D, Munteanu M, Chaput JC, Poynard T. Biomarkers for the prediction of liver fibrosis in patients with chronic alcoholic liver disease. Clin Gastroenterol Hepatol 2005 Feb; 3(2): 167-74.

[43] Cales P, Oberti F, Michalak S, Hubert-Fouchard I, Rousselet MC, Konate A, et al. A novel panel of blood markers to assess the degree of liver fibrosis. Hepatology 2005; 42: 1373–81.

[44] Cale P, Laine F, Boursier J, Deugnier Y, Moal V, Oberti F, Hunault G, Rousselet MC, Hubert I, Laafi J, Ducluzeaux PH, Lunel F. Comparison of blood tests for liver fibrosis specific or not to NAFLD. Journal of Hepatology 2009; 50: 165–73.

[45] Matthews DR, Hosker JP, Rudenski AS, Naylor BA, Treacher DF, Turner RC. Homeostasis model assessment: insulin resistance and beta-cell function from fasting plasma glucose and insulin concentrations in man. Diabetologia 1985; 28(7): 412-9.

[46] Sud A, Hui JM, Farrell GC, Bandara P, Kench JG, Fung C, Lin R, Samarasinghe D, Liddle C, McCaughan GW, George J. Improved prediction of fibrosis in chronic hepatitis C using measures of insulin resistance in a probability index. Hepatology 2004; 39:1239-47.

[47] Laurent Castera. Noninvasive Methods to Assess Liver Disease in Patients with Hepatitis B or C. Gastroenterology 2012; 142: 1293–1302.

[48] Forns X, Ampurdanes S, Llovet JM, et al. Identification of chronic hepatitis C patients without hepatic fibrosis by a simple predictive model. Hepatology 2002; 36: 986-92.

[49] Adams LA, Bulsara M, Rossi E, DeBoer B, Speers D, George J, et al. Hepascore: an accurate validated predictor of liver fibrosis in chronic hepatitis C infection. Clin Chem 2005; 51: 1867-73.

[50] Becker L, Salameh W, Sferruzza A, Zhang K, ng Chen R, Malik R, Reitz R, Nasser I, Afdhal NH. Validation of hepascore, compared with simple indices of fibrosis, in patients with chronic hepatitis C virus infection in United States. Clin Gastroenterol Hepatol 2009 Jun; 7(6): 696-701.

[51] Bourliere M, Penaranda G, Ouzan D, Renou C, Botta-Fridlund D, Tran A, et al. Optimized stepwise combination algorithms of non-invasive liver fibrosis scores including Hepascore in hepatitis C virus patients. Aliment Pharmacol Ther 2008; 28: 458-67.

[52] Hui AY, Chan HL, Wong VW, et al. Identification of chronic hepatitis B patients without significant liver fibrosis by a simple noninvasive predictive model. Am J Gastroenterol 2005; 100: 616–23.

[53] Leroy V, Monier F, Bottari S, Trocme C, Sturm N, Hilleret MN, Morel F,Zarski JP. Circulating matrix metalloproteinases 1, 2, 9 and their inhibitors TIMP-1 and TIMP-2 as serum markers of liver fibrosis in patients with chronic hepatitis C: comparison with PIIINP and hyaluronic acid. Am J Gastroenterol 2004; 99: 271-9.

[54] Lok AS, Ghany MG, Goodman ZD, et al. Predicting cirrhosis in patients with hepatitis C based on standard laboratory tests: results of the HALT-C cohort. Hepatology 2005; 42: 282–92.

[55] Castera L, Le Bail B, Roudot-Thoraval F, et al. Early detection in routine clinical practice of cirrhosis and oesophageal varices in chronic hepatitis C: comparison of transient elastography (FibroScan) with standard laboratory tests and non-invasive scores. J Hepatol 2009; 50: 59-68.

[56] Masuzaki R, Tateishi R, Yoshida H, Goto E, Sato T, Ohki T, Goto T, Yoshida H, Sugioka Y, Ikeda H, Kanai F, Hamamura K, Shiina S, Kawabe T and Omata M. M1570 Prospective Comparison of Liver Stiffness Measurement and Lok Index in Chronic Hepatitis C Patients. Gastroenterology 2008; 134: (4) Supplement 1: Page A-795.).

[57] Patel K, Gordon SC, Jacobson I, et al. Evaluation of a panel of non-invasive serum markers to differentiate mild from moderate-to-advanced liver fibrosis in chronic hepatitis C patients. J Hepatol 2004; 41: 935-42.

[58] Christensen C, Bruden D, Livingston S, Deubner H, Homan C, Smith K, et al. Diagnostic accuracy of a fibrosis serum panel (FIBROSpect II) compared with Knodell and Ishak liver biopsy scores in chronic hepatitis C patients. J Viral Hepat 2006; 13: 652-8.

[59] Poynard T, Aubert A, Bedossa P, Abella A, Naveau S, Paraf F, Chaput JC. A simple biological index for detection of alcoholic liver disease in drinkers. Gastroenterology 1991 May; 100(5 Pt 1): 1397-402.

[60] Teare JP, Sherman D, Greenfield SM, Simpson J, Bray G, Catterall AP, Murray-Lyon IM, Peters TJ, Williams R, Thompson RP. Comparison of serum procollagen III peptide concentrations and PGA index for assessment of hepatic hepatic fibrosis. Lancet 1993; 342: 895-8.

[61] Oberti F, Valsesia E, Pilette C, et al. Noninvasive diagnosis of hepatic fibrosis or cirrhosis. Gastroenterology 1997; 113: 1609–16.

[62] Kelleher TB, Mehta SH, Bhaskar R, Sulkowski M, Astemborski J, Thomas DL, Moore RE, Afdhal NH. Prediction of hepatic fibrosis in HIV/HCV co-infected patients using serum fibrosis markers: The SHASTA index. Journal of Hepatology 2005; 43: 78–84.

[63] Poynard T, Ratziu V, Naveau S, Thabut D, Charlotte F, Messous D, Capron D, Abella A, Massard J, Ngo Y, et al. The diagnostic value of biomarkers (SteatoTest) for the prediction of liver steatosis. Comp Hepatol 2005; 4: 10.

[64] Lassailly G, Caiazzo R, Hollebecque A, Buob D, Leteurtre E, Arnalsteen L, Louvet A, Pigeyre M, Raverdy V, Six MF, Verkindt H, Eberle C, Patrice A, Dharancy S, Romon M, Pattou F, Mathurin P. Validation of noninvasive biomarkers (FibroTest, SteatoTest, and NashTest) for prediction of liver injury in patients with morbid obesity. Eur J Gastroenterol Hepatol 2011 Jun; 23(6): 499-506.

[65] Angulo P, Hui JM, Marchesini G, Bugianesi E, George J, Farrell GC, et al. The NAFLD fibrosis score: a noninvasive system that identifies liver fibrosis in patients with NAFLD. Hepatology 2007; 45: 846–54.

[66] Kandemir O, Polat G, Saraçoğlu G, Taşdelen B. The predictive role of AST level, prothrombin time, and platelet count in the detection of liver fibrosis in patients with chronic hepatitis C. Turk J Med Sci 2009; 39 (6): 857-862.

[67] Cross TJS, Rizzi P, Berry PA, Bruce M, Portmann B, Harrison PM. King's Score: an accurate marker of cirrhosis in chronic hepatitis C. Eur J Gastroen Hepat. 2009; 21(7): 730-8 10.1097/ MEG.0b013e32830dfcb3.

[68] Cross TJS, Calvaruso V, Maimone S, Carey I, Chang TP, Pleguezuelo M, Manousou P, Quaglia A, Grillo F, Dhillon AP, Dusheiko GM, Burroughs AK and Harrison PM. Prospective comparison of Fibroscan, King score and liver biopsy for the assessment of cirrhosis in chronic hepatitis C infection. Journal of Viral Hepatitis 2010; 17: 546–54.

[69] Bota S, Sirli R, Sporea I, Focsa M, Popescu A, Danila M, et al. A new scoring system for prediction of fibrosis in chronic hepatitis C. Hepat Mon 2011; 11(7): 548-55.

[70] Parsian H, Alizadeh M, Negahdar H. Whould the Physicians Eventually Obsolete the Liver Biopsy for the Assessment of Liver Fibrosis? Hepat Mon 2012; 12(5): 353-4. DOI: 10.5812/hepatmon.6227.

[71] Pinzani M, Vizzutti F, Arena U, Marra F. Technology Insight: noninvasive assessment of liver fibrosis by biochemical scores and elastography. Nat Clin Pract Gastroenterol Hepatol. 2008 Feb;5(2):95-106.

Chapter 5

Radiologic Assessment of Liver Fibrosis – Present and Future

Luca Macarini and Luca P. Stoppino

Additional information is available at the end of the chapter

http://dx.doi.org/10.5772/55164

1. Introduction

Liver fibrosis results from chronic damage to the liver in conjunction with the accumulation of extracellular matrix (ECM) proteins including collagen, which is a characteristic of most types of chronic liver diseases (CLD) [1]. Hepatic fibrosis was historically thought to be a passive and irreversible process due to the collapse of the hepatic parenchyma and its substitution with a collagen-rich tissue [2, 3]. Currently, is recognised to be a dynamic process that can progress or regress over periods as short as months [4].

This process is associated with an inflammatory response and a limited deposition of ECM. If the hepatic injury persists, then eventually the liver regeneration fails, and hepatocytes are substituted with abundant ECM. The distribution of this fibrous material depends on the origin of the liver injury. In chronic viral hepatitis and chronic cholestatic disorders, the fibrotic tissue is initially located around portal tracts, while in alcohol-induced liver disease, it locates in pericentral and perisinusoidal areas [5]. As fibrotic liver diseases advance, the hepatic architecture is distorted by the accumulation of ECM proteins leading to the formation of a fibrous scar and the subsequent development of nodules of regenerating hepatocytes defines cirrhosis. Main event in this process is the activation of the hepatic stellate cells, the main collagen-producing cells, by fibrogenic cytokines. Other cells such as portal fibroblasts and bone marrow–derived cells may also be involved in the fibrogenic process [1].

Liver biopsy is considered the current clinical standard of reference for the assessment of liver fibrosis [6]. Histologic examination is useful in identifying the underlying cause of liver disease and assessing the necro-inflammatory grade and the stage of fibrosis. However, it represents an invasive procedure, with pain and major complications occurring in 40% and 0.5% of patients, respectively [7]. Further, liver biopsy can be associated with substantial sampling-error. Histologic examination is subject to intra- and inter-observer variation and does not predict disease progression [8]. Therefore, there is a need for reliable, simple, and non-invasive methods for assessing liver fibrosis. In recent years, a wide variety of imaging-based methods have been used for noninvasively assessing liver fibrosis, including ultrasound, CT and MRI.

In this chapter, we provide an overview of the newer imaging techniques used in the evaluation of liver fibrosis.

2. Epidemiology and natural history

Fibrosis leading to cirrhosis can accompany virtually any CLD that is characterized by the presence of architectural disruption and/or inflammation. Over many years the principle causes of CLD have been chronic viral hepatitis B and alcoholic liver disease. Other etiologies of liver disease include parasitic infestation (e.g. schistosomiasis), autoimmune attack on hepatocytes or biliary epithelium, neonatal liver disease, metabolic disorders including Wilson's disease, hemochromatosis and a variety of storage diseases, chronic inflammatory conditions (e.g. sarcoidosis), drug toxicity (e.g. methotrexate or hypervitaminosis A), and vascular derangements, either congenital or acquired. While rates of alcoholism and alcoholic liver disease are falling in many countries, hazardous drinking amongst young people is resulting in alarming rates of alcoholic liver disease in several northern European countries [9, 10]. Over the last few decades two other diseases have emerged to make a major contribution to the burden of CLD. Chronic hepatitis C and non-alcoholic fatty liver disease (NAFLD) are recognised to have already had a major impact on CLD incidence. Hepatitis C virus (HCV) is transmitted in blood and blood products through unsafe injection practices and the therapeutic use of infected blood products. It is thought that the world prevalence of chronic hepatitis C is nearly 200 million people [11, 12]. In the developed world with rapidly increasing rates of obesity, NAFLD is considered to represent a major cause of significant fibrosis. Although it appears that only a minority of patients with NAFLD (maybe 20%) develop significant fibrosis, due to the vast prevalence of the at-risk overweight population, NAFLD may give rise to an epidemic of liver fibrosis [13, 14].

Of the many causes of CLD, our understanding of natural history of fibrosis is most complete in HCV, with some information about HBV and steatohepatitic diseases, including alcoholic liver disease and NAFLD. Fibrosis associated with HCV can assume a variable course, from decades of viremia with tiny fibrosis to a rapid onset of cirrhosis within 10–15 years. It appears to be host factors rather than viral factors that correlate with fibrosis progression in HCV, such as older age at the time of infection, concurrent liver disease due to HBV or alcohol (>50g/day), male gender, increased body mass index (BMI) and HIV infection or immunosuppression [15, 16].

Information about fibrosis progression in other diseases is largely subjective, but the development of cirrhosis typically requires many years to decades. There are, however, some notable exceptions in which the development of cirrhosis can be greatly accelerated, possibly occurring within months rather than years: (1) neonatal liver disease – infants with biliary atresia may present at birth with severe fibrosis and marked parenchymal distortion; (2) HCV-infected patients after liver transplantation – a subset of patients who undergo liver transplantation for HCV cirrhosis may develop rapidly progressive cholestasis and recurrent cirrhosis within months, requiring retransplantation [17]; (3) patients with HIV/HCV co-infection – these patients have relatively rapid fibrosis compared to those with HCV alone [18], especially if the HIV is untreated; (4) severe delta hepatitis [19]; and (5) some cases of drug-induced liver disease. These examples of 'fulminant fibrosis' probably reflect dysregulation of several pathways, including defective immunity, massive inflammation and necrosis, and/or altered matrix resorption.

3. Assessment of stage of fibrosis

Liver biopsy is a common element of diagnostic workup in hepatic cirrhosis, and is the accepted diagnostic gold standard. Several systems for scoring liver fibrosis have been proposed in order to classify the progression of fibrosis to cirrhosis into discrete stages, each based on visual assessment of collagen staining of liver biopsy samples. The more frequently used systems are the histology activity index (HAI: Knodell score) [20], the Ishak modification of the HAI score [21], and the Metavir score [22].

The HAI system consists of the evaluation of two histopathological categories, necroinflammation and fibrosis. Furthermore, necroinflammation includes three subcategories: periportal necrosis and inflammation, scored from 0 to 10; intralobular necrosis and inflammation, scored from 0 to 4; and portal inflammation, scored from 0 to 4. Fibrosis is scored as 0, 1, 3, or 4, with 1 indicating portal fibrosis only, 3 indicating bridging fibrosis, and 4 indicating cirrhosis. The HAI score is the combined scores for necrosis, inflammation, and fibrosis, while the overall HAI scores can also be broken into individual components of necrosis, inflammation, and fibrosis to yield additional information [20]. Despite this system is widely used, is relatively insensitive to changes in fibrosis (lack of a score for stages between mild and severe), and has an intra- and inter-observer reproducibility relatively poor.

Ishak et al. [21] have proposed a modification of the HAI scoring system, which uses similar scores for necroinflammatory changes (activity: 0 to 18), but scores fibrosis on a scale from 0 to 6. Scores of 1 and 2 indicate portal fibrosis, 3 and 4 bridging fibrosis, 5 incomplete or early cirrhosis, and 6 established cirrhosis. The Ishak scale provides better discrimination in assessing small changes in fibrosis, permitting a better assessment of progression of disease, and possible effects of therapy. The intra- and interobserver variability of the Ishak scoring system has yet to be carefully defined.

The Metavir score [22] was developed in an attempt to address some of the problems with the Knodell score. The Metavir score is a semiquantitative classifications system and scores both necroinflammatory changes that fibrosis. The activity score is graded according to the intensity of necroinflammatory lesions (A0 = no activity, A1 = mild activity, A2 = moderate activity, A3 = severe activity). The fibrosis score is assessed on a five point scale (F0 = no fibrosis, F1 = portal fibrosis without septa, F2 = few septa, F3 = numerous septa without cirrhosis, F4 = cirrhosis) (Figure 1). Clinically significant fibrosis is generally defined by F2 involvement or greater. Compared to the Knodell fibrosis score (which has only four levels), the Metavir score permits recognition of subtler variation in the degree of fibrosis. The Metavir system has been carefully validated and shows good intra- and interobserver reproducibility. This system is commonly used in Europe. Table 1 compares the three systems described for evaluating the stage of fibrosis.

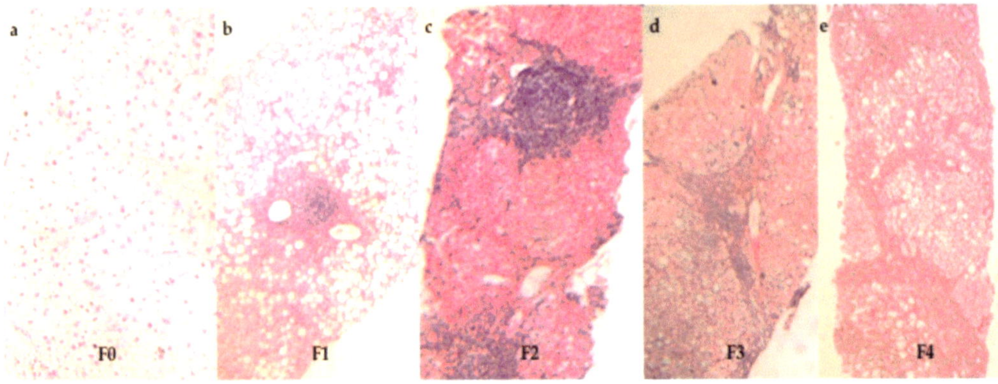

Figure 1. Progression of fibrosis from periportal fibrosis to cirrhosis according to the Metavir scoring system shown through photomicrographs (original magnification, ×10; Hematoxylin and Eosin stains) of histologic sections from liver biopsy specimens. **(a)** No fibrosis (stage F0). **(b)** Portal and periportal fibrosis only (stage F1). **(c)** Periportal fibrosis with few septa (stage F2). **(d)** Septal fibrosis and bridging without cirrhosis (stage F3). **(e)** Cirrhosis (stage F4) which appears as nodules of liver parenchyma separated by thick fibrous bands.

Stage of fibrosis	HAI (Knodell)	Ishak	Metavir*
0	No fibrosis	No fibrosis	No fibrosis
1	Portal fibrosis	Fibrosis of isolated portal areas with or without short septa	Portal fibrosis
2	n. d.	Increased fibrosis in most portal areas with or without short septa	Portal fibrosis with scattered septa
3	Portoportal or portocentral septa	Portal fibrosis with portoportal septa	Numerous septa without cirrhosis
4	Cirrhosis	Portal fibrosis Cirrhosis with marked porportoportal or portocentral septa	Cirrhosis
5	n. d.	Marked septum formation (portoportal or portocentral) with some nodule formation (incomplete cirrhosis)	n. d.
6	n. d.	Probable or definite cirrhosis	n. d.

n. d. = not defined;

* only validated in chronic hepatitis C

Table 1. Histological classification systems for evaluating the stage of fibrosis

According to the average size of the parenchymal nodules, *cirrhosis* may be classified into micronodular, macronodular, and mixed types. While micronodular cirrhosis is defined as nodules less than 0.3 cm in diameter, macronodular cirrhosis is defined as nodules larger than 0.3 cm. Micronodular cirrhosis is generally caused by diffuse liver injury, such as alcohol, other hepatotoxic agents, and metabolic disorders (nonalcoholic steatohepatitis), whereas macronodular cirrhosis is observed in disease processes where hepatocellular regeneration plays a significant role (chronic and autoimmune hepatitis) [23].

Although the scoring systems mentioned above for hepatic fibrosis are extremely useful in diagnosis and staging of liver fibrosis, all of these systems have important limitations. Hepatic fibrosis may not be homogenous throughout the liver, and the liver specimen obtained by the needle biopsy may not accurately reflect the overall average degree of fibrosis. A number of studies have demonstrated excessive rates of sampling error (25%-40%) resulting in poor reproducibility regardless of underlying liver disease origin [24]. The extent of variation from observer interpretation by expert histopathologists may be as high as 20% [25]. In addition, there is mounting evidence that liver biopsy has a number of limitations for its use in these roles as well. These include: (a) the effect of reduced biopsy size (<25 mm) and complete portal tract number (<11) on understaging fibrosis; (b) interobserver variation in histological interpretation; and (c) the qualitative nature of assessing fibrosis in 2 dimensions with descriptive staining techniques. Ultimately, the method of percutaneous liver biopsy is an invasive procedure with poor acceptance by patients. The associated morbidity from this technique is estimated at 3% with a mortality rate of 0.03% [26].

In summary, although liver biopsy is considered the standard of reference, it has several limitations (invasiveness, complications, sampling variability, subjectivity) that restrict its role as a method for screening and longitudinal assessment of liver fibrosis. New reproducible and reliable noninvasive techniques are required to evaluate disease progression in patients with CLD, and to monitor pharmacological treatment.

4. Imaging techniques

Since morphologic alterations and features of portal hypertension are present only in advanced CLD, routine examinations by ultrasound (US), computed tomography (CT) and magnetic resonance imaging (MRI) could produce specific findings, but with very limited sensitivity. The ability to detect early and intermediate stages of fibrosis using conventional ultrasound with Doppler assessment of the hepatic vasculature is unsatisfactory [27]. CT offers improved resolution of early morphological changes with cirrhosis but has low accuracy in fibrosis detection [28]. In fact, quantitative assessment of the density distribution of liver parenchyma showed that only diffuse steatosis and active alcoholic cirrhosis had significantly different mean hepatic attenuation values [29]. Moreover, most studies of contrast-enhanced CT involved patients with cirrhosis [30, 31] and it is thus unclear if changes in hepatic enhancement could be used to diagnose mild or moderate hepatic fibrosis. MRI identify specific features of cirrhosis such as hepatic vein narrowing, caudate to right lobe ratio, and expanded gallbladder fossa [32], but remains lacking in earlier stages of fibrosis [33]. Hence, assiduous efforts have been made to search for technological developments.

4.1. Sonography-based techniques for assessment of liver fibrosis

Recently, diverse sonography–based techniques have been used in assessment of liver fibrosis, including Transient Elastography, Real-Time Elastography, and Acoustic Radiation Force Imaging sonoelastography.

Transient Elastography. Transient Elastography (TE) (FibroScan®, Echosens, Paris, France) is a new imaging modality for detecting hepatic fibrosis. The measuring instrument comprises a computer driven control unit and a probe with an ultrasound transducer, which is located at the end of a vibrating piston. The piston generates a low frequency elastic wave (5 Mhz) that passes through the skin and liver tissue and is transmitted into hepatic tissue at a speed of around 1 m/s. The ultrasound then detects the propagation of the shear wave through the liver by measuring its velocity. The shear wave velocity is directly related to the tissue stiffness, with a higher velocity equating to higher tissue stiffness, corresponding to increasing severity of fibrosis.

TE is carried out with the patient supine, with his/her right arm behind their head. The measuring probe is positioned at the level of the xiphoid in the right mid-axillary line, at 90 degrees to the body. TE measures liver stiffness in a volume that approximates a cylinder 1 cm wide and 4 cm long, between 2,5 cm and 6,5 cm below the skin surface (Figure 2). Ten validated measurements are required, with the median value taken as the final result, which is expressed in units of kilopascals (kPa). The range of possible liver stiffness values obtained with this technique is from 2.5 to 75.0 kPa, with the normal liver stiffness value for healthy individuals being around 5.5 kPa (Figure 3) [34].

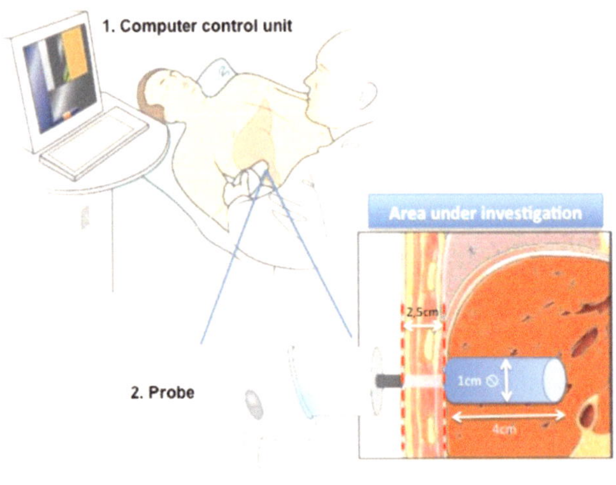

Figure 2. Illustration of the two different constituent of the measuring instrument and the positioning of the probe in relation to the area of liver under investigation.

The advantages of TE are that the results are immediately available, and the procedure is painless, rapid (~3 minutes per patient), and easy to perform. The interequipment, intraobserver (96–98%) and interobserver agreement (89–98%) of TE has been shown to be excellent, but the success rate depends on observer expertise, patient BMI and intercostal space [35-37]. Moreover, TE is a reliable method for the diagnosis of extensive fibrosis (Metavir F=3) and cirrhosis (F=4): positive and negative predictive values range from 70–95% and 77–95%, respectively [38-41]. The age of the subject does not affect liver stiffness, and males tend to have a slightly higher liver stiffness value compared to females [34]. One of the important aspects of liver stiffness measurements is the cut-off values that are adopted for different stages of fibrosis, with higher cut-off levels corresponding to higher fibrosis stages.

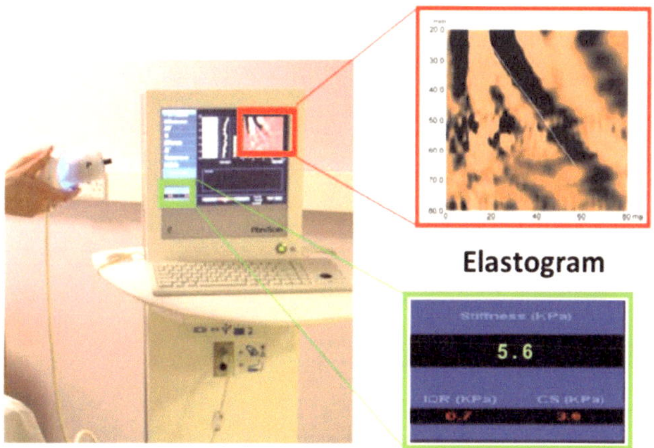

Figure 3. Example of shear wave propagation velocity in healthy subject with normal liver stifness.

The cut-off levels are also different for different diseases. Therefore it is important to interpret the results with the cut-off values specific for the underlying condition. Table 2 show a summary of the cut-off values used for specific liver diseases. For example, in HCV patients according to Castera et al. [42], liver stiffness cut-off values were 7.1 kPa for F≥2, 9.5 kPa for F≥3, and values ≥ 12.5 kPa for F=4 (defined according to Metavir system).

There are some physical limitations of TE, such as obesity (particularly the fatness of the chest wall), narrow intercostal space and ascites. Moreover, Fraquelli et al. found that TE reproducibility is significantly reduced in patients with steatosis, an increased BMI and lower degrees of hepatic fibrosis [35]. TE is an innovative and user-friendly technology for the assessment of hepatic fibrosis in patients with CLD. However, despite strong academic and commercial promotion, the key reason that TE cannot completely substitute a liver biopsy is that it is unable to diagnose liver disease and it only allows staging with the best diagnostic performances for severe fibrosis and cirrhosis. Assessment of pre-cirrhotic disease and the longitudinal assessment of change in fibrosis have not been fully evaluated.

Author	Disease	Cut-off F≥2 (kPa)	Cut-off F≥3 (kPa)	Cut-off F=4 (kPa)	Results
Castera et al. [42]	HCV	7.1	9.5	12.5	AUROC for F≥2: 0.80 AUROC for F≥3: 0.90 AUROC for F=4: 0.95
Marcellin et al. [43]	HBV	7.2	8.1	11.0	AUROC for F≥2: 0.81 AUROC for F≥3: 0.93 AUROC for F=4: 0.93
de Ledinghen et al. [44]	HIV/HCV coinfection	4.5	n.d.	11.8	AUROC for F≥2: 0.72 AUROC for F=4: 0.97
Yoneda M et al. [45]	NAFLD	6.6	9.8	17.5	AUROC for F≥2: 0.87 AUROC for F≥3: 0.90 AUROC for F=4: 0.99
Corpechot C et al. [46]	PBC or PSC	7.3	9.8	17.3	AUROC for F≥2: 0.92 AUROC for F≥3: 0.95 AUROC for F=4: 0.96

n. d. = not defined; PBC = primary biliary cirrhosis; PSC = primary sclerosing cholangitis.

Table 2. Diagnostic performance of TE for the diagnosis of cirrhosis according to liver disease

Real-Time Elastography. Real-Time Elastography (RTE) is an alternative method for measurement of tissue elasticity integrated in a sonography machine developed by Hitachi Medical Systems. This technique can reveal the physical property of tissue using conventional ultrasound probes during a routine sonography examination. Ophir et al. [47] first described the principle of this technique in 1991. To reduce the time-consuming calculations, Pesavento et al. [48] developed a fast cross-correlation technique that is the basis for RTE. The difference in hardness between diseased and surrounding tissue can be detected by RTE based on the physical properties of the tissue [49, 50]. In effect, this method measures the degree of tissue distortion (strain), mechanically induced, in the B mode image to quantify the elasticity of the tissue. By measuring the tissue strain induced by compression, it is possible to estimate the tissue hardness. The calculation of tissue elasticity distribution is assessed in real-time ultrasound imaging and depicted as color-coded images with the conventional B-mode image in the background [49, 51]. The color scale includes the following colors: red (soft tissue), green (intermediate, normal tissue), and blue (anelastic, hard tissue).

RTE is carried out with patients in a supine position with the right arm elevated above the head. Breathing does not cause any motion artifacts since each elastography image is obtained in a few milliseconds. The examination is performed on the right lobe of the liver through the intercostal space. 5-9 MHz probe is used because higher frequencies allow better analysis of areas close to the transducer. The measurement depth is between 20 and 50 mm (mean, 35 mm) with a 350–500 mm^2 area of measurement. The results are considered consistent only applying a pressure of

3–4 on a scale of 0–6 arbitrary units (Figure 4). Ten valid measurements are performed in each subject and the entire examination lasts approximately 5–10 minutes per patient.

Friedrich-Rust et al. first assessed real-time elastography for the detection of liver fibrosis [52], founding that the area under the receiver operating characteristic (AUROC), a measurement of the diagnostic accuracy of a test, was 0.75 for the diagnosis of significant fibrosis (F≥2). A significant increase in accuracy (AUROC = 0.93) was obtained by combining RTE score and two routine laboratory values (platelet count and GGT). In a recent paper Wang et al. [53] compared the overall elasticity determined by RTE in 55 patients with liver fibrosis and chronic hepatitis B and in 20 healthy volunteers. Using a new quantitative technology for diffuse histological lesion with 11 parameters characterizing the stiffness degree of tissue, the AUROC was 0.93 (F≥1, $p < 0.001$) for the diagnosis of liver fibrosis, 0.92 (F≥2, $p < 0.001$), 0.84 (F≥3, $p < 0.05$) and 0.66 (F=4, $p > 0.05$), respectively.

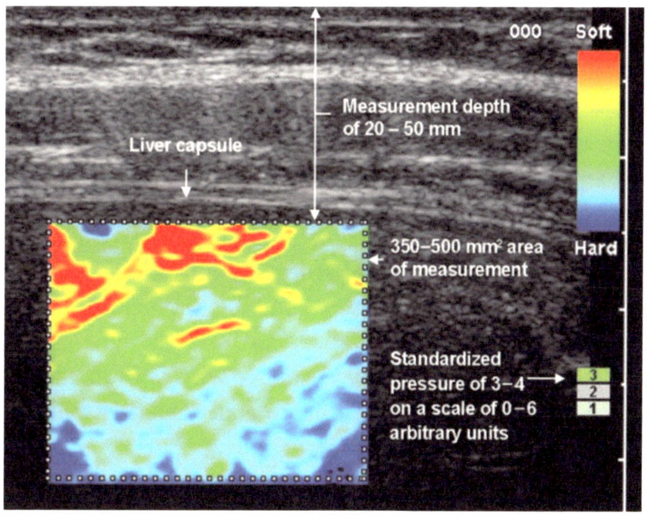

Figure 4. Example of tissue elasticity distribution in a helathy subject represented as color-coded images over conventional B-mode image.

As for TE even for RTE obesity, narrow intercostal space and ascites are potential physical limitations. More number of sample about chronic hepatitis with assessment by RTE is needed to performed to certify its advantages.

Acoustic Radiation Force Impulse Elastography. Acoustic Radiation Force Impulse (ARFI) imaging is a novel ultrasound-based elastography method that is integrated in a conventional ultrasound machine enabling the exact localization of measurement site. ARFI imaging involves the mechanical excitation of tissue using short-duration acoustic pulses (≈262 μsec) with a fixed transmit frequency of 2.67 MHz to generate localized, micron-scale displacements in tissue. The first available applications to implement this technology are Virtual Touch tissue imaging and Virtual Touch tissue quantification (Siemens, Erlangen, Germany). Unlike conventional B-mode sonography, which provides anatomical details based on differences in

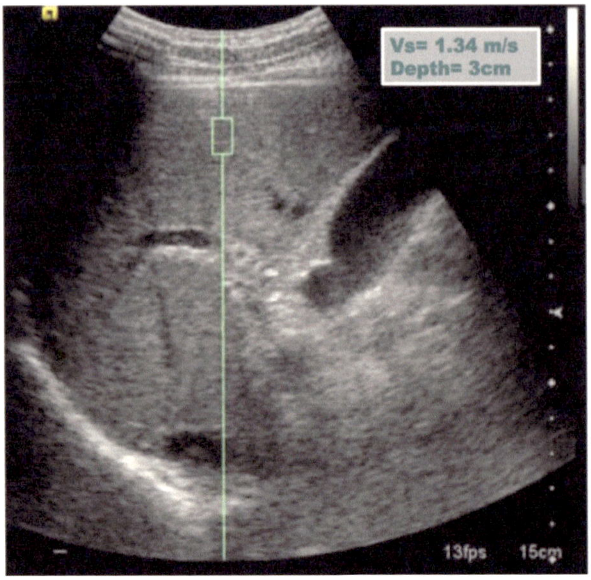

Figure 5. Measurement of the shear wave velocity with ARFI. The region of interest is placed 2–3 cm from the liver capsule at the right hepatic lobe, where the liver tissue is at least 5.5 cm thick.

acoustic impedance, Virtual Touch™ imaging describes relative physical tissue stiffness properties. In complement, Virtual Touch™ tissue quantification provides accurate numerical measurements related to tissue stiffness at user-defined anatomical locations. ARFI technology quantifies stiffness without manual compression since, using the Virtual Touch™ application, the tissue is compressed by acoustic energy. Virtual Touch tissue quantification is a quantitative assessment of tissue stiffness, through measurement of shear wave speed.

The system uses a standard ultrasonographic probe and offers elastography with a flexible metering box of 1 cm at variable depths (Figure 5). An acoustic push pulse transmitted by the transducer (3.5 MHz) toward the tissue induces an elastic shear wave that propagates through the tissue (Figure 6). The propagation of the shear wave is followed by detection pulses that are used to measure the velocity of shear wave propagation, which is directly related to tissue stiffness: speed increases with stiffness. The measurements were performed on the right lobe of the liver through the intercostal spaces, away from motion and portal/hepatic vessels, about 2 cm from the liver capsula, at a depth between 3.8 and 5.5 cm. Usually a total of 10 valid measurements per patient are performed. In difficult patients, to obtain better access to the liver without excessive pushing or breath holding, the measurements were performed on patients lying in the left lateral decubitus position, or using a subcostal approach to the left lobe. The results are expressed by the shear wave velocity - SWV (m/s). Thus, the measured SWV is an intrinsic and reproducible property of the tissue [54-56].

According to Sporea et al., [57] despite exhibiting a strong correlation with histological fibrosis, ARFI is an accurate test only for the prediction of severe fibrosis and cirrhosis (F=4) using 1.7 m/s as cut-off value (AUROC: 0.931, sensibility: 93%, specificity: 86.7%). Recently, a meta-

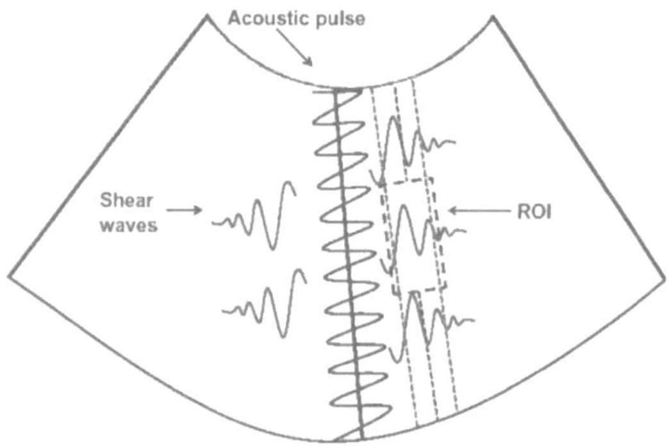

Figure 6. Principle of Acoustic Radiation Force Elastography. Transmission of short-duration acoustic pulses generates tissue displacement within a localized area of the liver, resulting in shear waves propagating away from the region of excitation. Shear wave velocity is measured in meters/s within a defined region of interest (ROI), and is proportional to the square root of tissue elasticity.

analysis was performed [58] including ARFI patient data obtained from eight studies for a total of 518 patients. The authors found that the AUROC was 0.87 for the diagnosis of significant fibrosis (F≥2), 0.91 for the diagnosis of severe fibrosis (F≥3), and 0.93 for the diagnosis of cirrhosis. The optimal cut-off for F≥2 was 1.34 m/s, for F≥3 1.55 m/s and for the diagnosis of liver cirrhosis 1.80 m/s, respectively.

Finally, Colombo et al. [59] performed a head-to-head comparison of TE, RTE, and ARFI imaging in the diagnosis of liver fibrosis, in a population consisting of 27 normal subjects and 54 patients with CLD. The three methods showed high correlation with fibrosis and poor correlation with necro-inflammatory activity, with TE showing the best performance (AUROC was 0.87 for F≥1 and 0.89 for F≥2, with the best cut-offs set at 6.3 kPa for fibrosis and 7.8 kPa for significant fibrosis). Only TE and ARFI exhibited high diagnostic accuracy (AUROC ≥ 0.9) in diagnosing cirrhosis (F=4). However, TE was unsuccessful in 15% of patients, mainly due to obesity. Nevertheless, the authors conclude that TE is probably the best method to screen for CLD patients in the general population and to identify significant fibrosis, but further studies are needed to fully explore the potential of RTE, since its technology and the equations used to calculate tissue elasticity are rapidly changing.

4.2. MR imaging-based techniques for assessment of liver fibrosis

In the last decade, the development of MRI scanner with high-performance magnetic field gradients made the introduction of three-dimensional sequences for liver imaging possible. Volumetric image acquisitions with near-isotropic voxels (1–3 mm in all three-dimensions) through the entire liver can be achieved in a single breath-hold or using respiratory triggering. In detail, several technological advances have been made for assessment of fibrosis, including Conventional MRI, Double contrast-material enhanced MRI, Diffusion-weighted MRI, MR elastography, perfusion MRI, and MR spectroscopy.

Unenhanced MRI. In patients with precirrhotic stages of liver fibrosis as well as patients with early cirrhosis, the liver parenchyma usually has a normal appearance or may reveal only subtle, generic heterogeneity on unenhanced MRI [60]. Conversely, in patients with advanced cirrhosis, fibrotic septa and bridges show low-signal-intensity reticulations on T1-weighted images and high signal-intensity reticulations on T2-weighted images (Figure 7) [61]. Dodd et al. [62] described four different patterns of diffuse fibrosis detectable on T2-weighted images: (1) patchy, poorly defined regions of high signal intensity, (2) thin perilobular bands of high signal intensity, (3) thick bridging bands of high signal intensity that surround regenerative nodules, and (4) diffuse fibrosis that causes perivascular (bull's-eye) cuffing. Although most forms of diffuse fibrosis can occur in any type of cirrhosis, thin perilobular bands and perivascular cuffing appear most commonly in primary biliary cirrhosis. The large water content of advanced fibrosis provides prolonged T2 relaxation times and may explain these signal intensity characteristics [63]. These reticulations frequently enclose regenerative nodules, which are <2 cm and isointense to hyperintense on T1-weighted images, isointense to hypointense on T2-weighted images. Lipid-containing nodules or steatotic nodules display signal loss on out-of-phase gradient echo (GRE) images in comparison with in-phase images. Iron containing nodules or siderotic nodules appear markedly hypointense on T2-weighted and T2*-weighted images [63].

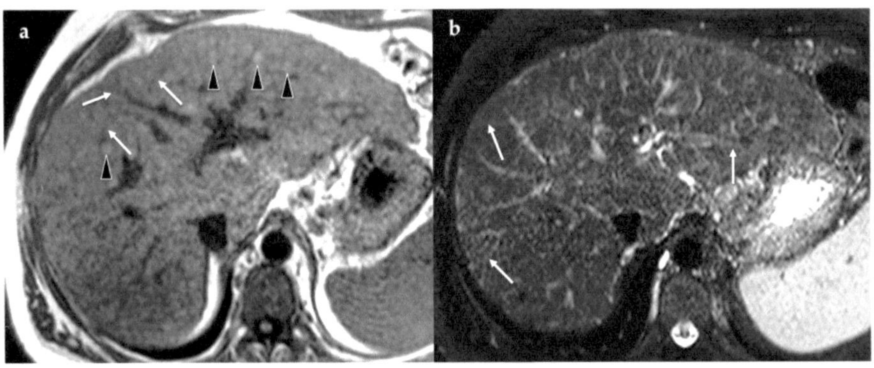

Figure 7. Unenhanced MR imaging in a in a 61-year-old man with alcohol-related cirrhosis. Unenhanced T1-weighted image (**a**) shows hypointense reticulations (arrows) and numerous regenerative nodules (arrowheads), which are iso- to hyperintense. Unenhanced T2-weighted fat-saturated image (**b**) allows a clearer visualization of the reticulations throughout the liver parenchyma visible as hyperintense septa (arrows).

Fibrotic scars up to several centimetres thick characterize *confluent fibrosis* with a mass-like appearance seen in approximately 15% of patients with advanced cirrhosis. Confluent fibrosis has similar signal intensity as fibrotic septa and bridges but is easier to visualize because of its size. This mass-like fibrosis typically has a wedge-shaped area, radiates from the portal hilum, contacts and retracts the liver capsule, and causes focal volume loss.

Furthermore, the cirrhotic liver develops characteristic morphologic alterations such as surface nodularity, widening of fissures, expansion of the gallbladder fossa, notching of the right lobe, atrophy of the right lobe, and relative enlargement of the lateral segments of the left lobe and caudate lobe (Figure 8) [62]. However, these signs of advanced disease have high specificity for cirrhosis but there are only few publications on unenhanced MRI for the staging of hepatic fibrosis.

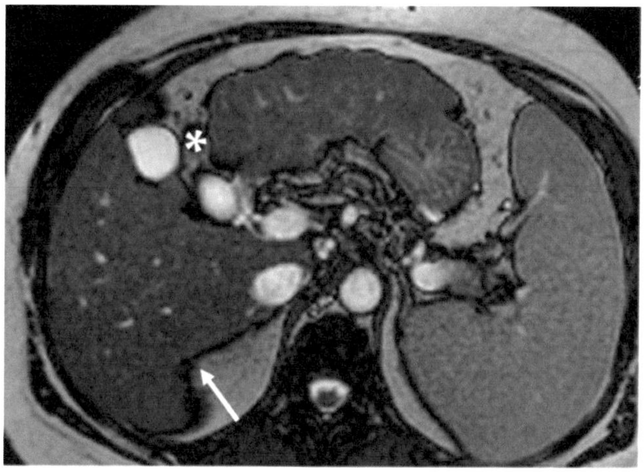

Figure 8. Axial Balanced fast field echo image in a 59-year-old man with alcoholic cirrhosis shows surface nodularity, hypertrophy of the left lobe, expanded gallbladder fossa (asterisk), and notching of the right lobe (arrow).

Contrast-enhanced MRI. The detection of liver fibrosis is improved by the administration of contrast agents. Three contrast agents are currently commercially available: gadolinium-based contrast agents; superparamagnetic iron oxide particles; Gd-EOB-DTPA.

Gadolinium-based contrast agents cause T1 shortening and signal enhancement on T1-weighted images. Most gadolinium-based contrast agent formulations freely equilibrate with the extracellular compartment and accumulate in tissues with large extracellular volumes such as liver fibrosis [64]. Thus, most gadolinium-based contrast agents preferentially enhance the signal of liver fibrosis on T1-weighted images. The reticulations enhance progressively after contrast agent administration. Although some of the reticulations are enhanced at the arterial phase, most are not enhanced until the more delayed images (late venous and equilibrium phases) (Figure 9). Similarly, the persistence of enhancement of the confluent fibrosis into the late phases associated with its characteristic morphology allows differentiation from HCC.

Superparamagnetic iron oxide particles (SPIO) are reticulo-endothelial-specific particulate MRI contrast agents which are cleared from the blood through phagocytosis and accumulate in the cells of the reticulo-endothelial system of the liver, spleen, and bone marrow, with approximately 80% taken up by the liver. SPIO markedly shorten T2 relaxation rates and signal loss is greatest with gradient recalled echoes because these are highly sensitive to T2*-shortening effects. Consequently, the signal intensity of the liver parenchyma decreases on T2-weighted sequences, except in the areas with reduced Kupffer cell density, like fibrosis within the liver, which accumulate less iron oxide and appear as high signal-intensity reticulations (Figure 10) [65]. Two SPIO particle formulations are clinically available, namely ferumoxides and ferucarbotran. Ferumoxides (Feridex IV, Berlex Laboratories; and Endorem, Guerbet) is a

SPIO colloid with low molecular weight dextran coating, with a particle size of 120-180 nm. This contrast agent is prepared as a dilution in 100 ml of 5% dextrose and administered as a drip infusion over about 30 min. At about 8 min following the intravenous injection, iron oxide particles are taken up by the reticulo-endothelial cells in the liver and in the spleen. Maximum signal loss is obtained after 1 h with an imaging window ranging from 30 min to 6 h after the injection. The recommended dosage of Endorem (ferumoxides injectable solution) is 0.56 milligrams of iron (0.05 mL Feridex IV) per kilogram of body weight. Ferucarbotran (Resovist, Bayer Healthcare) is a carboxydextrane-coated SPIO, with a hydrodynamic diameter ranging between 45 and 60 nm. Unlike Endorem, Resovist can be safely injected rapidly in a bolus fashion, and has an effect on the shortening of both T1 and T2 relaxation time. Dynamic T1-weighted GRE 3D sequences can be performed to acquire the perfusion properties of the lesion during the arterial and portal venous phases of the contrast agent. On dynamic MR imaging using T1-weighted GRE, enhancement was positive in the liver for at least 30 s after bolus injection of SPIO. On delayed images after 10 min, the T2/T2* effects are observed due to the reticulo-endothelial uptake in the liver. The recommended dose of Resovist is: for patients weighing less than 60 kg: 0.9 ml Resovist); for adults patients weighing 60 kg or more: 1.4 ml Resovist. Lucidarme et al. describe hypersignal intensities on the SPIO enhanced T2-weighted sequences in 76% of patients with chronic hepatitis and a Metavir score of F≥2 with good specificity (80%) [66]. It is hypothesized that reticulation patterns surrounding hypointense SPIO enhanced liver tissue correspond to fibrotic septa surrounding regenerative nodules [67].

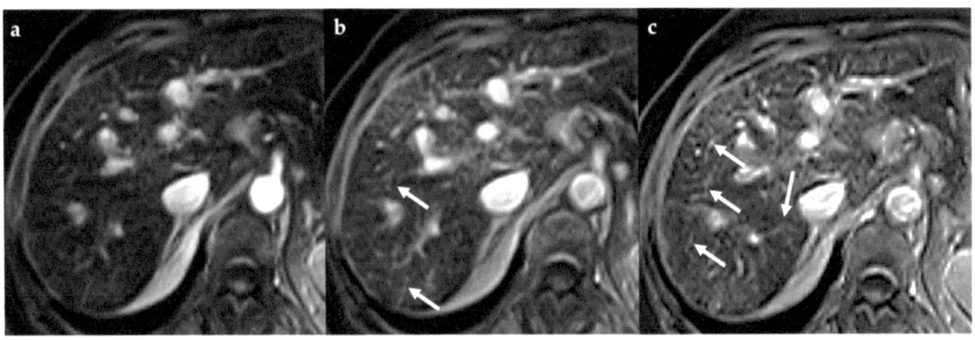

Figure 9. Dynamic enhancement patterns in fibrous tissue after administration of a gadolinium-based contrast agent. Axial 3D T1-weighted images obtained in the (**a**) arterial phase, (**b**) portal venous phase, and (**c**) 3 min after intravenous injection of a gadolinium-based contrast agent, show the progressive enhancement of the fibrotic reticulations in the liver parenchyma.

Gd-EOB-DTPA, a derivative of gadopentetate dimeglumine (Gd-DTPA), known generically as gadoxetic acid (Primovist, Bayer Schering, Berlin, Germany), is a recent hepatocyte-specific MR contrast agent and has been used to detect and characterize various hepatic tumors [68, 69]. Similar to Gd-DTPA, Gd-EOB-DTPA can be used as bolus injection. This contrast agent is actively transported from the sinusoidal space into liver cells and causes intense parenchymal enhancement, beginning within 1 or 2 min of contrast agent injection. The enhancement peaks at around 20 min and lasts for at least 2 h. Unlike Gd-DTPA, which will return into blood

http://dx.doi.org/10.5772/55164

vessels thereafter and is excreted entirely by kidneys, about 50% of Gd-EOB-DTPA is secreted through the biliary system, and the other 50% is secreted by kidney [70]. Deterioration of hepatic function would decrease the excretion of Gd-EOB-DTPA, because it needs adenosine triphosphate (ATP) for energy to secrete into the bile ducts by hepatocyte [71, 72]. In fact, in livers with good hepatic function, intense enhancement occurs. In livers without good function, due to cholestasis or hepatocellular dysfunction, enhancement of liver parenchyma may be weak. Using this contrast medium liver fibrosis can appear as an area of low signal intensity due to decreased hepatic function from fibrosis (Figure 11). Recent dynamic contrast-enhanced MRI studies have shown promising results using Gd-EOB-DTPA. Lee et al. [73] reported a significant alteration in signal intensity change between a group of patients with liver cirrhosis or chronic hepatitis and healthy subjects in the hepatocyte phase 20 min after contrast agent administration. In addition, Watanabe et al. [74] demonstrated that the contrast enhancement index significantly correlated with fibrosis stage. Clinical trials are currently under way to prospectively assess fibrosis staging with this contrast agent.

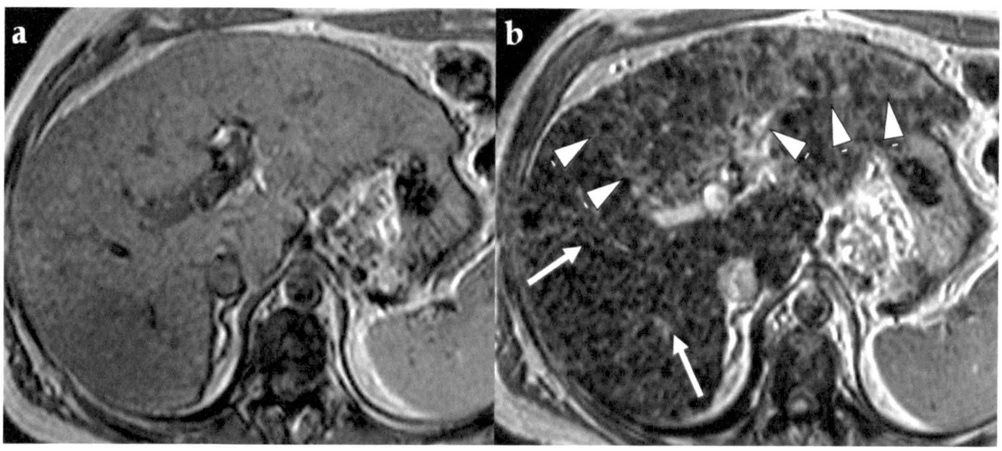

Figure 10. Advanced fibrosis and infiltrative HCC in a 46-year-old man with HCV-related cirrhosis. T2*-weighted gradient-echo images obtained before (**a**) and after (**b**) intravenous SPIO injection. After injection, fibrotic reticulations in the right lobe have diminished Kupffer cell density, do not accumulate iron oxides, and hence appear relatively hyperintense (arrows in **b**). The left lobe is expanded and shows a wedge-shaped mass with heterogeneous hyperintensity (arrowheads in **b**) in the hepatocellular phase, suggestive for infiltrative HCC.

Double-contrast enhanced MRI. Double-contrast MRI (DC-MRI) using extracellular contrast agents in combination with SPIO particles was shown to sensitively detect liver fibrosis and depict HCC in cirrhotic livers [75]. During DC-MRI, two contrast media boli with a synergistic effect are applied: 1) SPIO particles infusion to observe the accumulation of SPIO particles by Kupffer cells of normal liver parenchyma or by Kupffer cells located in benign liver lesions, which causes signal loss on T2*-weighted images followed by 2) Gadolinium chelates i.v. injection for analysis of delayed enhancement of hepatic septal and bridging fibrosis on T1-weighted images with fat suppression. The consequence is high image contrast between the low-signal-intensity liver parenchyma and high-signal-intensity fibrotic reticulations (Figure

12) [76]. Aguirre et al. [77] examined 101 CLD patients who underwent DC-MRI to detect hyperintense reticulations, which are postulated to represent septal fibrosis, and hypointense nodules thought to represent regenerating nodules. They achieved an accuracy of greater than 90% for the diagnosis of advanced hepatic fibrosis (F≥3) compared with histopathological analysis. Recently, Fischer et al. [78] assessed the performance of semiquantitative measurement of liver perfusion from analysis of SPIO induced signal-dynamics. In this study 31 patients, including 18 patients with biopsy proven liver cirrhosis, prospectively underwent DC-MRI with dynamic T2*-weighted gradient echo imaging after SPIO bolus injection measuring hepatic blood flow index (HBFI) and splenic blood flow index (SBFI). Significant inverse correlation was seen between HBFI and presence of liver cirrhosis resulting in a significant decrease of HBFI in patients suffering of cirrhosis compared with patients with healthy livers ($P < 0.05$).

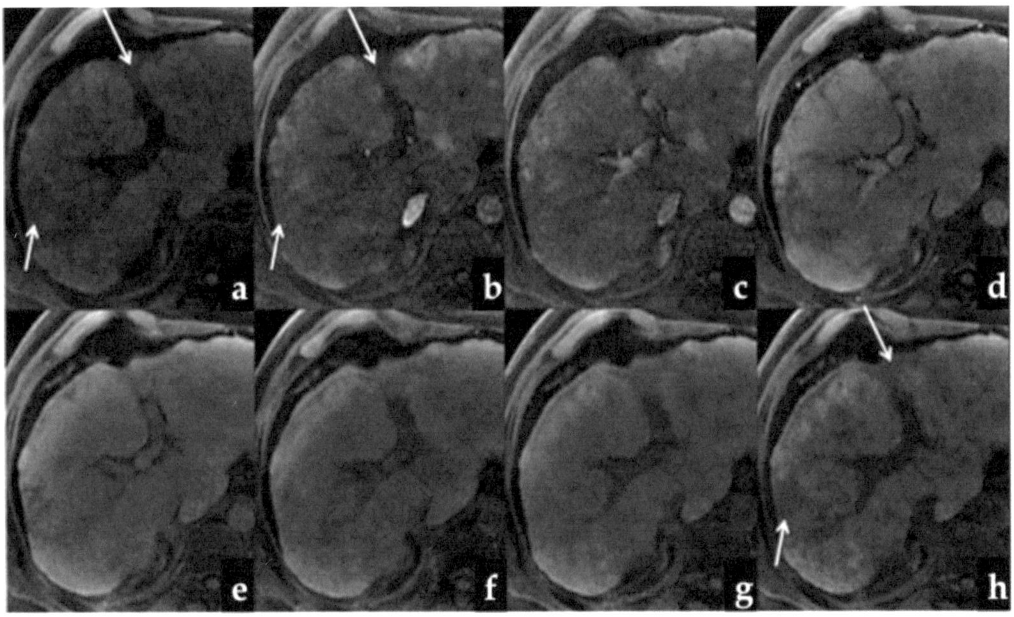

Figure 11. Confluent fibrosis in a 56-year-old man with cirrhosis. Precontrast (**a**), arterial phase (**b, c**), portal venous phase (**d**), 3 min (**e**), 5 min (**f**), 8 min (**g**), and hepatocellular phase (**h**). Wedge-shaped ill-defined areas associated with capsular retraction, with decreased enhancement in the dynamic phases and with no uptake of Gd-EOB-DTPA in the HCP (arrows).

An advantage of DC-MRI is that it works on routine imaging units and does not require specialized equipment. Computer-based texture analysis techniques may assess texture abnormalities qualitatively or quantitatively. The high cost and inconvenience associated with use of two contrast agents represent the main limitations of DC-MRI. Moreover, minor adverse events have been associated with use of SPIO, such as back pain, which has been reported in about 10% of cirrhotic patients during infusion of the particles. It is usually associated with rapid injection of SPIO and resolves after the injection is paused [79].

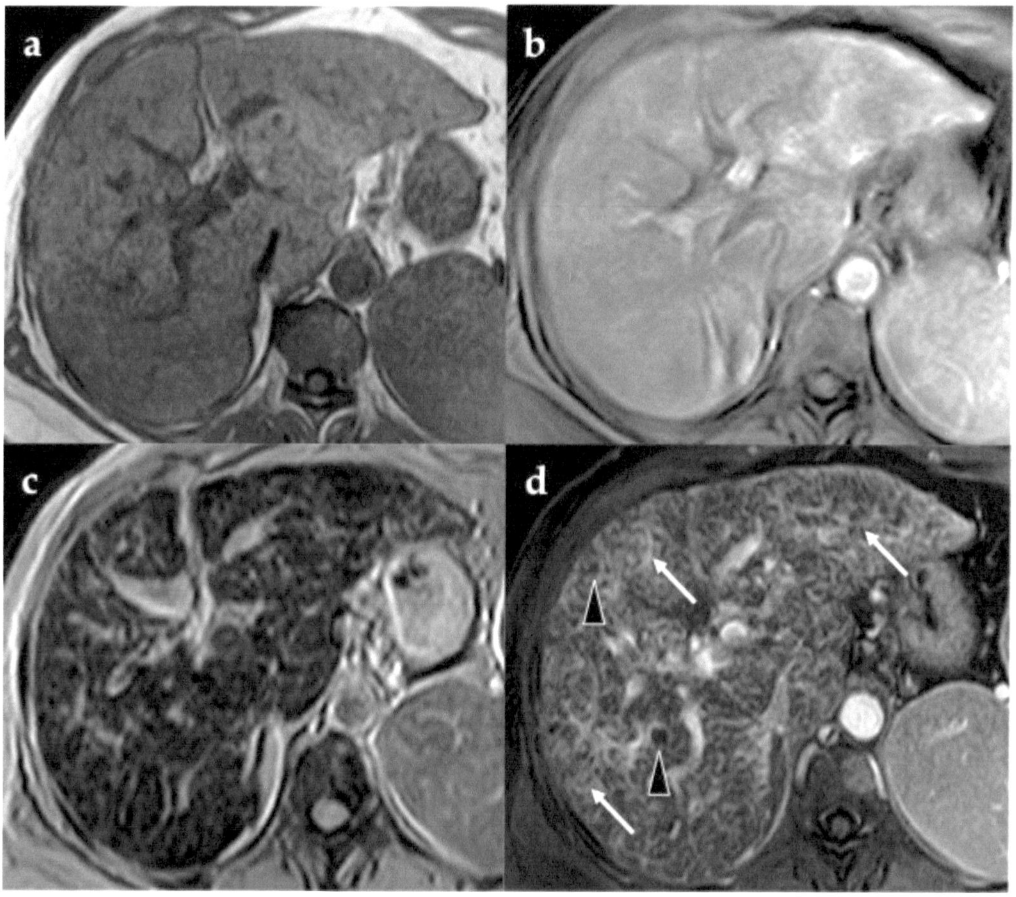

Figure 12. Double contrast-enhanced MR imaging appearance of cirrhosis in a 67-year-old woman with chronic HCV infection. Axial 2D T1-weighted unenhanced image (**a**); axial 3D T1-weighted enhanced image 30 sec after ferucarbotran injection, thus exploiting the shortening effect on T1 relaxation time; (**b**), T2*-weighted gradient-echo SPIO-enhanced image after 15 min (**c**); and axial 3D T1-weighted double contrast-enhanced image (**d**). SPIO and a gadolinium-based contrast agent are synergistic with better depiction of fibrotic reticulations (arrows in **d**) and regenerative nodules (arrowheads in **d**).

Diffusion weighted magnetic resonance imaging. Diffusion-weighted magnetic resonance imaging (DW-MRI) is a technique that assesses the freedom of diffusion of water protons in tissues and has been extensively applied for the early detection of cerebral ischemia. Recent advances have made it feasible to apply diffusion MRI techniques for abdominal imaging [80]. In liver fibrosis, extracellular collagen fibers, glycosaminoglycans and proteoglycans may inhibit molecular diffusion of water, which suggest that DWI can be an effective method for the evaluation of fibrosis.

In DW images the observed signal intensity of tissue varies inversely with the freedom of water proton diffusion. Tissues with reduced water proton diffusion will be brighter than those with normal water proton diffusion. The sensitivity of the imaging sequence to water diffusion can be altered by changing the b value, or b factor, which is dependent in a specific mathematical way on the diffusion encoding gradient waveforms [81] and increases with the duration and amplitude of the diffusion sensitizing gradients. If two or more DW images are obtained, then it is possible to calculate the apparent diffusion coefficient (ADC) of water protons in tissues, which is determined by the slope of the log intensity versus b value [82, 83]. Because of the relatively short T2 relaxation time of the normal liver parenchyma (approximately 46 msec at 1.5 T and 24 msec at 3.0 T) [84], the b values used for clinical imaging are typically no higher than 1000 sec/mm^2. Applying a small diffusion weighting of b less than 100–150 sec/mm^2 nulls the intrahepatic vascular signal, creating the so-called black-blood images, which improves detection of focal liver lesions [85, 86], while higher b values ($\geq$ 500 sec/mm^2) give diffusion information that helps assessment of liver cirrhosis and focal liver lesion characterization [87]. The calculated ADC values can be displayed as an image and quantitative analysis can be performed by placing measuring the mean value within a region of interest, which is typically positioned in the right hepatic parenchyma to avoid major vascular structures and cardiac motion artifacts (Figure 13).

Because DW images were acquired using different b values and protocols and likely different patient populations, ADC values of cirrhosis are not consistent throughout the literature. Examples include ADC cutoff values of 1.41×10^{-3} mm^2/s by Taouli et al. [88], 0.88×10^{-3} mm^2/s by Kim et al. [89], 1.11×10^{-3} mm^2/s by Girometti et al. [90], and more recently 1.63×10^{-3} mm^2/s by Kovač et al. [91]. Although there are various ADC values for the diagnosis of cirrhosis, the cirrhotic liver tissues consistently have significantly lower ADC values compared with liver tissues with no fibrosis as seen in prior studies [92-94]. Previously published studies with DWI showed moderate sensitivity and specificity in distinguishing advanced fibrosis to cirrhosis (F3–F4) from lesser degrees of fibrosis. However, considerable overlap in ADC values between tissues with cirrhosis and with no to moderate fibrosis was also observed.

In a recent study, Bakan et al. [95] performed DWI with b-factors of 0, 500 and 1000 s/mm^2 in order to investigate the relationship between ADC values and liver inflammation (HAI scores). They found that as HAI scores increased there was a statistically significant decrease in ADC values ($P<0.01$). However, differences in MRI equipment and sequence parameters make it difficult to compare studies. In addition, despite technical improvements in DWI, the method remains sensitive to susceptibility and motion-related artifacts, and it is difficult to obtain images with sufficient quality for reliable quantitative analysis on a consistent basis. Further studies are required to create a standard setup for DWI to make studies comparable and to evaluate how various ADC values of liver tissue other than fibrosis may be influenced by other factors associated with chronic liver diseases.

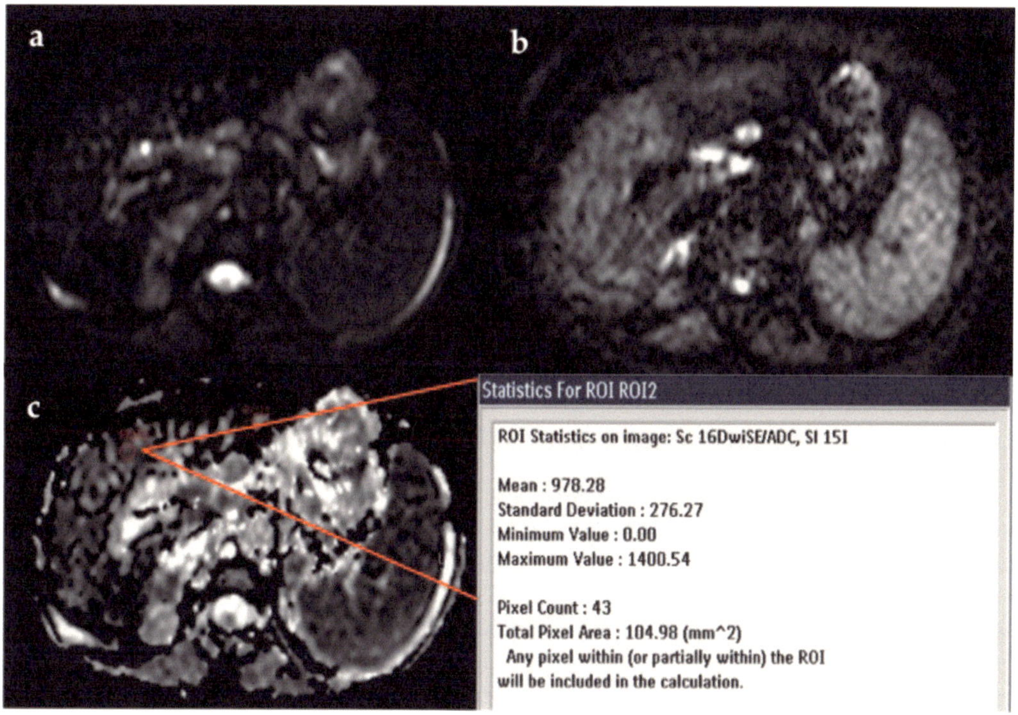

Figure 13. year-old man with biopsy-proven hepatitis C and related stage III fibrosis. Diffusion-weighted images obtained with b value of 0 (**a**) and 800 (**b**) s/mm^2 and apparent diffusion coefficient (ADC) map (**c**) are shown. Mean ADC value was 0.98 × 10^{-3} mm^2/s.

MR Elastography. A new option for assessing shear stiffness in various tissue types, including liver fibrosis, is MR Elastography (MRE) [96]. MRE uses a modified phase contrast technique to sensitively image the propagation characteristics of acoustic shear waves that are generated with the organ of interest [97]. This system consisted of an acoustic driver system, a gradient-echo MRE pulse sequence, and special software for data analysis. A 19cm diameter, 1.5cm thick cylindrical passive driver is placed against the right chest wall over the liver with the center of the driver at the level of the xiphoid of the sternum (Figure 14). The passive driver is held in place with an abdominal binder. Continuous acoustic vibration at frequencies between 40 and 120 Hz transmits from an active driver to the passive driver through a flexible vinyl tube was used to produce propagating shear waves in the liver [98-100]. When the pneumatic device is activated, the patient will feel vibrations in the rib cage due to the pressure waves. MR images are acquired with a gradient-echo sequence as the waves propagate through the liver. The velocity and wavelength of the waves propagating in the abdomen depend on the stiffness of the tissue (velocity and wavelength increase with greater tissue stiffness), enabling the stiffness estimation [101].

A specialized phase-contrast MRI sequence is then used to image the propagating waves in the liver. This sequence uses motion-encoding gradients that are oscillated synchronously with the applied vibrations, allowing waves with amplitudes in the micron range to be readily imaged. Each MRE acquisition provides an image that represents the displacement caused by shear wave propagation in the medium. The wave images are then processed using a specially developed inversion algorithm to generate quantitative images called elastograms [96]. Elastograms are maps of tissue stiffness shown on a color scale ranging from soft to hard. Mean elasticity values measured in regions of interest within the liver are obtained. The unit of measurement for elasticity is kilopascal (kPa), as it is with ultrasound-based transient elastography (TE) (Figure 15). Each MRE examination is performed during a single breath-hold of 10 to 30 seconds to allow imaging of wave propagation, in addition to the standard 30-40 minute MRI examination of the abdomen [102].

Initial studies in patients with a spectrum of liver disease types have shown that liver stiffness as measured with MRE increases as the stage of fibrosis advances. The differences in stiffness between patients with early stages of fibrosis (F0 vs F1 vs F2) are small and there is overlap between groups, but the differences between groups with higher stages (F2 vs F3 vs F4) are large, with little overlap between groups [99, 102].

As for ADC values in DWI examinations, a variety of MRE cutoff values are observed throughout the literature. In a recent study, to identify fibrosis stage ≥ 2 (F2–F4) and stage ≥ 3 (F3–F4), Wang et al. [103] reported sensitivity of 91% and 92% and specificity of 97% and 95% with cutoff values of 5.37 and 5.97 kPa, respectively. Huwart et al. [104] showed similar high sensitivity of 98% and 95% and specificity of 100% and 100% for discrimination, although relatively lower cutoff values of 2.5 kPa and 3.1 kPa were used. The variability of cutoff values observed may be potentially explained by MRE different scanner manufacturers, case mixes, imaging protocols, and post-processing procedures.

As reported by Rustogi et al. [105] stiffness measurements are repeatable with high overall inter-reader agreement (P=0.74); thus, MRE shows potential for longitudinal monitoring of patients. Furthermore, Yin et al. found that this technique has a high negative predictive value (97%) for excluding the presence of fibrosis, suggesting that MRE could have a role for improving the ability to risk-stratify patients for liver biopsy [102].

MRE benefits from the intrinsic advantages of MR imaging, such as freely oriented field of view, no "acoustical window" requirement, the ability to quantify steatosis, operator independence, and the ability to perform conventional liver MRI at the same time. In addition, MRE is relatively unaffected by the patient's body habitus and the presence of ascites, as shear waves generated in vivo in MRE have good hepatic penetration.

Nevertheless MRE has some limitations. The most important one is that MRE measures a surrogate of liver fibrosis (tissue stiffness) rather than fibrosis itself. A variety of factors may confound MRE assessment of liver fibrosis, including hepatic inflammation, steatosis, hepatic vascular congestion, cholestasis, and portal hypertension. Moreover, the selection of significant regions of interest is subjective and requires judgment and experience. As with the other techniques, efforts to standardize the equipment and techniques used for MRE should be practiced to maximize diagnostic accuracy and enable comparison of results in different settings. Further prospective evaluation is required for characterizing the diagnostic performance of MRE.

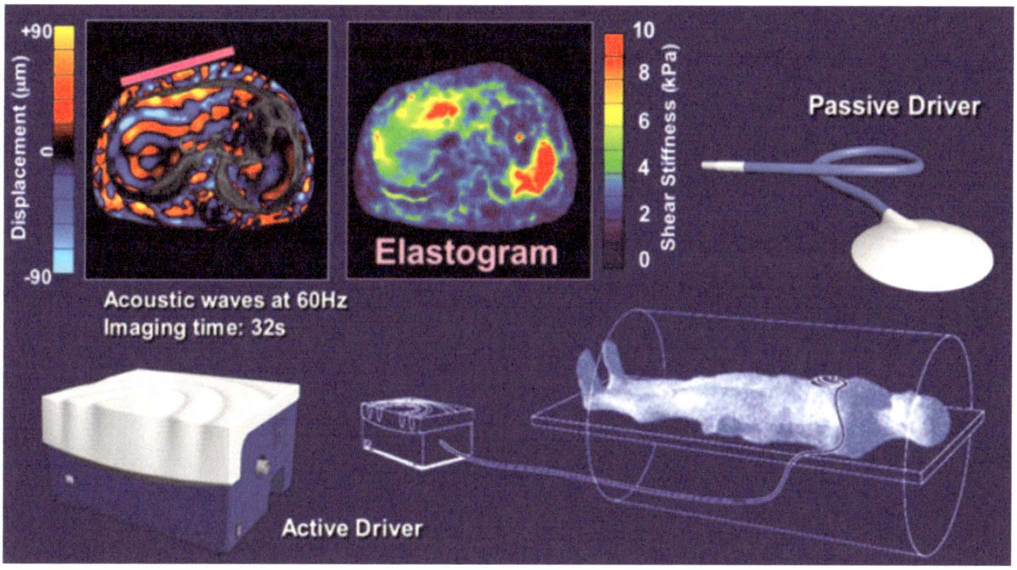

Figure 14. A remote acoustic driver pumps air into a pneumatic device strapped onto the patient's body, eliciting tissue displacement, which is measured by MRE and used to derive images showing tissue stiffness.

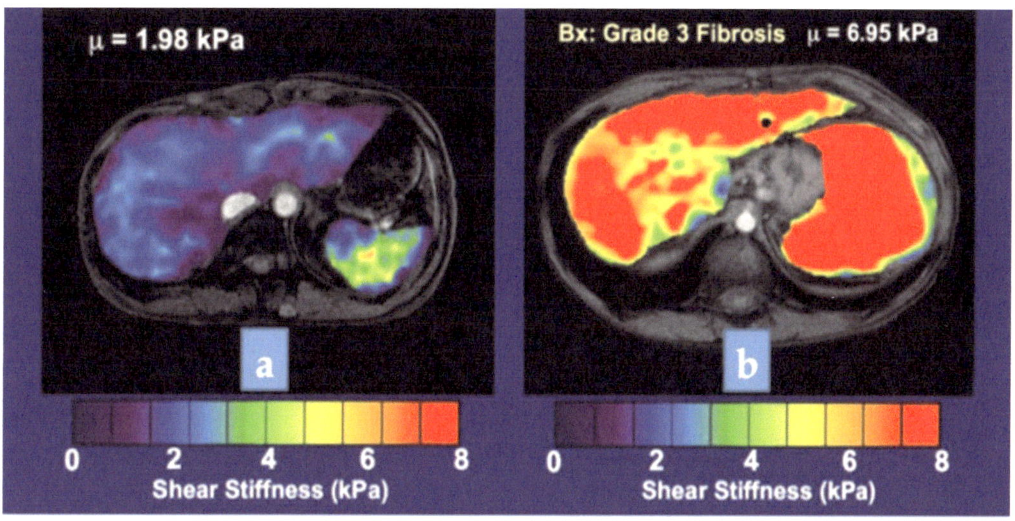

Figure 15. An elastogram of a healthy liver (**a**) showing a post processed value of 1.98 kPa corresponding to normal tissue stiffness. An elastogram of the liver of a patient with Grade 3 fibrosis (**b**), with a shear stiffness value of 6.95 kPa.

Perfusion MRI. Perfusion MRI provides a method of measuring perfusion changes in the liver. Liver fibrosis gradually led to a loss of normal fenestrae, due to deposition of basement membrane and new formation of capillary tight junctions along the sinusoids (phenomenon of capillarization). There is also deposition of fibers by activated hepatic stellate cells, which results in enlargement of the Space of Disse. Consequently, intrahepatic vessels and sinusoids obliteration reduces passage of blood through the parenchyma, producing increase in hepatic arterial perfusion and decrease in portal venous perfusion. Several studies have shown that careful kinetic modeling of dynamic contrast-enhanced (DCE) MR images can noninvasively quantify regional and global changes in hepatic perfusion associated with liver cirrhosis and fibrosis [106-109].

For perfusion MRI of the liver, a rapid injection of a low-molecular-weight gadolinium-chelate contrast is necessary, using a programmable pump injector. Is recommended the intravenous administration of Gd-DTPA (0.1-0.2 mmol of contrast medium/kg body weight) followed by a 20ml saline flush, at an injection rate of 3–5 ml/s. T1-weighted 3D spoiled gradient echo sequence is typically performed, with whole liver coverage and high temporal resolution (i.e. repeated imaging of the same area in the liver about every 4 s). An oblique imaging plane (oblique coronal) is particularly useful in order to include the aorta and the portal vein in the same image sections. Patients are generally instructed to fast for 4–6 h prior to the scan, given the potential changes in portal venous flow occurring in the post-prandial state.

The analysis can be performed by semi-quantitative or quantitative techniques. One semi-quantitative description of liver vascularity is the hepatic perfusion index (HPI), which describes the relative contribution of arterial vs portovenous flow to the total liver perfusion. The HPI has been investigated using different imaging techniques, and appears to provide biologically meaningful information despite its relative simplicity [110]. For quantitative methods, regions of interest (ROIs) are placed over the area of interest to generate signal intensity (SI) versus time curve. Typically, arterial input function is obtained by placing a ROI on the abdominal aorta. Portal input function is obtained from a ROI placed on the main portal trunk, and a ROI at the level of hepatic parenchyma to measure the time–activity curve. Several kinetic models are currently in use for the assessment of liver perfusion. Single-input models assume that the vascular input is derived from the hepatic artery only, whereas dual-input models assume that the vascular input is derived from both the hepatic artery and the portal vein. Single compartment models assume that the contrast is confined to only one compartment (i.e. vascular space), whereas dual compartment models assume that there is dynamic distribution of contrast between two compartments (i.e. the vascular space and the interstitial space). Therefore, numerous perfusion parameters can be estimated, including absolute portal venous blood flow, absolute arterial blood flow, absolute total liver blood flow, portal venous fraction, arterial fraction, distribution volume (DV), and mean transit time (MTT) [111].

In a previous study, Annet et al. [106] have investigated a dual-input single compartment model and have demonstrated altered arterial, portal and total liver perfusion, as well as increased MTT in cirrhotic livers compared to non-cirrhotic livers, and found a correlation with severity of disease as assessed by the Child-Pugh class and degree of portal hypertension. In a recent study, Leporq et al. [112] applied dual-input single-compartment model and quantitative perfusion parameters for the noninvasive assessment of liver fibrosis. HPI, arterial and portal perfusion, tissue blood volume, and MTT showed a significant difference between nonadvanced fibrosis (F0–F2) and advanced fibrosis (F3–F4). In addition, HPI and portal perfusion showed a strong correlation with the fibrosis score ($P < 0.001$). Chen et al. performed a prospective study using Gd-EOB-DTPA in patients with chronic hepatitis to calculate perfusion parameters by applying a dual-input single compartment model. They found a significant increase in arterial perfusion at 60 s and 100 s in patients compared with healthy subjects and a significant difference in arterial perfusion when three different fibrotic subgroups (none, mild and advanced) were compared at 60 s [113].

Several factors limit the correlation between perfusion parameters and fibrosis, such as cardiac status, fasting state, hepatic congestion, hepatic inflammation, hepatic lesions, and portal venous flow. Other limitations include differences in technical parameters, imaging system, and use of different pharmacokinetic models [114]. In addition, relevant is the laborious post-processing required to obtain quantitative perfusion parameters. However, standardization of imaging acquisition and analysis techniques need to be actively addressed for the technique to be widely adopted.

MR Spectroscopy. MR spectroscopy (MRS) enables the non-invasive measurement of concentrations of different chemical components within tissues, which are displayed as a spectrum with peaks consistent with the various chemicals detected. The liver is considered an ideal organ for MRS investigation due to its anatomical location and increased metabolic demands [115,116]. MRS of the liver is performed using a whole body MRI system at field strengths of 1.5 Tesla (T) or higher. The patient lies supine on the MRI table with RF coils positioned appropriately. After a standard MR imaging for localization, special MR pulse sequences are applied to generate spectroscopic data within the appropriate anatomical location and volume (defined by voxels) of interest. A typical examination will take 45 to 60 minutes. The spectral analysis of data requires processing to reduce noise and perform analysis. Metabolite concentrations can be expressed in absolute or relative terms. In general, the peak area of a metabolite signal is directly related to its concentration. Whereas a number of in vivo studies have explored the diagnostic performance of MRS for characterizing hepatic lesions [117], more recently there has been some interest in the role of MRS for detecting hepatic fibrosis. MRS is most commonly used to assess signals from hydrogen (^{1}H) and phosphorus (^{31}P).

^{1}H-based MRS is widely used for the quantification of hepatic lipid. In vitro MRS studies of oils [118] and intact liver tissue [119] have demonstrated that lipid resonances might be quantified to derive indices of lipid composition, including saturation and polyunsaturation. These compositional indices differed between obese patients with and without hepatic steatosis. Indices of lipid composition using in vivo proton (^{1}H) MRS at 1.5 Tesla have been shown to delineate the severity of fibrosis in patients with chronic hepatitis C (in whom hepatic steatosis is prevalent) [120]. In patients with chronic HCV infection, as fibrosis advances, steatosis tends to recede [121]. McPherson et al. [122] confirmed this inverse relation and found that with ^{1}H-MRS, the percentage of steatotic hepatocytes in patients with more advanced fibrosis tended to be underestimated. However, because ^{1}H-MRS yields an estimate of proton density fat fraction and not a measure of the degree of hepatocellular involvement, this result would be expected. When ROCs were generated for the diagnosis of steatosis with ^{1}H-MRS according to fibrosis stage, the values were only slightly lower in cases of more advanced fibrosis (AUC, 0.97 for F=0–1 vs 0.95 for F=2–3). More recently, Georgoff et al. [123] also found only a small decrease in the ROC for ^{1}H-MRS in subjects with fibrosis (AUC, 0.96 for F=0 vs 0.92 for F=1–4).

^{31}P-based MRS has also shown promise as a method of assessing the degree of hepatic fibrosis, in particular through analysis of the phosphomonoester/phosphodiester (PME/PDE) ratio [124]. As the stage of fibrosis increases, the PME peak may represent extensive membrane remodeling due to elevated levels of cell membrane precursors (such as phosphocholine and phosphoethanolamine). At the same time, there is a reduction in the PDE peak owing to reduced levels of membrane degradation products such as glycerophosphorylethanolamine and glycerylphosphorylcholine. Therefore, changes in the PME/PDE ratio are thought to reflect an increase in the regenerative efforts made by the damaged liver [125]. Moreover, ^{31}P-MRS had a sensitivity and specificity of 82% and 81% respectively for cirrhosis and showed statistically significant differences between mild hepatitis, moderate hepatitis, and cirrhosis [126].

Several limitations with current MRS approaches, however, are observed. The major problem in obtaining MRS signals from abdominal organs is sensitivity to physiologic movement during the scan time usually exceeding several minutes. Various methods of reducing movement, such as breath holding and placing patients in the prone position during signal acquisition, have been used [127]. Furthermore MRS requires considerable operator skills (sequence programming, shimming, analysis of spectra) and access to special equipment. Most studies contain small numbers of patients from heterogeneous populations assessed by varying MRS methods. In addition, the variation in reproducibility of data acquisition from healthy volunteers can range between 4% and 20% for both subject and examination. Ultimately, the role of in vivo MRS for detecting hepatic fibrosis requires assessment in larger diagnostic accuracy studies among patients with various hepatobiliary disorders.

5. Conclusion and future directions

A fast, safe and reliable technique to assess fibrosis of CLD and to follow up progression or regression of fibrosis during treatment is required. Ultrasound is still a widespread, low cost, user-friendly, and accurate technique. However, it may not have a high specificity due to limitations related to the patient or operator and its role is probably more oriented to patient's selection and follow-up. MRI is a more "challenging" method for radiologists and especially for patients, with limitations related to: the availability of high performance scanner; the presence of experienced personnel; the examination's timing and to its less tolerability. MRI may, however, represent the one-stop shop technique, allowing the diagnosis and characterization of fibrosis but also the overall assessment of CLD. In addition, MRI is more research-oriented, since its multiparametric potential, allows not only distinguishing the various fibro-steatosic alterations but also performing metabolic assessments. This last feature permits studies on the pathogenetic mechanisms and on drug therapies studies.

The diagnostic performances of all described noninvasive radiologic modalities were better in distinguishing patients with cirrhosis from lesser degrees of fibrosis. However, staging of fibrosis was rarely achieved reliably. In conclusion, to date, the most promising techniques appear to be Transient Elastography [59] and MRE [128, 129] since they provide reliable results in detecting severe fibrosis and future developments promise to increase the reliability and

http://dx.doi.org/10.5772/55164

accuracy of staging of hepatic fibrosis. In the future, MRI technical development and new contrast agents could permit imaging of fibrogenesis.

Author details

Luca Macarini and Luca P. Stoppino

Department of Surgical Sciences, Section of Diagnostic Imaging, Foggia University School of Medicine, Azienda Ospedaliero-universitaria "Ospedali Riuniti", Foggia, Italy

References

[1] Friedman SL. Hepatic fibrosis: overview. Toxicology 2008;254(3):120-129.

[2] Popper H, Uenfriend S. Hepatic fibrosis. Correlation of biochemical and morphologic investigations. Am J Med 1970;49:707-721.

[3] Schaffner F, Klion FM. Chronic hepatitis. Annu Rev Med 1968;19:25-38.

[4] Soyer MT, Ceballos R, Aldrete JS. Reversibility of severe hepatic damage caused by jejunoileal bypass after re-establishment of normal intestinal continuity. Surgery 1976;79:601-604.

[5] Pinzani M. Liver fibrosis. Springer Semin Immunopathol 1999;21:475-490.

[6] Afdhal NH, Nunes D. Evaluation of liver fibrosis: a concise review. Am J Gastroenterol 2004;99:1160–1174.

[7] Thampanitchawong P, Piratvisuth T. Liver biopsy: complications and risk factors. World J Gastroenterol 1999;5:301-304.

[8] Regev A, Berho M, Jeffers LJ, et al. Sampling error and intra-observer variation in liver biopsy in patients with chronic HCV infection. Am J Gastroenterol 2002;97:2614-2618.

[9] Leon DA, McCambridge J. Liver cirrhosis mortality rates in Britain, 1950 to 2002. Lancet 2006;367(9511):645.

[10] Leon DA, Saburova L, Tomkins S, et al. Hazardous alcohol drinking and premature mortality in Russia: a population based case-control study Lancet 2007;369(9578): 2001-2009.

[11] World Health Organisation. Hepatitis C. WHO Fact Sheet 2000;164:1-4.

[12] Shepard CW, Finelli L, Alter MJ. Global epidemiology of hepatitis C virus infection. Lancet Infect Dis 2005;5:558-567.

[13] Farrell GC LC. Nonalcoholic fatty liver disease: from steatosis to cirrhosis. Hepatology 2006;43:S99-S112.

[14] Day CP. Natural History of NAFLD: Remarkably benign in the absence of cirrhosis. Gastroenterology 2005;129:375-377.

[15] Powell EE, Edwards-Smith CJ, Hay JL, et al. Host genetic factors influence disease progression in chronic hepatitis C. Hepatology 2000;31:828-833.

[16] Monto A, Patel K, Bostrom A, et al. Risks of a range of alcohol intake on hepatitis C-related fibrosis. Hepatology 2004;39:826-834.

[17] Schiano TD, Kim-Schluger L, Gondolesi G, Miller CM. Adult living donor liver transplantation: the hepatologist's perspective. Hepatology 2001;33:3-9.

[18] Benhamou Y, Di Martino V, Bochet M, et al. Factors affecting liver fibrosis in human immunodeficiency virus- and hepatitis C virus-coinfected patients: impact of protease inhibitor therapy. Hepatology 2001;34:283-287.

[19] Farci P, Roskams T, Chessa L, et al. Long-term benefit of interferon alpha therapy of chronic hepatitis D: regression of advanced hepatic fibrosis. Gastroenterology 2004;126:1740-1749.

[20] Knodell RG, Ishak KG, Black WC, et al. Formulation and application of a numeral scoring system for assessing histological activity in asymptomatic chronic active hepatitis. Hepatology 1981;1:431-435.

[21] Ishak K, Baptista A, Bianchi L, et al. Histologic grading and staging of chronic hepatitis. J Hepatol 1995; 22:696-699.

[22] Bedossa P, Poynard T. The METAVIR cooperative study group. An algorithm for the grading of activity in chronic hepatitis C. Hepatology 1996;24:289-293.

[23] Thiese ND, Bodenheimer HC, Ferrell LD. Acute and chronic viral hepatitis. In: Burt AD, Portmann BC, Ferrell LD, eds. MacSween's pathology of the liver. 5th ed. Edinburgh, Scotland: Churchill Livingstone, 2006; chap 8.

[24] Ratziu V, Charlotte F, Heurtier A, et al. Sampling variability of liver biopsy in nonalcoholic fatty liver disease. Gastroenterology 2005;128:1898-1906.

[25] Bravo AA, Sheth SG, Chopra S. Liver biopsy. N Engl J Med 2001;344:495-500.

[26] Piccinino F, Sagnelli E, Pasquale G, Giusti G. Complications following percutaneous liver biopsy: a multicentre retrospective study on 68,276 biopsies. J Hepatol 1986;2:165-173.

[27] Colli A, Fraquelli M, Andreoletti M, et al. Severe liver fibrosis or cirrhosis: accuracy of US for detection—analysis of 300 cases. Radiology 2003;227:89-94.

[28] Cohen EI, Wilck EJ, Shapiro RS. Hepatic imaging in the 21st century. Semin Liver Dis 2006;26:363-372.

[29] Fritz GA, Schoellnast H, Deutschmann HA, et al. Density histogram analysis of unenhanced hepatic computed tomography in patients with diffuse liver diseases. J Comput Assist Tomogr 2006;30:201-205.

[30] Colagrande S, Centi N, Galdiero R, Ragozzino A. Transient hepatic intensity differences: part 2, those not associated with focal lesions. AJR Am J Roentgenol 2007;188:160-166.

[31] Partanen KP. Dynamic CT of liver cirrhosis. Invest Radiol 1984;19:303-308.

[32] Ito K, Mitchell DG, Gabata T, Hussain SM. Expanded gallbladder fossa: simple MR imaging sign of cirrhosis. Radiology 1999;211:723-726.

[33] Hussain SM, Semelka RC. Hepatic imaging: comparison of modalities. Radiol Clin North Am 2005;43:929-947.

[34] Roulot D, Czernichow S, Le Clesiau H, et al. Liver stiffness values in apparently healthy subjects: Influence of gender and metabolic syndrome. J Hepatol 2008;48:606-613.

[35] Fraquelli M, Rigamonti C, Casazza G, et al. Reproducibility of transient elastography in the evaluation of liver fibrosis in patients with chronic liver disease. Gut 2007;56:968-973.

[36] Sandrin L, Fourquet B, Hasquenoph JM, et al. Transient elastography: A new noninvasive method for assessment of hepatic fibrosis. Ultrasound Med Biol 2003;29:1705-1713.

[37] Konate A, Boursier J, Reaud S, et al. Liver stiffness measurement by transient elastography: predictive factors of accuracy, success and reproducibility. J Hepatol 2006;44:S195.

[38] Ziol M, Handra-Luca A, Kettaneh A, et al. Non-invasive assessment of liver fibrosis by measurement of stiffness in patients with chronic hepatitis C. Hepatology 2005;41:48-54.

[39] Carrion JA, Navasa M, Bosch J, et al. Transient elastography for diagnosis of advanced fibrosis and portal hypertension in patients with hepatitis C recurrence after liver transplantation. Liver Transpl 2006;12:1791-1798.

[40] Foucher J, Chanteloup E, Vergniol J, et al. Diagnosis of cirrhosis by transient elastography (FibroScan): a prospective study. Gut 2006;55:403-408.

[41] Nguyen-Khac E. Results and place of fibroscan in the noninvasive diagnosis of hepatic fibrosis. Rev Med Interne 2007;28:94-102.

[42] Castera L, Vergniol J, Foucher J, et al. Prospective comparison of transient elastography, Fibrotest, APRI, and liver biopsy for the assessment of fibrosis in chronic hepatitis C. Gastroenterology 2005;12:343-350.

[43] Marcellin P, Ziol M, Bedossa P, et al. Non-invasive assessment of liver fibrosis by stiffness measurement in patients with chronic hepatitis B. Liver Int 2009;29:242-247.

[44] de Ledinghen V, Douvin C, Kettaneh A, et al. Diagnosis of hepatic fibrosis and cirrhosis by transient elastography in HIV/hepatitis C viruscoinfected patients. J Acquir Immune Defic Syndr 2006;41:175-179.

[45] Yoneda M, Yoneda M, Mawatari H, et al. Noninvasive assessment of liver fibrosis by measurement of stiffness in patients with nonalcoholic fatty liver disease (NAFLD). Dig Liver Dis 2008;40:371-378.

[46] Corpechot C, El Naggar A, Poujol-Robert A, et al. Assessment of biliary fibrosis by transient elastography in patients with PBC and PSC. Hepatology 2006;43:1118-1124.

[47] Ophir J, Cespedes I, Ponnekanti H, Yazdi Y, Li X. Elastography: a quantitative method for imaging the elasticity of biological tissues. Ultrason Imaging 1991;13:111-134.

[48] Pesavento A, Krueger C, Ermert H. A time efficient and accurate strain estimation concept for ultrasonic elastography using interactive phase zero estimation. IEEE Trans an Ultrason Ferroelect Freq Contr 1999;46:1057-1067.

[49] Frey H. Realtime elastography. A new ultrasound procedure for the reconstruction of tissue elasticity Radiologe 2003; 43:850-855.

[50] Itoh A, Ueno E, Tohno E, Kamma H, Takahashi H, Shiina T, Yamakawa M, Matsumura T. Breast disease: clinical application of US elastography for diagnosis. Radiology 2006; 239:341-350.

[51] Srinivasan S, Kallel F, Ophir J. The effects of digitization on the elastographic signal-to-noise ratio. Ultrasound Med Biol 2002; 28:1521-1534.

[52] Friedrich-Rust M, Ong MF, Herrmann E et al. Real-time elastography for noninvasive assessment of liver fibrosis in chronic viral hepatitis. AJR Am J Roentgenol 2007;188:758-764.

[53] Wang J, Guo L, Shi X, et al. Real-time elastography with a novel quantitative technology for assessment of liver fibrosis in chronic hepatitis B. Eur J Radiol 2012;81:e31-e36.

[54] Zhai L, Palmeri ML, Bouchard RR, et al. An integrated indenter-ARFI imaging system for tissue stiffness quantification. Ultrason Imaging 2008;30:95-111.

[55] Nightingale K, Soo MS, Nightingale R, Trahey G. Acoustic radiation force impulse imaging: in vivo demonstration of clinical feasibility. Ultrasound Med Biol 2002;28:227-235.

[56] Mauldin FW Jr, Zhu HT, Behler RH, et al. Robust principal component analysis and clustering methods for automated classification of tissue response to ARFI excitation. Ultrasound Med Biol 2008;34: 309-325.

[57] Sporea I, Badea R, Sirli R, et al. How efficient is acoustic radiation force impulse elastography for the evaluation of liver stiffness? Hepat Mon. 2011;11:532-538.

[58] Friedrich-Rust M, Nierhoff J, Lupsor M, et al. Performance of Acoustic Radiation Force Impulse imaging for the staging of liver fibrosis: a pooled meta-analysis. J Viral Hepat 2012;19:e212-219.

[59] Colombo S, Buonocore M, Del Poggio A, et al. Head-to-head comparison of transient elastography (TE), real-time tissue elastography (RTE), and acoustic radiation force impulse (ARFI) imaging in the diagnosis of liver fibrosis. J Gastroenterol 2012;47:461-469.

[60] Martin DR. Magnetic resonance imaging of diffuse liver diseases. Top Magn Reson Imaging 2002;13:151-163.

[61] Ito K, Mitchell DG, Siegelman ES. Cirrhosis: MR imaging features. Magn Reson Imaging Clin N Am 2002;10:75-92.

[62] Dodd GDI, Baron RL, Oliver JHI, Federle MP: Spectrum of imaging findings of the liver in end-stage cirrhosis: Part I. Gross morphology and diffuse abnormalities. AJR Am J Roentgenol 1999;173:1031-1036.

[63] Brancatelli G, Federle MP, Ambrosini R, et al. Cirrhosis: CT and MR imaging evaluation. Eur J Radiol 2007;61:57-69.

[64] Balci NC, Semelka RC. Contrast agents for MR imaging of the liver. Radiol Clin North Am 2005;43:887-898.

[65] Hundt W, Petsch R, Helmberger T, Reiser M. Signal changes in liver and spleen after Endorem administration in patients with and without liver cirrhosis. Eur Radiol 2000;10:409.

[66] Lucidarme O, Baleston F, Cadi M, et al. Non-invasive detection of liver fibrosis: is superparamagnetic iron oxide particle-enhanced MR imaging a contributive technique? Eur Radiol 2003;13:467-474.

[67] Elizondo G, Weissleder R, Stark DD, et al. Hepatic cirrhosis and hepatitis: MR imaging enhanced with superparamagnetic iron oxide. Radiology 1990;174:797-801.

[68] Ahn SS, Kim MJ, Lim JS, et al. Added value of gadoxetic acid-enhanced hepatobiliary phase MR imaging in the diagnosis of hepatocellular carcinoma. Radiology 2010;255:459-466.

[69] Ichikawa T, Saito K, Yoshioka N, et al. Detection and characterization of focal liver lesions: a Japanese phase III, multicenter comparison between gadoxetic acid disodium-enhanced magnetic resonance imaging and contrast-enhanced computed tomography predominantly in patients with hepatocellular carcinoma and chronic liver disease. Invest Radiol 2010;45:133-141.

[70] Reimer P, Rummeny EJ, Shamsi K, et al. Phase II clinical evaluation of Gd-EOB-DTPA: dose, safety aspects, and pulse sequence. Radiology 1996;199:177-183.

[71] Tsuda N, Matsui O. Cirrhotic rat liver: reference to transporter activity and morphologic changes in bile canaliculi– gadoxetic acid-enhanced MR imaging. Radiology 2010;256:767-773.

[72] Nilsson H, Nordell A, Vargas R, et al. Assessment of hepatic extraction fraction and input relative blood flow using dynamic hepatocyte-specific contrast-enhanced MRI. J Magn Reson Imaging 2009:29:1323-1331.

[73] Lee WJ, Cha SH, Kim MY, et al. Quantitative evaluation of the hepatic parenchymal change in patients with chronic liver disease using Gd-EOB-DTPA-enhanced MRI: comparison with normal liver. J Korean Soc Radiol 2011;64:49-55.

[74] Watanabe H, Kanematsu M, Goshima S, et al. Staging hepatic fibrosis: comparison of gadoxetate disodium-enhanced and diffusion-weighted MR imaging–preliminary observations. Radiology 2011;259:142-150.

[75] Macarini L, Marini S, Milillo P, et al. Double-contrast MRI (DC-MRI) in the study of the cirrhotic liver: Utility of administering Gd-DTPA as a complement to examinations in which SPIO liver uptake and distribution alterations (SPIO-LUDA) are present and in the identification and characterisation of focal lesions. Radiol Med 2006; 111:1087-1102.

[76] Hughes-Cassidy F, Chavez AD, Schlang A, et al. Superparamagnetic iron oxides and low molecular weight gadolinium chelates are synergistic for direct visualization of advanced liver fibrosis. J Magn Reson Imaging 2007;26:728-737.

[77] Aguirre DA, Behling CA, Alpert E, et al. Liver fibrosis: noninvasive diagnosis with double contrast material enhanced MR imaging. Radiology 2006;239:425-437.

[78] Fischer MA, Donati OF, Reiner CS, et al. Feasibility of semiquantitative liver perfusion assessment by ferucarbotran bolus injection in double-contrast hepatic MRI. J Magn Reson Imaging 2012;36:168-176.

[79] Helmberger T, Semelka RC. New contrast agents for imaging the liver. Magn Reson Imaging Clin N Am 2001;9(4):745–766.

[80] Naganawa S, Kawai H, Fukatsu H, et al. Diffusion-weighted imaging of the liver: technical challenges and prospects for the future. Magn Reson Med Sci 2005;4:175-186.

[81] Le Bihan D. Molecular diffusion nuclear magnetic resonance imaging. Magn Reson Q 1991;7:1-30.

[82] Girometti R, Furlan A, Bazzocchi M, et al. Diffusion-weighted MRI in evaluating liver fibrosis: a feasibility study in cirrhotic patients. Radiol Med 2007;112:394-408.

[83] Koinuma M, Ohashi I, Hanafusa K, Shibuya H. Apparent diffusion coefficient measurements with diffusion-weighted magnetic resonance imaging for evaluation of hepatic fibrosis. J Magn Reson Imaging 2005;22:80-85.

[84] de Bazelaire CM , Duhamel GD , Rofsky NM , Alsop DC. MR imaging relaxation times of abdominal and pelvic tissues measured in vivo at 3.0 T: preliminary results. Radiology 2004;230:652-659.

[85] Okada Y, Ohtomo K, Kiryu S, Sasaki Y. Breath-hold T2-weighted MRI of hepatic tumors: value of echo planar imaging with diffusion-sensitizing gradient. J Comput Assist Tomogr 1998; 22:364-371.

[86] Hussain SM, De Becker J, Hop WC, et al. Can a single shot black-blood T2-weighted spin-echo echo-planar imaging sequence with sensitivity encoding replace the respiratorytriggered turbo spin-echo sequence for the liver? An optimization and feasibility study. J Magn Reson Imaging 2005;21:219-229.

[87] Taouli B, Koh DW. Diffusion-weighted MR Imaging of the Liver. Radiology 2010;254:47-66.

[88] Taouli B, Tolia AJ, Losada M, et al. Diffusion weighted MRI for quantification of liver fibrosis: preliminary experience. AJR Am J Roentgenol 2007; 189:799-806.

[89] Kim T, Murakami T, Takahashi S, et al. Diffusion-weighted single-shot echoplanar MR imaging for liver disease. AJR Am J Roentgenol 1999;173:393-398.

[90] Girometti R, Furlan A, Esposito G, et al. Relevance of b-values in evaluating liver fibrosis: a study in healthy and cirrhotic subjects using two single-shot spin-echo echoplanar diffusionweighted sequences. J Magn Reson Imaging 2008;28:411-419.

[91] Kovač JD, Daković M, Stanisavljević D, et al. Diffusion-weighted MRI versus transient elastography in quantification of liver fibrosis in patients with chronic cholestatic liver diseases. Eur Radiol 2011;17 [Epub ahead of print].

[92] Luciani A, Vignaud A, Cavet M, et al. Liver cirrhosis: intravoxel incoherent motion MR imaging— pilot study. Radiology 2008;249:891-899.

[93] Lewin M, Poujol-Robert A, Boelle PY, et al. Diffusion-weighted magnetic resonance imaging for the assessment of fibrosis in chronic hepatitis C. Hepatology 2007;46:658-665.

[94] Sandrasegaran K, Akışık FM, Lin C, et al. Value of diffusion-weighted MRI for assessing liver fibrosis and cirrhosis. AJR Am J Roentgenol 2009;193:1556-1560.

[95] Bakan AA, Inci E, Bakan S, et al. Utility of diffusion-weighted imaging in the evaluation of liver fibrosis. Eur Radiol 2012;22:682-687.

[96] Manduca A, Oliphant TE, Dresner MA, et al. Magnetic resonance elastography: noninvasive mapping of tissue elasticity. Med Image Anal 2001;5:237-254.

[97] Kruse SA, Smith JA, Lawrence AJ, et al. Tissue characterization using magnetic resonance elastography: preliminary results. Phys Med Biol 2000;45:1579-1590.

[98] Huwart L, Peeters F, Sinkus R, et al. Liver fibrosis: non-invasive assessment with MR elastography. NMR Biomed 2006;19:173-179.

[99] Rouviere O, Yin M, Dresner MA, et al. MR elastography of the liver: preliminary results. Radiology 2006;240:440-448.

[100] Klatt D, Asbach P, Rump J, et al. In vivo determination of hepatic stiffness using steady-state free precision magnetic resonance elastography. Invest Radiol 2006;41:841-848.

[101] Talwalkar JA, Yin M, Fidler JL, et al. Magnetic resonance imaging of hepatic fibrosis: emerging clinical applications. Hepatology 2008;47:332-342.

[102] Yin M, Talwalkar JA, Glaser KJ, et al. Assessment of hepatic fibrosis with magnetic resonance elastography. Clin Gastro Hep 2007;5:1207-1213.

[103] Wang Y, Ganger DR, Levitsky J, et al. Assessment of chronic hepatitis and fibrosis: comparison of MR elastography and diffusion-weighted imaging. AJR Am J Roentgenol 2011;196:553-561.

[104] Huwart L, Sempoux C, Salameh N, et al. Liver fibrosis: noninvasive assessment with MR elastography versus aspartate aminotransferase-to-platelet ratio index. Radiology 2007;245:458-466.

[105] Rustogi R, Horowitz J, Harmath C, et al. Accuracy of MR Elastography and Anatomic MR Imaging Features in the Diagnosis of Severe Hepatic Fibrosis and Cirrhosis. J Magn Reson Imaging 2012;35:1356-1364.

[106] Annet L, Materne R, Danse E, et al. Hepatic flow parameters measured with MR imaging and Doppler US: correlations with degree of cirrhosis and portal hypertension. Radiology 2003;229:409-414.

[107] Materne R, Smith AM, Peeters F, et al. Assessment of hepatic perfusion parameters with dynamic MRI. Magn Reson Med 2002;47:135-142.

[108] Van Beers BE, Materne R, Annet L, et al. Capillarization of the sinusoids in liver fibrosis: noninvasive assessment with contrastenhanced MRI in the rabbit. Magn Reson Med 2003;49:692-699.

[109] Hagiwara M RH, Lee VS, Losada M, et al. Advanced liver fibrosis: diagnosis with 3D whole liver perfusion MR imaging initial experience. Radiology 2008;246:926-934.

[110] Thng CH, Koh TS, Collins DJ, Koh DM. Perfusion magnetic resonance imaging of the liver. World J Gastroenterol 2010;16:1598-1609.

[111] Hagiwara M RH, Lee VS, Losada M, et al. Advanced liver fibrosis: diagnosis with 3D whole liver perfusion MR imaging initial experience. Radiology 2008;246:926-934.

[112] Leporq B, Dumortier J, Pilleul F, Beuf O. 3D-Liver Perfusion MRI With the MS-325 Blood Pool Agent: A Noninvasive Protocol to Asses Liver Fibrosis. J Magn Reson Imaging 2012;35:1380-1387.

[113] Chen BB, Hsu CY, Yu CW, et al. Dynamic contrast-enhanced magnetic resonance imaging with Gd-EOB-DTPA for the evaluation of liver fibrosis in chronic hepatitis patients. Eur Radiol 2012;22:171-180.

[114] Chandarana H, Taouli B. Diffusion and perfusion imaging of the liver. Eur J Radiol 2010;76:348-358.

[115] Khan SA, Cox IJ, Hamilton G, Thomas HC, Taylor-Robinson SD. In vivo and in vitro nuclear magnetic resonance spectroscopy as a tool for investigating hepatobiliary disease: a review of H and P MRS applications. Liver Int 2005;25:273-281.

[116] Solga SF, Horska A, Clark JM, Diehl AM. Hepatic 31P magnetic resonance spectroscopy: a hepatologist's user guide. Liver Int 2005;25:490-500.

[117] Khan SA, Cox IJ, Hamilton G, Thomas HC, Taylor-Robinson SD. In vivo and in vitro nuclear magnetic resonance spectroscopy as a tool for investigating hepatobiliary disease: a review of H and P MRS applications. Liver Int 2005;25:273-281.

[118] Johnson NA, Walton DW, Sachinwalla T et al. Noninvasive assessment of hepatic lipid composition: advancing understanding and management of fatty liver disorders. Hepatology 2008;47:1513-23.

[119] Cobbold JF, Anstee QM, Goldin RD et al. Phenotyping murine models of non-alcoholic fatty liver disease through metabolic profiling of intact liver tissue. Clin Sci 2009;116:403-13.

[120] Cobbold JF, Patel JH, Goldin RD et al. Hepatic lipid profiling in chronic hepatitis C: an in vitro and in vivo proton magnetic resonance spectroscopy study. J Hepatol 2010;52:16-24.

[121] Lok AS, Everhart JE, Chung RT, et al. Evolution of hepatic steatosis in patients with advanced hepatitis C: results from the hepatitis C antiviral long-term treatment against cirrhosis (HALT-C) trial. Hepatology 2009;49:1828-1837.

[122] McPherson S, Jonsson JR, Cowin GJ, et al. Magnetic resonance imaging and spectroscopy accurately estimate the severity of steatosis provided the stage of fibrosis is considered. J Hepatol 2009;51:389-397.

[123] Georgoff P, Thomasson D, Louie A, et al. Hydrogen-1 MR Spectroscopy for Measurement and Diagnosis of Hepatic Steatosis. AJR Am J Roentgenol 2012;199:2-7.

[124] Noren B, Dahlqvist O, Lundberg P, et al. Separation of advanced from mild fibrosis in diffuse liver disease using 31P magnetic resonance spectroscopy. Eur J Radiol 2008;66:313-320.

[125] Taylor-Robinson SD. Applications of magnetic resonance spectroscopy to chronic liver disease. Clin Med 2001;1:54-60.

[126] Lim AK, Patel N, Hamilton G, et al. The relationship of in vivo 31P MR spectroscopy to histology in chronic hepatitis C. Hepatology 2003;37:788-794.

[127] Sijens PE, Oudkerk M. Clinical magnetic resonance spectroscopy. Imaging Decisions MRI 2005;9:23-38.

[128] Wang QB, Zhu H, Liu HL, Zhang B. Performance of Magnetic Resonance Elastography and Diffusion-Weighted Imaging for the Staging of Hepatic Fibrosis: A Meta-Analysis. Hepatology 2012;56:239-247.

[129] Godfrey EM, Patterson AJ, Priest N, et al. A comparison of MR elastography and 31P MR spectroscopy with histological staging of liver fibrosis. Eur Radiol 2012 [Epub ahead of print].

Chapter 6

Current Concepts on Management of Chronic Hepatitis B

Teresa Santantonio and Massimo Fasano

Additional information is available at the end of the chapter

http://dx.doi.org/10.5772/54759

1. Introduction

An estimated 400 million people are chronically infected with hepatitis B virus (HBV), worldwide, and over 500,000 chronic hepatitis B (CHB) patients die annually because of cirrhosis and hepatocellular carcinoma (HCC) [1,2]. Clinical care for patients with CHB has advanced considerably during the last decades as a result of growing knowledge about the mechanisms of disease, diagnostic procedures and advances in therapeutic options.

Since the introduction of interferon alpha as first antiviral therapy at the end of the 1980s, management of CHB has dramatically evolved due to the availability of direct antivirals which greatly increased the therapeutic options, thus permitting treatment of patients previously excluded from IFN treatment. In particular, new oral antivirals have been developed and used in clinical practice, leading to a substantial improvement in antiviral efficacy, mainly due to their increased potency and higher barrier to resistance. On the other hand, the expanding molecular and clinical knowledge of HBV infection and evolution of therapy have made the management of CHB patients much more complex. Therefore, within the recent past, several guidelines have been issued by many organizations and professional expert panels in order to better define diagnostic criteria and improve therapeutic decisions.

This chapter focuses on the current management of chronic hepatitis B patients and reviews up-to-date studies and concepts regarding antiviral treatment.

2. Pre-therapeutic assessment

Chronic HBV infection is not necessarily accompanied by progressive liver disease requiring antiviral therapy. Therefore, as a first step, an accurate evaluation of all HBsAg-positive carriers is required in order to identify: a) the phase of infection, b) the subjects with chronic liver damage, c) the stage of liver disease, d) the concurrent causes of liver disease, and e) patients requiring treatment.

The natural history of chronic HBV infection can be divided into five, not necessarily sequential, phases (Figure 1). Firstly, the (i) *immune-tolerant phase* is characterized by high levels of serum HBV DNA, HBeAg positivity, normal ALT levels, and mild or absent liver necroinflammation. In patients who remain in the immune-tolerant phase, disease progression is minimal [3]. After a variable time depending on the age at acquisition of HBV infection, immune-tolerance to the virus is lost and the immune system mounts an attack on the infected hepatocytes, thus entering into the (ii) *immune-reactive phase*.This phase is characterized by fluctuating, but progressively decreasing, HBV-DNA levels, elevated ALT and hepatic necroinflammation *(HBeAg-positive CHB)*. A prolonged immune-reactive phase with multiple ALT flares may result in progressive liver fibrosis, leading to cirrhosis. An important outcome of the *immune-reactive* phase is the seroconversion from HBeAg to anti-HBe, thus marking the transition to the (iii) *immune-control phase*, characterized by low (<2000 IU/ml) or undetectable serum HBV DNA, normal ALT levels, and disappearance of liver necroinflammation (*inactive carrier state*). The estimated annual incidence of spontaneous HBeAg seroconversion is 2%-15%, depending on factors such as age, ALT levels, and HBV genotype [2]. In a minority of patients, despite HBe seroconversion, reactivation of HBV replication may occur due to the selection of HBeAg defective HBV mutants. This (iv) *reactivation phase* is characterized by positivity for anti-HBe antibodies, fluctuating HBV DNA and ALT levels and a high risk of progression to severe hepatic fibrosis (*HBeAg-negative CHB*). In patients with periodic ALT flares and normalization, HBV-DNA levels can fall below the inactive carrier cut-off (2000 IU/ml), making differential diagnosis between active CHB and the inactive carrier status problematic. Therefore, to warrant an accurate differential diagnosis, it is mandatory to monitor serum HBV-DNA by sensitive and quantitative polymerase chain reaction (PCR) assays and ALT levels over a period of at least 1 year. A recent study, however, demonstrated that a single-point combined quantification of HBV-DNA (<2000 IU/ml) and HBsAg (<1000 IU/mL) permits to identify inactive HBV genotype D carriers with a very high diagnostic accuracy which is comparable to that of 1-year monthly monitoring [4]. In the (V) "*HBsAg-negative phase*" after HBsAg loss, low-level HBV replication may persist with detectable HBV DNA in the liver [5]. In patients with "*occult*" HBV infection the persistence of an efficient HBV immunological control has been demonstrated [6], and it is now well known that immunosuppression may lead to HBV reactivation in these patients.

On the basis of the serological and virological profile, three distinct HBsAg carrier types can be identified, each characterized by a distinct natural course, prognosis, and treatment indications: 1) immune tolerant carrier, 2) inactive carrier, 3) carrier with CHB (HBeAg-positive and HBeAg-negative CHB). In both tolerant and inactive HBV carriers, treatment is not indicated, but an appropriate longitudinal follow-up is crucial. Immunotolerant patients should be subjected to ALT measurements every 3-6 months and should be tested for the presence of HBeAg every 6 months. In the inactive carriers, ALT and HBV DNA levels should be assessed every 3 months during the first year, and then every 6 months [7-9]. Patients with serum HBV DNA <2000 IU/ml and levels of HBsAg less than 1000 IU/ml, may require less frequent monitoring due to a very low probability of disease reactivation [7].

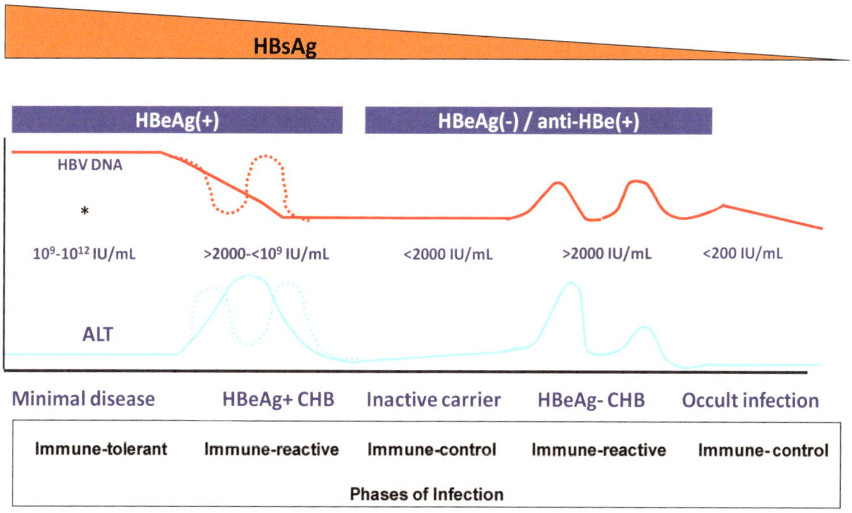

Figure 1. Natural history of chronic HBV infection

In the HBsAg carriers with CHB, the diagnostic work-up must be continued and the severity of liver disease should be assessed by laboratory tests, and hepatic ultrasound examination. A liver biopsy would be useful for determining the grade of necroinflammation and stage of fibrosis. Prognosis and management of CHB greatly depend on the stage and progression of liver fibrosis and thus the risk of developing cirrhosis. In addition, liver biopsy may help to clarify diagnosis when ALT and HBV DNA levels are discordant and to exclude other coexistent causes of liver disease (e.g. fatty liver or alcoholic liver disease).

Liver biopsy has traditionally been considered the "gold standard" to measure fibrosis. However, liver biopsy is an invasive procedure which can be painful, and carries a small risk of complications; it is also costly and prone to sampling errors. To provide a reliable estimation of grading and staging of liver disease, liver biopsy specimens should be at least 20-25 mm long and/or containing more than 11 complete portal tracts [10]. Recently, non-invasive methods, including serum markers and transient elastography, are being increasingly utilized to assess liver fibrosis [10]. Transient elastography (FibroScan) is a rapid, noninvasive, and reproducible method for measuring liver stiffness, which correlates with the degree of liver fibrosis. It has demonstrated a high diagnostic accuracy for the detection of cirrhosis, but transient elastography might be inaccurate in discriminating between the different stages of intermediate fibrosis (F1 *vs* F2), F2 being considered the threshold for initiating antiviral therapy. Moreover, stiffness measurement may be influenced by potential confounding factors such as additional space-occupying tissue abnormalities (e.g. oedema and inflammation, cholestasis).

Lastly, in the diagnostic work-up of CHB, the presence of other possible liver damaging cofactors (co-infections with HDV, HCV and HIV, co-morbidities including alcoholism, autoimmune or metabolic liver disease) which would increase the risk of progression to cirrhosis or HCC should be assessed [11].

3. Treatment indications

Candidates for treatment are the HBsAg carriers with CHB and, consequently, those with active viral replication, increased ALT levels and evidence of liver disease at liver biopsy or other non-invasive methods.

According to the 2012 HBV guidelines of the European Association for the Study of the Liver (EASL), patients should be considered for treatment when they present HBV DNA levels above 2000 IU/ml, serum ALT levels above the upper limit of normal (ULN) and a liver biopsy showing moderate to severe necroinflammation and/or at least moderate fibrosis using a standardized score system. The comparison between EASL guidelines and American Association for the Study of Liver Diseases (AASLD) guidelines and Asian Pacific Association for the Study of the Liver (APASL) guidelines can be found in Table 1.

However, patients with compensated or decompensated cirrhosis and detectable HBV DNA should be considered for treatment, independent of ALT levels. Moreover, treatment indications should also take into account the patient's age, health status, family history of HCC or cirrhosis and extrahepatic manifestations.

Criteria	EASL 2012(Ref.7)	AASLD 2009(Ref.8)	APASL 2008(Ref.9)
HBV DNA treatment threshold			
- HBeAg(+) (IU/mL)	2,000	20,000	20,000
- HBeAg(-) (IU/mL)	2,000	2,000–20,000	2,000
ALT treatment threshold	>ULN	>2 x ULN	>2 x ULN
Liver Biopsy	Moderate to severe necroinflammation or fibrosis	Not applicable (Consider in certain groups)	

Table 1. EASL guidelines compared to other international guidelines

4. Goal of therapy and end-points

The ultimate goal of CHB therapy is the prevention of cirrhosis, hepatic decompensation and/or HCC [7-9]. This goal can be achieved if HBV replication can be suppressed in a sustained manner, thus leading to biochemical remission, HBe seroconversion in HBeAg-positive patients, histological improvement and prevention of cirrhosis and its complications. Several studies have demonstrated that undetectable or low levels of HBV DNA are associated with a lower risk to develop cirrhosis [12-14].

Loss of HBsAg from serum with or without seroconversion to anti-HBs is considered the ideal end-point of therapy, as it is associated with remission of chronic hepatitis B activity and an improved long-term outcome [11]. The loss of HBsAg, however, is infrequently achieved with currently available anti-HBV agents. Hence, a more realistic end-point is the induction of a sustained or maintained virological response. It must be emphasized that a complete eradication of HBV infection is impossible to achieve due to the persistence of the so-called covalently-closed-circular DNA (cccDNA), the transcriptionally active HBV mini-cromosome in the nucleus of infected hepatocytes; that is to say, that an HBV infected patient can be "cured" but the HBV infection cannot be eradicated and continues to persist as an occult infection.

5. Anti-HBV drugs

Two different types of drugs have been approved for the treatment of CHB: conventional interferon alpha (IFN) and its pegylated form (Peg-IFN), and 5 nucleoside/nucleotide analogues (NAs) (Figure 2). Currently, IFN has been replaced by Peg-IFN due to the more convenient administration (once weekly). There are two pegylated-IFN formulations: Peg-IFN alpha-2a and Peg-IFN alpha-2b which have shown similar efficacy in clinical trials, but only the former is globally licensed for treatment of CHB, while Peg-IFN alpha-2b has been approved in only a few countries. Among the nucleoside analogues with anti-HBV activity, emtricitabine is not licensed for HBV treatment in most European countries and its combination with tenofovir in one tablet (*Truvada*) has been licensed only for treatment of human HIV infection.

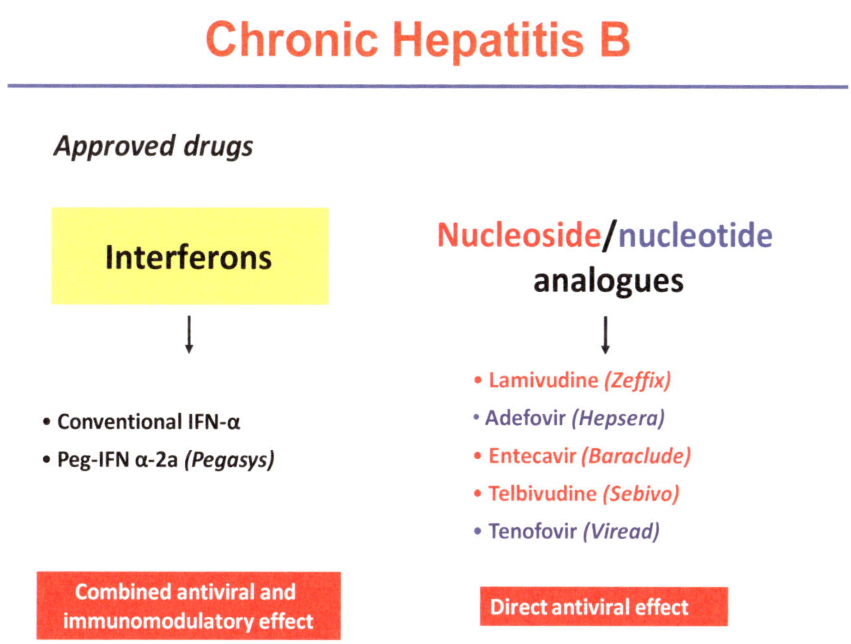

Figure 2. Approved drugs for therapy of chronic hepatitis B

6. Peg-interferon

Peg-IFN is a cytochine with a dual antiviral and immunomodulatory activity and is administered by subcutaneous injections. After binding with receptors located on the surface of several different cells, it induces the activation of at least 40 cellular genes, encoding for several antiviral proteins. Peg-IFN suppresses HBV virion budding, HBV entry and synthesis of the nucleocapsid; moreover, this cytochine enhances the interaction between the antigen-presenting cells and CD4, and between CD8 and infected hepatocytes. Therefore, Peg-IFN has the potential for an immune-mediated control of HBV infection, thus providing the opportunity to obtain a sustained virological response after treatment discontinuation, and the possibility of inducing HBsAg loss in patients who achieve and maintain undetectable HBV DNA. IFN-based treatment, however, is often complicated by the occurrence of side effects, such as influenza-like symptoms, fatigue, neutropenia, thrombocytopenia, and depression, which sometimes require dose modification and cause premature cessation of treatment [15]. Moreover, Peg-IFN is contraindicated in patients with decompensated HBV-related cirrhosis or autoimmune disease, in patients with uncontrolled severe depression or psychosis, in patients receiving immunosuppressive therapy or chemotherapy, and in female patients during pregnancy [7].

7. Nucleoside/nucleotide analogues

NAs are oral direct antiviral agents which specifically inhibit the viral polymerase/reverse transcriptase, an enzyme with a crucial role in the HBV life cycle. As a result, NAs block the production of new virions and progressively reduce serum HBV DNA to undetectable levels, but they have little or no effect on the cccDNA present in the nucleous of the infected hepatocytes. The persistence of the intrahepatic cccDNA determines the reactivation of HBV replication after stopping NA treatment and therefore justifies the need for a long-term (potentially life-long) therapy for a sustained viral replication control.

After lamivudine (LAM), the first nucleoside analogue approved for the treatment of CHB, another two nucleosides, telbivudine (LdT) and entecavir (ETV), and two nucleotide analogues, adefovir (ADV) and tenofovir (TDF) have become gradually available in recent years. NAs are characterized by a different antiviral potency and drug-resistance pattern. Entecavir and tenofovir are the two most potent analogues with a high barrier to resistance development. Resistance rates in NA-naïve patients treated with monotherapy are shown in Figure 3.

The main advantages and disadvantages of Peg-IFN and NAs in the treatment of CHB are shown in the following Table 2.

8. Treatment strategies

There are two different therapeutic strategies for both HBeAg-positive and HBeAg-negative CHB patients: short-term or "curative" treatment and long-term or "suppressive" treatment

(Figure 4). The first strategy aims to obtain a sustained suppression of viral replication off-treatment by inducing an immune controll status of HBV infection. The immune control status corresponds to the profile of an inactive carrier: normal ALT levels coupled with HBV DNA <2000 IU/ml and anti-HBe positivity. This strategy is IFN-based (Peg-IFN administered for 48 weeks); a finite treatment with NA is possible only in HBeAg-positive patients. The second strategy aims to obtain a rapid and long-term maintained viral suppression (HBV DNA <10-15 IU/ml). This strategy is exclusively based on NAs.

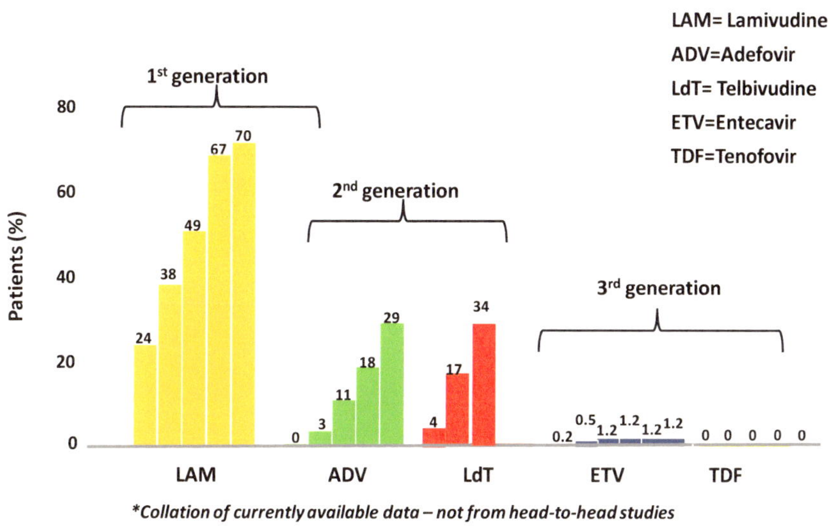

EASL 2012 HBV Guidelines (Ref. 7)

Figure 3. Incidence of Resistance in NA-naïve patients

	Peg-IFN	NAs
Advantages	• Finite duration • Higher rates of anti-HBe & anti-HBs seroconversion with 12 mos of therapy • Absence of resistance	• Potent antiviral effect • Good tolerance • Oral administration
Disadvantages	• Moderate antiviral effect • Inferior tolerability • Risk of adverse events • Subcutaneous injections	• Indefinite duration • Risk of resistance • Unknown long-term safety

EASL 2012 HBV Guidelines (Ref. 7)

Table 2. Main advantages and disadvantages of Peg-IFN and Nucleos(t)ides analogues (NAs) in chronic hepatitis B

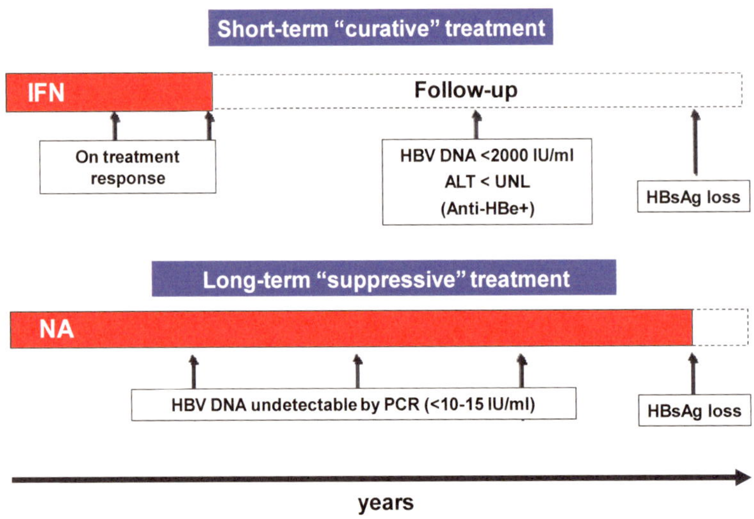

Figure 4. Therapeutic strategies for chronic hepatitis B

9. First-line monotherapy

Peg-IFN, entecavir or tenofovir are recommended as first-line monotherapy by all major guidelines in patients with CHB or compensated cirrhosis [7-9]. The choice of first-line monotherapy should be based on several factors including host, virus and drug related factors (Figure 5). The most favourable candidates for Peg-IFN are those with low HBV DNA levels, high ALT and HBV genotype A or B rather than C or D, and those without advanced disease. Peg-IFN alpha-2a is administered as subcutaneous injections at the dose of 180 μg once weekly for 48 weeks.

Entecavir or tenofovir are the only therapeutic options in patients with decompensated liver disease, in patients undergoing immunosuppressive treatment, in patients with controindications or unwilling to receive Peg-IFN. The licensed entecavir dose for patients with decompensated cirrhosis is 1 mg (instead of 0.5 mg for patients with CHB or compensated liver disease) once daily. Tenofovir is administered orally at dosage of 245 mg/die.

For oral antiviral agents, in HBeAg-positive patients, treatment can be discontinued after a 12 month-consolidation therapy from documented HBeAg seroconversion with undetectable HBV DNA. Close monitoring for relapse is required following therapy discontinuation. In HBeAg-negative patients, long-term treatment is necessary and can be stopped when confirmed HBsAg loss occurs [7,8].

As Peg-IFN can achieve a sustained off-therapy response in only a minority of cases, and a proportion of patients cannot tolerate or present controindications to IFN or do not wish to be treated with Peg-IFN, long-term treatment with NAs is the most commonly used treatment strategy.

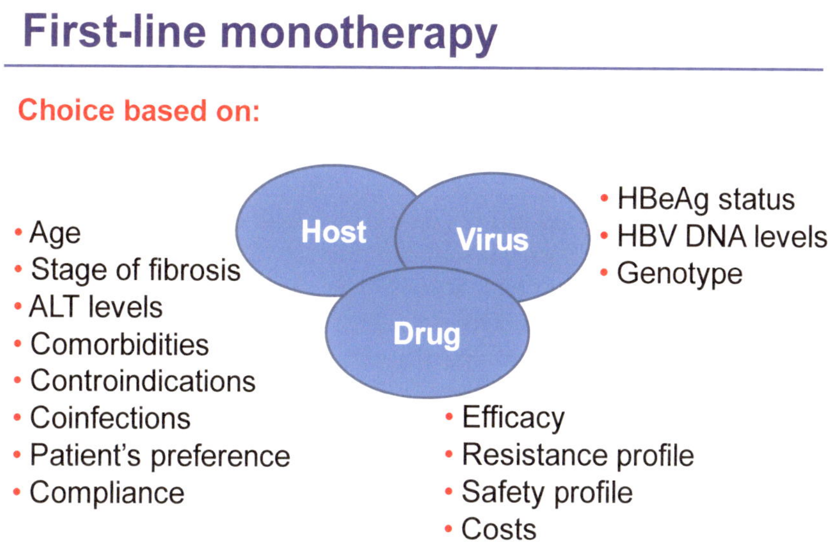

Figure 5. Factors influencing the choice of first-line monotherapy

10. Virological and non-virological monitoring

During Peg-IFN therapy, full blood counts and serum ALT levels should be monitored monthly and TSH should be assessed every 3 months. All patients should be monitored for safety throughout the 12 months of treatment. Serum HBV DNA levels should be assessed by real-time PCR at 3, 6, 12 months during treatment and at 6 and 12 months post-treatment. Quantitative determination of serum HBsAg levels should be checked after 3 months of therapy in order to identify patients with a low probability of response in whom IFN therapy discontinuation should be considered [7]. In HBeAg-positive patients, HBeAg and anti-HBe should be tested every 6 months. Lastly, in all responder patients, HBsAg should be checked at 12-month intervals [7].

In patients treated with NAs, HBV DNA levels should be monitored at month-3 to ascertain virological response, and thereafter, every 3-6 months. In patients treated with ETV or TDF, the frequency of DNA measurements may be decreased once patient compliance and treatment efficacy are confirmed. In HBeAg-positive patients, HBeAg and anti-HBe should be tested every 6 months. HBsAg should be checked at intervals of 12 months in all patients with undetectable HBV DNA by real-time PCR [7].

All NAs are cleared by the kidneys, therefore all patients should be tested for serum creatinine levels and estimated creatinine clearance at baseline to identify the need for dose adjustments. As the nephrotoxic potential damage seems to be higher for nucleotide analogues, it is recommended for patients treated with ADV or TDF renal monitoring, including serum phosphate levels every three months during the first year and every 6 months thereafter. In patients at high renal risk or in those who develop clearance creatinine <60 ml/min or serum phosphate <2 mg/dl, a closer renal monitoring is required [7].

11. IFN-based therapy: Update

Published data have demonstrated that in patients with HBeAg-positive CHB, Peg-IFN achieves a more than 30% HBeAg seroconversion rate after one year of treatment [7]. In a registration trial, Peg-IFN alpha-2a provided a sustained immune control which increased post-therapy; in fact, the HBeAg seroconversion rate continued to increase from 27% at the end of treatment to 32% during the six months after discontinuing treatment, and to 42% after 1 year post-treatment [16,17]. Moreover, the seroconversion remained stable over time in >80% of Peg-IFN alpha-2b treated patients achieving this end-point at the end of therapy [18]. Peg-IFN also determined HBsAg seroconversion in up to 30% of patients with a long-term follow-up [19].

In patients with HBeAg-negative CHB, Peg-IFN alpha-2a demonstrated a sustained immune control (HBV DNA <2000 IU/ml) in 31% of patients after 1-year post-treatment. Among these, 88% maintained this response up to 5-year follow-up, and remarkably 28% achieved HBsAg clearance after 5-years post-treatment [20].

Thus, Peg-IFN treatment remains an attractive therapeutic option, since it provides higher rates of off-therapy immune control, including HBsAg clearance, when compared with NAs. However, IFN is effective in only a minority of patients (20-30%), has a poor tolerability and significant costs. Therefore, the improvement of Peg-IFN efficacy is a major challenge. Several attempts have been made to optimize the cost-effectiveness of IFN-based therapy, including combination therapy, duration of therapy, pre-treatment predictors of response, and on-treatment predictors of response. De novo combination therapy with NAs, did not improve sustained response in either HBeAg-positive or HBeAg-negative patients [16,21-23]. Regarding duration of therapy, the NEPTUNE study conducted in patients with HBeAg-positive CHB reported that dose and duration are important because the highest sustained response was obtained with 180 μg and 48 weeks compared to 90 μg and 24 weeks [24]. A recent study has demonstrated that extended treatment with Peg-IFN alpha-2a to 96 weeks was well-tolerated and improved the rates of sustained virological response (29% vs 12%) in HBeAg-negative genotype D patients when compared to the current standard of care of 48 weeks. In addition, after 1-year post-treatment, HBsAg clearance (6%) was observed only in the extended therapy group [25].

There have been many attempts to identify pretreatment predictors of response, resulting in the identification of high ALT levels, low HBV DNA, and virus genotype as significant predictors [7-9]. When combining data from the two largest clinical trials regarding HBeAg-positive CHB patients [16,26], Buster et al. found that the best candidates for a sustained response to Peg-IFN were genotype A patients with high levels of ALT (ALT≥2xULN) or low levels of HBV DNA (<9 $\log_{10}$ copies/ml), and genotypes B and C patients who have both high levels of ALT and low HBV DNA. Genotype D patients have a low chance of sustained response [19]. However, these factors cannot accurately predict response at the individual level; furthermore, ALT and HBV DNA levels are time-dependent and thus their use in clinical practice is difficult.

To obtain additional insight into the individual patient's probability of achieving response to Peg-IFN, the presence of precore and basal core promoter mutants before treatment has been correlated to the serological and virological response in HBeAg-positive CHB patients [27]. Data from this study demonstrated that the presence of a wild-type virus at baseline was an independent predictor of response to Peg-IFN and can assist in improving patient selection for this treatment option [27]. Lastly, the role of IL28B polymorphisms, clearly indicated as a baseline host factor predictor of response in patients with chronic hepatitis C, has been also investigated in CHB patients. Studies in HBeAg-positive patients provided conflicting results, while, in the only study carried out in HBeAg-negative genotype D patients, the rs12979860 genotype in the IL28B locus independently predicted both virological and serological responses [28-31]. Therefore, further studies are necessary to define the role of IL28B polymorphisms as a baseline factor to improve pretreatment patient selection.

A promising approach to improve the cost-effectiveness of Peg-IFN therapy is a response-guided treatment, based on HBsAg kinetics which permit early identification of either responders, for whom continuation of treatment to week 48 could be beneficial, or non-responders who should discontinue IFN treatment.

Two stopping rules at week 12 have been proposed for HBeAg-positive patients: 1) no HBsAg decline, 2) HBsAg levels >20 000 IU/ml [24,32,33]. The negative predictive value (NPV) for a sustained response ranged from 82% to 100%, depending on prevalence of HBV genotypes in the various studies. In HBeAg-negative genotype D patients, no HBsAg decline and <2 log copies/ml HBV DNA decline at week 12 has been proposed as a stopping rule and independently validated with a 100% NPV [34,35]. Overall, therapy with Peg-IFN could be discontinued at week 12 in the 20% of primary non-responders, who are therefore candidates for suppressive therapy with NAs.

12. NA-based therapy: Update

Entecavir and tenofovir are the third-generation NAs recommended as first line therapy for CHB NA-naïve patients by all international guidelines. In registration trials, both antivirals demonstrated a long-lasting efficacy (viral suppression in more than 95% of patients over 5 years) associated with prevention of developing cirrhosis and to a greater extent, with fibrosis regression [36-40]. Moreover, these studies reported a minimal risk of drug resistance (1.2% with ETV after six years and 0% with TDF after 5 years) and a favourable safety profile [39-43]. However, as registration trials are conducted under standardized conditions in well-selected and compliant patients, long-term efficacy and safety of ETV and TDF remain to be confirmed in real-life patients who generally have a more complex clinical profile as they are usually older with a higher prevalence of cirrhosis and comorbidities treated with several concomitant medications.

13. Entecavir in real-life practice

Currently, 2,736 CHB naïve patients have been treated with ETV monotherapy in six real-life studies and 4-year efficacy and safety data are available for two of these. In a multicenter Italian study, 418 consecutive NA-naïve patients initiating treatment with ETV 0.5 mg/die were enrolled. In this cohort, at baseline patients were older (median age 58 years), were predominately infected with HBV genotype D (90%), presented a diagnosis of cirrhosis in 49% and concomitant disease in 56%. Viral suppression was achieved in 100% of patients over 48 months of therapy, independent of HBeAg status. Only one patient with a partial virological response at week 48 developed resistance at year 3 of treatment with a cumulative rate of 0.2%. In HBeAg-positive patients, the 4-year cumulative probability of HBeAg seroconversion and HBsAg loss were 56% and 21%, respectively. However, despite persistent suppression of viral replication, HCC developed in cirrhotic patients at 2.5% yearly rates, making continuous surveillance for liver cancer mandatory [44].

A cohort from Hong Kong included 222 NA-naïve patients who demonstrated a 96% 4-year cumulative rate of virological response [45]. Only one patient developed resistance, corresponding to a 0.6% cumulative resistance rate up to year-4.

The safety profile of ETV in real-life studies has been excellent, as there have been no reports of drug-related adverse reactions, discontinuation, or renal toxicity [44-46].

In the VIRGIL multicenter study including 243 consecutive NA-naïve patients receiving ETV monotherapy, the cumulative probability of achieving a virological response at week 144 was 90% in HBeAg-positive patients and 99% in HBeAg-negative patients [47]. In this cohort, 81% of patients with partial virological response at 48 weeks reached a virological response during prolonged ETV monotherapy and no patient developed ETV resistance. When stratifying patients according to their viral load at week 48, 95% of patients with HBV DNA<1000 IU/ml and 57% of patients with HBV DNA>1000 IU/ml achieved a virological response without treatment adaptation during the prolonged treatment period beyond week 48. Therefore, the authors concluded that no treatment adaptation is needed in the majority of NA-naïve patients treated with ETV and obtaining partial virological response, particularly in those with HBV DNA <1000 IU/mL at week 48. In addition, data from the Virgil cohort demonstrated that in cirrhotic patients, virological response to ETV is associated with a lower probability of developing a clinical event and disease progression [48].

14. Tenofovir in real-life practice

A total of 1,203 CHB patients, including both NA-naïve and experienced, were treated with TDF monotherapy in real-life. In the multicenter European cohort study, 302 consecutive NA-

naïve patients receiving tenofovir (245mg/die) were retrospectively and prospectively followed for a median period of 28 months. At baseline, median age was 55 years, 35% of patients had cirrhosis, and concomitant diseases were present in 43% [49]. By month 36, virological response was reached in 86% of HBeAg-positive patients and 98% of HBeAg-negative patients. No patient developed drug resistance and, in HBeAg-positive patients, cumulative probability of HBeAg seroconversion at 30 month was 33%. Most partial virological responders at week 48 achieved undetectable HBV DNA during additional treatment. Data from this European cohort confirmed the safety profile of TDF reported in the registration studies. Discontinuation therapy was reported in 9 patients (3%) including renal-related adverse events in two. The TDF dose was reduced in ten patients (3%) because of a decline in the estimated glomerular filtration rate [49].

15. Antiviral treatment failure

All patients receiving NA-therapy for CHB should be closely monitored for virologic response defined as undetectable HBV DNA by a sensitive PCR assay. Failure of antiviral therapy may be due to several reasons and three types of treatment failure can be identified: 1) Primary Non Response; 2) Partial Virologic Response; 3) Virologic Breakthrough [50] (Figure 6).

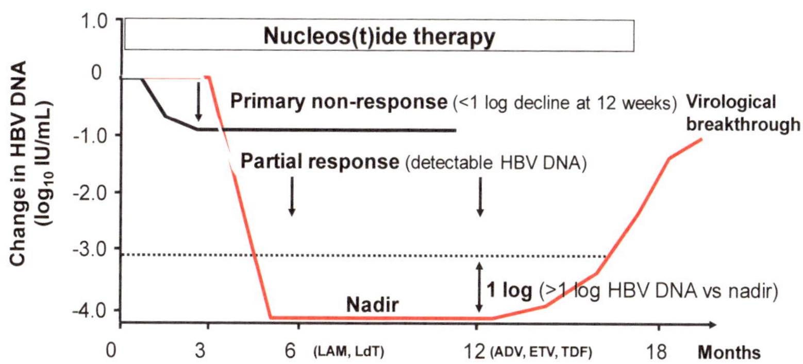

EASL 2012 HBV Guidelines (Ref. 7)

Figure 6. Antiviral treatment failure in patients receiving NA-therapy

Primary non response is defined as less than 1 log_{10} IU/ml decrease in HBV DNA level from baseline after 3 months of therapy; the cause might be attributed to lack of compliance or to reduced drug susceptibility in a particular individual. Primary non response seems to be more frequent with Adefovir than with other NAs because of sub-optimal antiviral efficacy. When a primary non response is identified antiviral treatment should be modified to prevent disease progression and drug resistant development. In a compliant patient HBV genotyping for the identification of possible resistant mutations should be performed and a switch to a more potent NA is recommended [7].

Partial virological response is defined as a decrease in HBV DNA of more than 1 $\log_{10}$ IU/ml, but detectable HBV DNA after 24 weeks of therapy in compliant patients treated with low genetic barrier NAs (LAM, LdT) and after 48 weeks in patients receiving ADV.

Several studies demonstrated that in patients with persisting viremia after 24 weeks of LAM therapy or 48 weeks of ADV therapy, there is a greater risk of resistance development with further treatment, compared to patients with undetectable HBV DNA. Therefore, an alternative treatment should be considered in these patients before emergence of genotypic resistance and a change to a more potent drug (entecavir or tenofovir) without cross-resistance is recommended [7]. With the more potent and high genetic barrier drugs, such as ETV and TDF, it has been shown that the rate of viral suppression continues to increase even after one year of treatment, without evidence of drug-resistance [7]. These data suggest that a modification of therapy is not necessary in patients with partial virological response under entecavir or tenofovir, especially in those with declining serum HBV DNA levels. However, in patients with persisting low viremia or when HBV DNA levels do not continue to decline, treatment should be adapted (switching or adding the other drug) in order to maximize viral suppression and prevent long-term resistance [7].

Virological breakthrough is defined as a confirmed increase in HBV DNA level of more than 1 $\log_{10}$ IU/ml compared to the lowest value (nadir) achieved during treatment. In all patients with a virological breakthrough, treatment compliance should be assessed. In compliant patients, virological breakthrough is related to the selection of HBV drug-resistant mutants [50].

16. Antiviral drug-resistance

Antiviral drug-resistance is defined as the reduced susceptibility of a virus to the inhibitory effect of a drug due to adaptive mutations selected under the selective pressure of antiviral therapy. In CHB patients treated with NAs, antiviral drug-resistance is due to mutations within the Polymerase gene of HBV, thus resulting in amino acid substitutions within the polymerase/reverse transcriptase, target of all NAs. These amino acid changes reduce the affinity of the enzyme for the antiviral drug, in favor of natural substrates. Moreover, the resistance-associated mutations selected by a particular NA confer at least some degree of cross-resistance to other members of its structural group but may also diminish the sensitivity to NAs from a different chemical group, thus limiting future treatment options (Figure 7).

Development of antiviral drug-resistance is a complex and multistep phenomenon. Figure 8 shows the chronology of events.

Initially, during antiviral therapy, there is the emergence of mutants containing the primary mutations which are known to confer resistance to the antiviral drug (genotypic resistance). If treatment is continued, resistant mutants are selected under the selective pressure of the drug, and over time become the dominant viral species, producing the progressive increase in serum HBV DNA levels. The virological breakthrough is then followed by a biochemical breakthrough, defined as elevation in serum alanine aminotransferase, after achieving normalization. The time span between virological and biochemical breakthrough may vary from weeks to years.

HBV variant	LVD	LdT	ETV	ADV	TDF
Wild-type	S	S	S	S	S
M204I/V	R	R	I	S	S
L180M+M204V	R	R	I	S	S
A181T/V	R	R	S	R	I
N236T	S	S	S	R	I
A181T/V + N236T	R	R	S	R	R
L180M+M204V/I ± I169T ± T184G ± S202I/G ± M250I/V	R	R	R	S	S

S= sensitive, I= intermediate/reduced susceptibility, R= resistant

Zoulim and Locarnini. J. Hepatol 2012 (Ref. 50)

Figure 7. Cross-resistance data for the most frequent resistant HBV variants

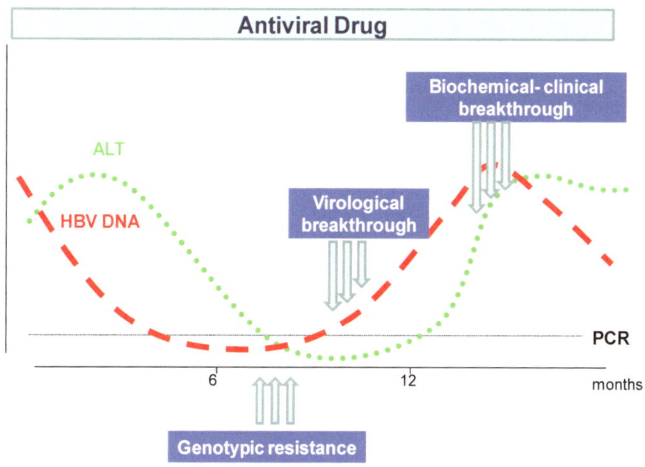

Figure 8. Chronology of events in patients developing antiviral drug-resistance

Development of antiviral drug-resistance has important clinical implications, as it provokes the loss of clinical benefits due to treatment. The selection of drug-resistant mutants was one of the most important concerns with the first and second generation NAs, especially with LAM (Figure 3). Currently, the availability of most potent antivirals with a high barrier to resistance, such as entecavir and tenofovir, significantly reduced the rates of resistance. Consequently, the correct choice of a first-line monotherapy provides the best chance of preventing treatment failure and drug resistance.

In clinical practice, the early identification of the virologic breakthrough permits an effective timely rescue therapy, before the biochemical breakthrough, thus avoiding disease progression, decompensation in patients with advanced cirrhosis, and accumulation of secondary mutations which may improve viral fitness and may become the basis for cross-resistance with other NAs.

In all patients with a virological breakthrough, genotypic resistance testing should be performed to confirm genotypic resistance and to determine the pattern of mutations. There are two commercially available methods for detection of resistance mutations: a direct PCR-based sequencing, which detects all mutations present in a resistant mutant if it is present in ≥20% of the viral quasispecies, and a hybridization-based genotyping method, which can detect only known nucleotide mutations, but is more sensitive, allowing for detection of mutants when they constitute 5% or more of the total viral population.

The management of treatment failure has changed significantly in recent years, due to the availability of potent antivirals. An appropriate rescue therapy should be initiated with the most effective antiviral drug without cross-resistance to reduce the risk of selecting multiple drug-resistant viral strains. The *add-on* strategy is the therapeutic approach recommended by guidelines, in order to prevent the emergence of multi-drug resistant strains and raise the resistance barrier. However, with the availability of more potent drugs, such as entecavir and tenofovir, there is a trend to recommend a *switch* to a complementary drug having a high barrier to resistance. Both options are considered in the recent EASL guidelines [7]. Recommendations for treatment adaptation in CHB-resistant patients are showed in Table 3. The switch strategy does not apply to patients who have been exposed to multiple monotherapies; these patients should be treated with add-on strategies in order to minimize the risk of subsequent treatment failure.

Resistance	Action
LAM resistance	Switch to TDF (add ADV if TDF not available)
ADV resistance	If patient was NA naive before ADV: Switch to ETV or TDF; ETV may be preferred in such patients with high viraemia If patient had prior LAM resistance: Switch to TDF and add a nucleoside analogue
LdT resistance	Switch to or add TDF (add ADV if TDF not available)
ETV resistance	Switch to or add TDF (add ADV if TDF not available)
TDF resistance	TDF resistance not detected to date: add a nucleoside analogue. Switch to ETV if patient had no prior LAM resistance

EASL 2012 HBV Guidelines (Ref. 7)

Table 3. EASL 2012 Guidelines recommendations in patients with antiviral resistance

17. Summary and conclusions

Chronic hepatitis B remains a serious clinical problem because of its worldwide distribution and potential progression of liver damage. Over the last decades, treatment of CHB has greatly advanced due to the availability of safe and effective drugs and guidelines have been developed. Both Peg-IFN and two NAs, entecavir and tenofovir, can currently be indicated as first-line therapies for CHB.

Peg-IFN treatment is a short-term treatment strategy which provides a significant off-treatment sustained responses, including loss of HBsAg. However, as Peg-IFN is effective in 20-30% of patients, it should, therefore, be considered only for patients with an elevated possibility of response based on pre-treatment and on-treatment factors. In particular quantitative HBV-DNA and HBsAg may be suitable to early identify patients who are unlikely to benefit from Peg-IFN early during the treatment course, thereby avoiding unnecessary treatment. Nevertheless, despite this individualised and response-guided approach, increasing the cost-effectiveness of Peg-IFN therapy remains a clinical challenge. Combining Peg-IFN with NA appears to be the most appealing approach to increase the efficacy of antiviral therapy and new trials on a combination of Peg-IFN with ETV or TDF are required.

Currently, nucleos(t)ides analogues represent the treatment option used in the majority of CHB patients due to their potent antiviral effect, oral administration (one oral tablet daily) and optimum tolerance. In registration trials, entecavir and tenofovir, third-generation potent antivirals with a high barrier to resistance, showed long-term HBV-DNA suppression, low rise of resistance, potential reversion of fibrosis and no progression to cirrhosis, and lower risk of adverse clinical events in cirrhotic patients, except for HCC development. Real life studies have confirmed the long-term efficacy and safety of these two first-line NAs. However, NAs require a long-term, perhaps indefinite, treatment thus raising several concerns: patient's commitment to lifelong treatment, adherence, long-term safety, drug resistance in the long-term and costs. Combination of IFN and NAs might achieve an antiviral synergy and provide new opportunities to increase HBsAg clearance rates and shorten treatment duration. New studies exploring different strategies of combining Peg-IFN with ETV or TDF are required to further improve the treatment of chronic hepatitis B.

Author details

Teresa Santantonio* and Massimo Fasano

*Address all correspondence to: t.santantonio@unifg.it

Department of Clinical and Experimental Medicine, University of Foggia, Foggia, Italy

References

[1] Lavanchy, D. Hepatitis B virus epidemiology, disease burden, treatment, and current and emerging prevention and control measures. J Viral Hepat (2004). , 11, 97-107.

[2] Fattovich, G. Natural history and prognosis of hepatitis B. Semin Liver Dis (2003). , 23, 47-58.

[3] Hui, C. K, Leung, N, Yuen, S. T, Zhang, H. Y, Leung, K. W, Lu, L, et al. Natural History and Disease Progression in Chinese Chronic Hepatitis B Patients in Immune-tolerant Phase. Hepatology (2007). , 46, 395-401.

[4] Brunetto, M. R, Oliveri, F, Colombatto, P, Moriconi, F, Ciccorossi, P, Coco, B, et al. Hepatitis B surface antigen serum levels help to distinguish active from inactive hepatitis B virus genotype D carriers. Gastroenterology (2010). , 139, 483-490.

[5] Raimondo, G, Allain, J. P, Brunetto, M. R, Buendia, M. A, Chen, D. S, Colombo, M, et al. Statements from the Taormina expert meeting on occult hepatitis B virus infection. J Hepatol (2008). , 49, 652-657.

[6] Zerbini, A, Pilli, M, Boni, C, Fisicaro, P, Penna, A, Di Vincenzo, P, et al. The characteristics of the cell-mediated immune response identify different profiles of occult hepatitis B virus infection. Gastroenterology (2008). , 134, 1470-1481.

[7] European Association for the Study of the Liver. EASL Clinical Practice Guidelines: Management of chronic hepatitis B virus infection. J Hepatol (2012). , 57, 167-185.

[8] Lok, A. S, & McMahon, B. J. Chronic hepatitis B: Update 2009. Hepatology (2009). , 50, 661-662.

[9] Liaw, Y. F, Leung, N, Kao, J. H, Piratvisuth, T, Gane, E, Han, K. H, et al. Asian-Pacific consensus statement on the management of chronic hepatitis B: a 2008 update. Hepatol Int (2008). , 2, 263-283.

[10] Castera, L. Non invasive methods to assess liver disease in patients with hepatitis B or C. Gastroenterology (2012). , 142, 1293-1302.

[11] Fattovich, G, Bortolotti, F, & Donato, F. Natural history of chronic hepatitis B: special emphasis on disease progression and prognostic factors. J Hepatol (2008). , 48, 335-352.

[12] Yang, H. I, Lu, S. N, Liaw, Y. F, You, S. L, Sun, C. A, Wang, L. Y, et al. Hepatitis B e antigen and the risk of hepatocellular carcinoma. N Engl J Med (2002). , 347, 168-174.

[13] Iloeje, U. H, Yang, H. I, Su, J, Jen, C. L, You, S. L, Chen, S. J, et al. Predicting cirrhosis risk based on the level of circulating hepatitis B viral load. Gastroenterology (2006). , 130, 678-686.

[14] Chen, C. J, Yang, H. I, Su, J, Jen, C. L, You, S. L, Lu, S. N, et al. Risk of hepatocellular carcinoma across a biological gradient of serum hepatitis B virus DNA level. JAMA (2006). , 295, 65-73.

[15] Van Zonneveld, M, Flink, H. J, Verhey, E, Senturk, H, Zeuzem, S, Akarca, U. S, et al. The safety of pegylated interferon alpha-2b in the treatment of chronic hepatitis B: predictive factors for dose reduction and treatment discontinuation. Aliment Pharmacol Ther (2005). , 21, 1163-1171.

[16] Lau, G. K, Piratvisuth, T, Luo, K. X, Marcellin, P, Thongsawat, S, Cooksley, G, et al. Peginterferon alpha-2a, Lamivudine, and the combination for HBeAg-positive chronic hepatitis B. N Engl J Med (2005). , 352, 2682-2695.

[17] Lau, G. K, Piratvisuth, T, Luo, H. X, Marcellin, P, Thongsawat, S, Cooksley, G, et al. Durabilty of response and occurrence of late response to peginterferon alpha-2a (40KD) [Pegasys] one year post-treatment in patients with HBeAg-posive chronic hepatitis B. J Hepatol (2006). Abs 50.

[18] Buster, E. H, Flink, H. J, Cakaloglu, Y, Simon, K, Trojan, J, Tabak, F, et al. Sustained HBeAg and HBsAg loss after long-term follow-up of HBeAg positive patients treated with peginterferon alpha-2b. Gastroenterology (2008). , 135, 459-467.

[19] Buster EHCJ, Hansen BE, Lau GK, Piratvisuth T, Zeuzem S, Steyerberg EW, et al. Factors that predict response of patients with hepatitis B e antigen-positive chronic hepatitis B to peginterferon-alfa. Gastroenterology (2009). , 137, 2002-2009.

[20] Piratvisuth, T, et al. Sustained Immune Control 1 Year Post-Treatment With Peginterferon Alfa-2a [40KD] (PEGASYS) is Durable up to 5 Years Post-Treatment and is Associated With a High Rate of HBsAg Clearance in HBeAg-Negative Chronic Hepatitis B. Hepatol Int (2010). Abs210.

[21] Marcellin, P, Lau, G. K, Bonino, F, et al. Peginterferon alfa-2a alone, lamivudine alone, and the two in combination in patients with HBeAg-negative chronic hepatitis B. N Engl J Med (2004). , 351, 1206-1217.

[22] Piccolo, P, Lenci, I, Demelia, L, Bandiera, F, Piras, M. R, Antonucci, G, et al. A randomized controlled trial of pegylated interferon-alpha2a plus adefovir dipivoxil for hepatitis B e antigen-negative chronic hepatitis B. Antivir Ther (2009). , 14, 1165-1174.

[23] Rijckborst V, ter Borg MJ, Cakaloglu Y, Ferenci P, Tabak F, Akdogan M, et al. A randomized trial of peginterferon alpha-2a with or without ribavirin for HBeAg-negative chronic hepatitis B. Am J Gastroenterol. (2010). , 105, 1762-1769.

[24] Liaw, Y. F, Jia, J. D, Chan, H. L, Han, K. H, Tanwandee, T, Chuang, W. L, et al. Shorter durations and lower doses of peginterferon alfa-2a are associated with inferior hepatitis B e antigen seroconversion rates in hepatitis B virus genotypes B or C. Hepatology. (2011). , 54, 1591-1599.

[25] Lampertico P, Viganò M, Di Costanzo GG, Sagnelli E, Fasano M, Di Marco V, et al. Randomised study comparison 48 and 96 weeks peginterferon α-2a therapy in genotype D HBeAg-negative chronic hepatitis B. Gut (2012). Epub ahead of print]

[26] Janssen HLA, van Zonneveld M, Senturk H, Zeuzem S, Akarca US, Cakaloglu Y, et al. Pegylated interferon alfa-2b alone or in combination with lamivudine for HBeAg-positive chronic hepatitis B: a randomized trial. Lancet (2005). , 365, 123-129.

[27] Sonneveld, M. J, Rijckborst, V, Zeuzem, S, Heathcote, E. J, Simon, K, Senturk, H, Pas, S. D, Hansen, B. E, & Janssen, H. Presence of precore and core promoter mutants limits the probability of response to peginterferon in hepatitis B e antigen-positive chronic hepatitis B. Hepatology (2012). , 56, 67-74.

[28] Tseng, T. C, Yu, M. L, Liu, C. J, Lin, C. L, Huang, Y. W, Hsu, C. S, et al. Effect of host and viral factors on hepatitis B e antigen-positive chronic hepatitis B patients receiving pegylated interferon alpha-2a therapy. Antivir Ther (2011). , 16, 629-637.

[29] Sonneveld, M. J, Wong, V. W, Woltman, A. M, Wong, G. L, Cakaloglu, Y, Zeuzem, S, et al. Polymorphisms near IL28B and serological response to peginterferon in HBeAg-positive patients with chronic hepatitis B. Gastroenterology (2012). , 142, 513-520.

[30] Wu, X, Xin, Z, Zhu, X, Pan, L, Li, Z, Li, H, et al. Evaluation of susceptibility locus for response to interferon-alpha based therapy in chronic hepatitis B patients in Chinese. Antiviral Res (2012). , 93, 297-300.

[31] Lampertico, P, Viganò, M, Cheroni, C, Facchetti, F, Invernizzi, F, Valveri, V, et al. IL28B polymorphisms predict interferon-related HBsAg seroclearance in genotype D HBeAg-negative patients with chronic hepatitis B. Hepatology (2012). Epub ahead of print]

[32] Sonneveld, M. J, Rijckborst, V, Boucher, C. A, Hansen, B. E, & Janssen, H. L. Prediction of sustained response to peginterferon alpha-2b for hepatitis B e antigen-positive chronic hepatitis B using on-treatment hepatitis B surface antigen decline. Hepatology (2010). , 52, 1251-1257.

[33] Piratvisuth, T, Marcellin, P, Popescu, M, Kapprell, H. P, Rothe, V, & Lu, Z. M. Hepatitis B surface antigen: association with sustained response to peginterferon alfa-2a in hepatitis B e antigen-positive patients. Hepatol Int (2011). Epub ahead of print]

[34] Rijckborst, V, Hansen, B. E, Cakaloglu, Y, Ferenci, P, Tabak, F, Akdogan, M, et al. Early on-treatment prediction of response to peginterferon alpha-2a for HBeAg-negative chronic hepatitis B using HBsAg and HBV DNA levels. Hepatology (2010). , 52, 454-461.

[35] Rijckborst, V, Hansen, B. E, Ferenci, P, Brunetto, M. R, Tabak, F, Cakaloglu, Y, et al. Validation of a stopping rule at week 12 using HBsAg and HBV DNA for HBeAg-negative patients treated with peginterferon alfa-2a. J Hepatol (2012). , 56, 1006-1011.

[36] Chang TT, Lai CL, Kew Yoon S, Lee SS, Coelho HS, Carrilho FJ, et al. Entecavir treatment for up to 5 years in patients with hepatitis B e antigen-positive chronic hepatitis B. Hepatology (2010). , 51, 422-430.

[37] Shouval, D, Lai, C. L, Chang, T. T, Gadano, A, Wu, S. S, Halota, W, et al. Three years of entecavir (ETV) re-treatment of HBeAg(-) ETV patients who previously discontinued ETV treatment: results from study ETV-901. Hepatology (2008). Abs 927.

[38] Marcellin, P, Heathcote, E. J, Buti, M, Gane, E, De Man, R. A, Krastev, Z, et al. Tenofovir disoproxil fumarate versus adefovir dipivoxil for chronic hepatitis B. N Engl J Med. (2008). , 359, 2442-2455.

[39] Heathcote, E. J, Marcellin, P, Buti, M, Gane, E, De Man, R. A, Krastev, Z, et al. Three-year efficacy and safety of tenofovir disoproxil fumarate treatment for chronic hepatitis B. Gastroenterology (2011). , 140, 132-43.

[40] Marcellin, P, Buti, M, Gane, E. J, Krastev, Z, Flisiak, R, Germanidis, G, et al. Five years of treatment with tenofovir DF (TDF) for chronic hepatitis B (CHB) infection is associated with sustained viral suppression and significant regression of histological fibrosis and cirrhosis. Hepatology (2011). Suppl 1):1011A-1012A. Abs 1375.

[41] Tenney, D. J, Rose, R. E, Baldick, C. J, Pokornowski, K. A, Eggers, B. J, Fang, J, et al. Long-term monitoring shows hepatitis B virus resistance to entecavir in nucleoside-naive patients is rare through 5 years of therapy. Hepatology (2009). , 49, 1503-1514.

[42] Snow-lampart, A, Chappell, B, Curtis, M, Zhu, Y, Myrick, F, Schawalder, J, et al. No resistance to tenofovir disoproxil fumarate detected after up to 144 weeks of therapy in patients monoinfected with chronic hepatitis B virus. Hepatology (2011). , 53, 763-773.

[43] Manns, M, Akarca, U. S, Chang, T. T, Sievert, W, Yoon, S-K, Tsai, N, et al. Low rates of nucleos(t)ide-associated adverse events in the long-term experience with entecavir. J Hepatol (2010). S393. Abs 1016.

[44] Lampertico, P, Soffredini, R, Invernizzi, F, Vigano, M, Facchetti, F, Minola, E, et al. Maintained viral suppression and excellent safety profile of Entecavir monotherapy in 418 NUC-naïve patients with chronic hepatitis B: a 4-year field practice, multicenter study. J Hepatol (2012). S206. Abs 522.

[45] Seto WK, Lai CL, Fung J, Yuen DKH, Wong M, Yuen MF. Outcome of 4-year treatment of entecavir for treatment-naive chronic hepatitis B. J Hepatol (2011). S301. Abs 748.

[46] Buti, M, Morillas, R. M, Prieto, M, Diago, M, Pérez, J, Solà, R, et al. Efficacy and safety of entecavir in clinical practice in treatment-naive Caucasian chronic hepatitis B patients. Eur J Gastroenterol Hepatol (2012). , 24, 535-542.

[47] Zoutendjik, R, Reijnders, J. G, Brown, A, et al. Entecavir treatment for chronic hepatitis B: adaptation is not needed for the majority of naïve patients with a partial virologic response. Hepatology (2011). , 54, 443-451.

[48] Zoutendijk, R, Reijnders, J, Zoulim, F, Brown, B, Mutimer, D, Deterding, K, et al. Virological response to Entecavir is associated with a better clinical outcome in chronic hepatitis B patients. Gut (2012). Epub ahead of print]

[49] Lampertico, P, Soffredini, R, Vigano, M, Yurdaydin, C, Idilman, R, Papatheodoridis, G. V, et al. Tenofovir monotherapy for naïve patients with chronic hepatitis B: a

multicenter European study in clinical practice in 302 patients followed for 30 months. J Hepatol (2012). S208. Abs 525.

[50] Zoulim, F, & Locarnini, S. Management of treatment failure in chronic hepatitis B. J Hepatol (2012). Suppl 1:S, 112-122.

Chapter 7

Treatment of Chronic HCV Infection in the Era of Protease Inhibitors

R. Villani, F. Bellanti and G. Serviddio

Additional information is available at the end of the chapter

http://dx.doi.org/10.5772/56139

1. Introduction

Hepatitis C virus infection represents the most common cause of chronic hepatitis with potential evolution into cirrhosis and hepatocellular carcinoma [1]. The infected population appears heterogeneous for age, modalities of infection, and disease duration [2]. To date the standard of care of treatment (SOC) has been pegylated interferon alpha 2a or alpha 2b associated with ribavirin. The main goal of the therapy is the achievement of a sustained virological response (SVR) defined as undetectable HCV RNA 24 weeks after stopping treatment.

Several factors influence therapeutic schedules. First of all, HCV genotype 1 (G1) and 4 require longer treatment as compared to G2 and G3.

Early virologic negativization after starting therapy, together with virus genotype, are the most important predictors of sustained virological response.

The absence of a virologic response by week 12 has the highest negative predictive value for all genotypes suggesting that HCV RNA disappearance should be achieved as soon as possible [3].

Many other factors such as age, gender, degree of fibrosis and viral load influence SVR; more recently, the single nucleotide polymorphism (SNPs) of the IL28B gene has been demonstrated to be a good predictor of response [4].

The analysis of large cohorts demonstrates that, even in patients treated for 48 weeks, almost half of G1 infected patients does not reach a SVR, as compared to 20% of G2/3 [5].

Treatment failure is defined on the basis of the virological response to treatment, as follows:

a. **null responders**, if the reduction of HCV RNA is less than 1 log_{10} at week 12 of therapy;

b. **virological nonresponse** is considered when the serum HCV RNA level remains above the limit of detection throughout treatment and is defined as less than 2 log10 decline in HCV RNA between baseline and week 12;

c. **partial responders** if the reduction of HCV RNA is at least 2 $\log_{10}$ at 12 weeks but it is still detectable at week 24;

d. **relapsers** if HCV RNA decreases and remains below the limit of detection (<50 IU/mL) during treatment but becomes detectable after cessation of treatment [6].

HCV infection is often characterized by extrahepatic associated diseases. HCV is considered a stimulus for B-cell clonal expansion underlying benign and malignant B-cell dyscrasias including a subgroup of B-cells non Hodgkin's lymphomas. In this context, we must consider that HCV infection is also characterized by several extrahepatic manifestations. The most common and well characterized is mixed cryoglobulinemia. This condition, as well as some B-cell non Hodgkin's lymphomas, is the result of B-cell clonal expansion due to viral persistence [7].

Accordingly, the treatment of HCV chronic infection should be addressed not only to the treatment of chronic liver disease, but also to the prevention of HCV-associated diseases.

It is estimated that 25% of HCC worldwide is related to HCV [8].

If the rate of response to antiviral therapy increases to 80%, over the next ten years, the treatment of half of HCV-infected persons would reduce cirrhosis by 15%, hepatocellular carcinoma by 30% and death for liver disease by 34%. [9].

The application of the most effective therapy should be a common strategy to block permanently viral replication and avoid the progression to cirrhosis and the development of hepatocellular carcinoma.

Boceprevir and telaprevir are HCV protease inhibitors, recently approved for antiviral therapy in HCV infected patients, are effective to control the viral replication.

2. Target of protease inhibitors

HCV genome is a single strand RNA of 9000-9100 nucleotide encoding for three stuctural (C, E1, E2), seven non structural (xlink, NS3, NS4A, NS4B, NS5A, NS5B, p7) and F proteins whose role is unknown [10] (Fig 1).

HCV replicative cycle involves the translation of the HCV RNA into a single polyprotein that is subsequently cleaved to obtain every single structural and non structural proteins.

NS3 is a serine protease while NS4 serves as cofactor. NS3 and NS4A must be assembled in order to become active in catalyzing the cleavage of the other NS proteins from the HCV polyprotein at the NS3/NS4A, NS4A/NS4B, NS4B/NS5A and NS5A/NS5B junctions, a condition required for viral replication.

HCV virions turn over rapidly (with a half-life of about 3 h), and up to 10^{12} viruses are produced per day in an infected person [11].

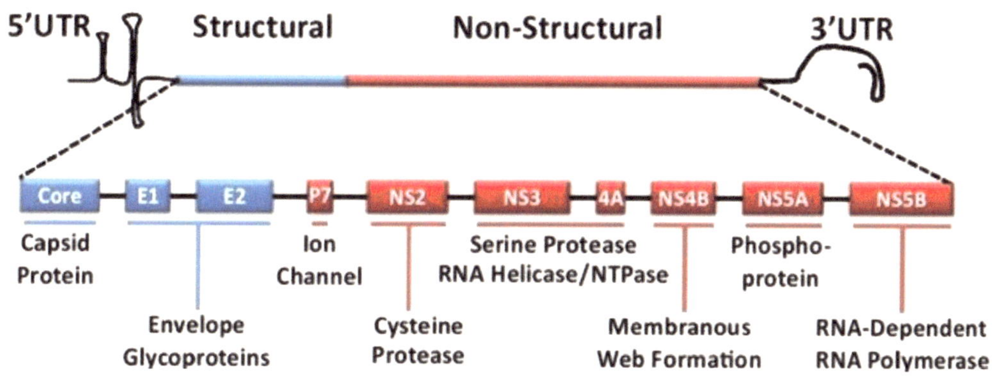

Figure 1. Genomic organization of hepatitis C polyprotein. The HCV genome (about 9000 nucleotides) is translated in a single polypeptide of 3000 aminoacids. Then the polypeptide is cleved to produce ten proteins whose role is explained below. During an alternative splicing within the core, a new protein (F protein) can be produced (this one not represented) (From :Poordad F, Dieterich D. Treating hepatitis C: current standard of care and emerging direct-acting antiviral agents. J Viral Hepat 2012 Jul;19(7):449-464)..

Boceprevir and Telaprevir link to NS3/NS4A enzymatic complex in a covalent and reversible manner to disrupt the processing of the HCV polyprotein.

Even if the protease inhibitors are potent antiviral agent, their administration without interferon and ribavirin is characterized by rapid selection of resistant variants of the virus [12]. Accordingly boceprevir and telaprevir need to be administered in a regimen with pegylated-interferon and ribavirin, commonly named "triple therapy".

During the initial 2 weeks of triple therapy the viral load decline is rapid and unaffected by ribavirin. However, beyond 2 weeks, viral breakthrough occurs if ribavirin is not administered. After 12 weeks, breakthrough occurs in 24% of patients treated with peg-interferon and telaprevir.

Ribavirin also affects the rate of viral relapse. In regimens without ribavirin, relapse occurs in 48% of patients as compared to 14-30% of patients treated with ribavirin [13].

3. Management of antiviral therapy in naive patients

Three trials (SPRINT-2, ADVANCE, ILLUMINATE) examined the efficacy of boceprevir and telaprevir in naïve patients.

Telaprevir obtained a SVR rate of 75% as compared to 44% of the SOC with peg-interferon plus ribavirin.

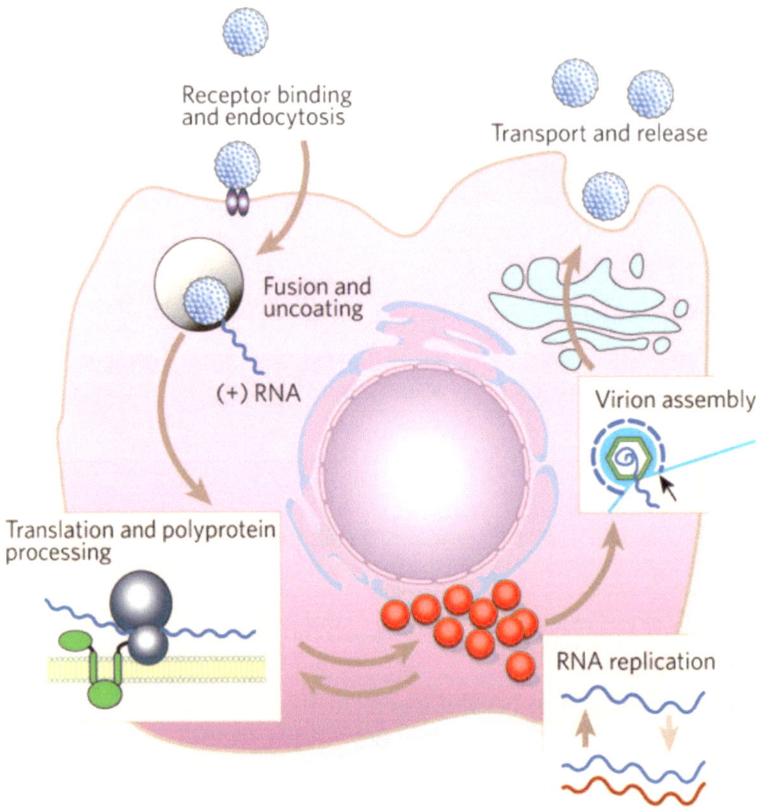

Figure 2. The nucleocapsid of the HCV genome is surrounded by an envelope that facilitates attachment and penetration into host cells. Upon entry into the host cell by endocytosis, the virus undergoes undergoes a fusion and uncoating step. Its RNA is translated into a polyprotein of approximately 3,000 aminoacids that is processed by cellular and viral proteases (including NS3) to yield structural and non structural proteins. Boceprevir and telaprevir block the polyprotein processing by stopping activity of NS3/NS4A complex, which has protease activity on the polypeptide (From Lindenbach BD, Rice CM. Unravelling hepatitis C virus replication from genome to function. Nature 2005;436:933-938; Manns MP, Foster GR, Rockstroh JK, Zeuzem S, Zoulim F, Houghton M. The way forward in HCV treatment--finding the right path. Nat Rev Drug Discov 2007 Dec;6(12):991-1000).

The schedule includes triple therapy (telaprevir + peg-interferon + ribavirin) for the first 12 weeks and peg-interferon+ribavirin for additional 36 weeks (fig 3). Telaprevir is administered at the dose of 750 mg thrice daily.

The tablets should be taken with high fat (>20 g) meal or snack for optimal adsorption (table 2).

Patients with undetectable HCV RNA at week 4 (rapid virological response, RVR) and 12 (extended rapid virological response, eRVR) can stop therapy after 24 weeks of treatment (response-guided therapy, RGT) [14].

In the contrast, telaprevir should be stopped when:

a. HCV RNA is more than 1000 UI/ml at week 4 or 12 or

b. HCV RNA is detectable at week 24

Boceprevir was differently studied in black and non-black populations.

The SVR rate was 53% and 68% in black and not-black population, respectively.

Boceprevir requires a "lead-in" phase with peg-interferon and ribavirin for 4 weeks and triple therapy (boceprevir + peg-interferon + ribavirin) for 24 or 32 weeks and again a dual therapy with peg-interferon and ribavirin for the last 4 weeks (fig 4).

The lead-in in phase is useful in naïve patients to assess the responsiveness to peg-interferon and ribavirin.

In fact, lower SVR rates and development of boceprevir-resistant mutants are more common in patients with HCV RNA reduction less than 1 $\log_{10}$ at week 4 independently from the treatment scheme [15].

The recommended dose of boceprevir is 800 mg thrice daily. Meal seems not influence the absorption as much as observed in telaprevir regimens.

In patients with RVR after the "lead-in" phase, SOC is still recommended since SVR is observed in 88% after 48 weeks of therapy [16].

Accordingly to the response-guided therapy, RGT, patients treated with boceprevir with undetectable HCV RNA at weeks 8 and 24 can stop therapy after 36 weeks of treatment.

If HCV RNA is detectable at week 8, the treatment should continue to 48 weeks.

Boceprevir should be stopped when:

a. HCV RNA is more than 100 UI/ml at week 12 or

b. HCV RNA is detectable at week 24.

4. Management of antiviral therapy in null responders

Retreatment of null responders with peg-interferon and ribavirin is effective in less than 5% of patients [17].

Telaprevir increases SVR to 31%.

The schedule requires 48 weeks of treatment, with the first 12 weeks of triple and the remaining 36 weeks with peg-interferon and ribavirin.

The stopping rules are the same of naïve patients.

Boceprevir trials did not include null responders and, to date, it is not recommended in such patients.

5. Management of antiviral therapy in partial responders

Retreatment of partial responders with SOC is effective in 7-15% of patients [17, 18].

Triple therapy with boceprevir or telaprevir may increase the rate of SVR to 52% and 57%, respectively.

Response-guided therapy is not recommended since 48 weeks are commonly requested.

6. Management of antiviral therapy in relapsers

Retreatment of relapsers with SOC induces a SVR in less than 1/3 of patients [17, 18].

Telaprevir is administered for the first 12 weeks and SOC for the further 36 weeks with a SVR rate of 86%.

Boceprevir requires the "lead-in" phase of SOC and triple therapy for the additional 44 weeks with a SVR of 75%.

If HCV RNA is not detected at weeks 8 and 24, the therapy may be stopped at week 32.

STUDY	Drug	Population	Treatment arms	Intervention SVR	SOC SVR	Main findings
SPRINT-2	Boceprevir	Naive	Black-RGT Black- 48 week Non Black RGT Non Black- 48 week	42% 53% 67% 68%	23% 40%	RGT therapy as effective as 48 weeks of therapy for non black patients. About 50% of patients elegible for RGT
ADVANCE	Telaprevir	Naive	T8 (pooled 24- and 48-week total therapy) T12 (pooled 24- and 48-week total therapy)	69% 75%	44%	12-week telaprevir regiment preferable to 8-week regimen
ILLUMINATE	Telaprevir	Naive	T12 overall eRVR+24-week therapy eRVR+48-week therapy	75% 92% 88%	N/A	24-week total therapy for eRVR patients non inferior to 48 weeks of therapy. About 75% of patients eligible for shorter duration of therapy

STUDY	Drug	Population	Treatment arms	Intervention SVR	SOC SVR	Main findings
RESPOND-2	Boceprevir	Treatment experienced	RGT- prior relapser RGT-Prior non responder 48 weeks-relapsers 48week-non responders	69% 40% 75% 52%	29% 7%	Null responders excluded. Relapsers had similar outcomes as naive population
REALIZE	Telaprevir	Treatment experienced	T12 (48-week total therapy) Prior relapsers Prior partial responders Prior null responders	86% 57% 31%	24% 15% 5%	Relapers had similar outcomes as naive population

Table 1. Summary of phase 3 clinical trials for boceprevir and telaprevir.eRVR, extended rapid virologic response; RGT, response guided therapy; SOC, standard of care; SVR, sustained virologic response; T8, 8-week telaprevir arm; T12, 12-week telaprevir arm (From: Barritt AS, Fried MW. Maximizing opportunities and avoiding mistakes in triple therapy for hepatitis C virus. Gastroenterology 2012 May;142(6):1314-1323).

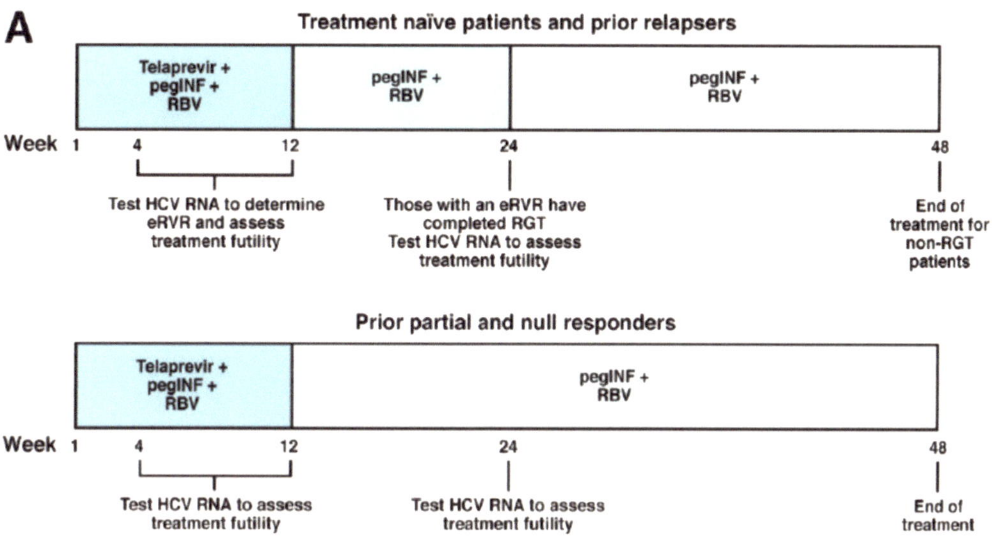

Figure 3. Telaprevir schedule. In naïve and prior relapser patients telaprevir should be administered for the first 12 weeks and peg-interferon plus ribavirin for 12 or 36 weeks additional. In case of eRVR (HCV RNA not detected at week 4 and 12 the treatment may be stopped after 24 weeks. If HCV RNA is still detected at week 12, peg-interferon and ribavirin should be continued for additional 36 weeks. In any case if HCV RNA is detectable at week 24 or results > 1000 UI/ml between 4 and 12 weeks, the treatment should be stopped. RBV, ribavirin; eRVR, extended rapid virologic

Examples of food containing at least 20 g of fat
Bagel with cream cheese
½ cup of nuts
3 tablespoons of peanut butter
1 cup of ice cream
60 g of American or cheddar cheese
60 g of potato chips
½ cup of trail mix
33 g of granola
3 slices of homemade French toast
2 cups 3.3% whole milk
60 g of chocolate candy bar with almonds or peanuts
Two 60 g plain doughnuts
1 slice pecan pie
1 medium avocado
100 g of lean hamburger in bun
100 g of salami
4 slices of bologna
100 g of broiled pork chop
Three 100 g sausage patties
2 cup chow mein noodles
200 g of fried chicken breast
2 small roasted chicken legs

Table 2. Food containing at least 20 g of fat (From: Kiser JJ, Burton JR, Anderson PL, Everson GT. Review and management of drug interactions with boceprevir and telaprevir. Hepatology 2012 May;55(5):1620-1628.)

response (From: Barritt AS, Fried MW. Maximizing opportunities and avoiding mistakes in triple therapy for hepatitis C virus. Gastroenterology 2012 May;142(6):1314-1323.)

7. Management of side effect of antiviral therapy

Even if only 2% are severe, almost all patients treated with boceprevir or telaprevir report side effects. Among all, anaemia is the most common, occurring in 50% of patients treated with protease inhibitor as compared to 20% of peg-interferon and ribavirin.

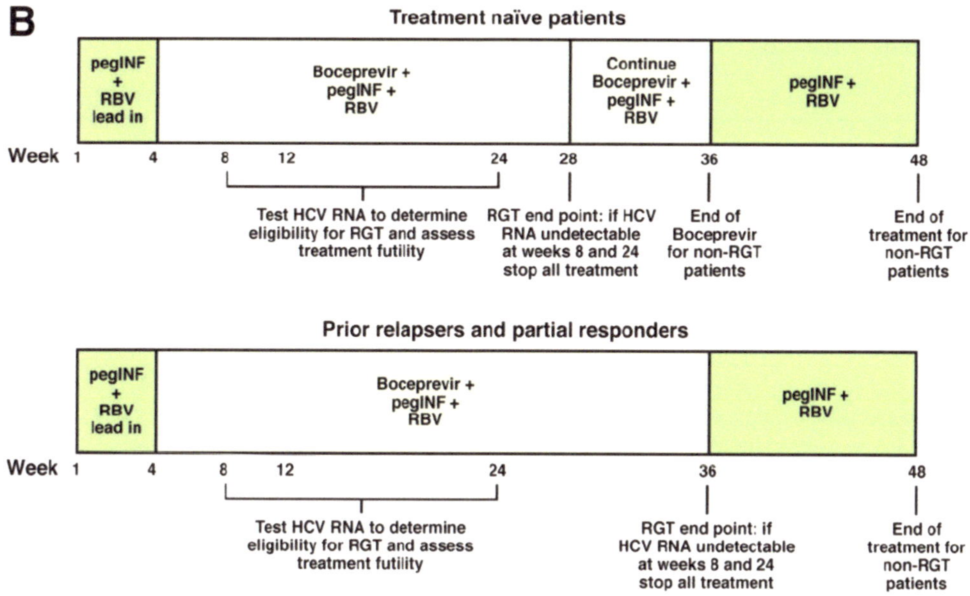

Figure 4. Boceprevir schedule. A "lead in" phase (4 weeks of peg-interferon and ribavirin before the beginning of the triple therapy) is considered for all patients. In naïve patients boceprevir should be administered for a minimum of 24 weeks. If HCV RNA is negative at week 8 and 24 all drugs must be stopped at week 28. If HCV RNA is detectable at week 8 o 24, boceprevir should be administrated for 32 weeks and peg-interferon plus ribavirin for additional 12 weeks.In prior relapsers and partial responders boceprevir should be administered for 32 weeks and peg-interferon plus ribavirin for additional 12 weeks. In any case, if HCV RNA is detectable at week 24 or HCV RNA is >100 UI/ml at week 12, the treatment should be stopped (From: Barritt AS, Fried MW. Maximizing opportunities and avoiding mistakes in triple therapy for hepatitis C virus. Gastroenterology 2012 May;142(6):1314-1323.).

Blood count should be monitored during the first 4 weeks to identify those who will need support.

In patients treated with boceprevir, SVR has been observed more frequently in those who develop anaemia [19].

Administration of subcutaneous alpha-erythropoietin 40.000 UI once a week is effective in controlling anaemia induced by peg-interferon and ribavirin as well as protease inhibitors trying to maintain the blood level around 100 g/L.

If ineffective, ribavirin may be reduced and blood transfusion considered.

It has been reported that, in triple therapy regimen, ribavirin may be safely reduced without affecting the SVR rate.

When this strategy is insufficient and anaemia becomes more severe, blood transfusion is required.

Neutropenia occurs in 70-80% of patients treated with triple therapy and this is more commonly observed in those developing anaemia [20].

Filgrastim 30 MU subcutaneous one to three times a week usually maintains the count of neutrophils > 1000/μL.

	Boceprevir	*Telaprevir*
Complete blood count	Baseline week 2 and 4 weekly for the first month of triple therapy (from week 4 to 8) then monthly or as necessary	Baseline weekly for the first month of triple therapy Every three weeks until the end of triple then monthly during the left dual therapy or as necessary
Liver function tests	Baseline week 4-6 and 8 then monthly	Baseline Week 2-4 and 8 Then monthly
Serum electrolytes Creatinine Uric acid	Baseline week 2 then monthly	Baseline week 2 then monthly
TSH	Baseline week 12 and 24 then as necessary	Baseline week 12 and 24 then as necessary
Cholesterol Tryglicerides	Baseline week 12 and 24 then as necessary	Baseline week 12 and 24 then as necessary

Table 3. Proposal for blood monitoring during triple therapy

HEMATOLOGICAL SIDE EFFECT	**CHANGE DURING THERAPY**	
Anemia	< 100 g/L	Erythropoietin 40.000 UI once a week
	< 90 g/L	Ribavirin dose reduction + Erythropoietin
	< 80 g/L	Blood transfusion
Thrombocytopenia	≥ 100.000/μL	No change
	≥ 50.000/μL	Weekly control then monthly
	< 50.000/μL	Peg-interferon dose reduction
	< 25.000/μL	Stop therapy
Neutropenia	< 1000/μL	Filgrastim 30 MU once/ twice/ thrice a week
	< 750/μL	Peg-interferon dose reduction

Table 4. Management of haematological side effects during triple therapy.

The adverse effects described during peg-interferon and ribavirin therapy such as rush, flu like and gastrointestinal symptoms are more commonly observed during triple therapy.

http://dx.doi.org/10.5772/56139

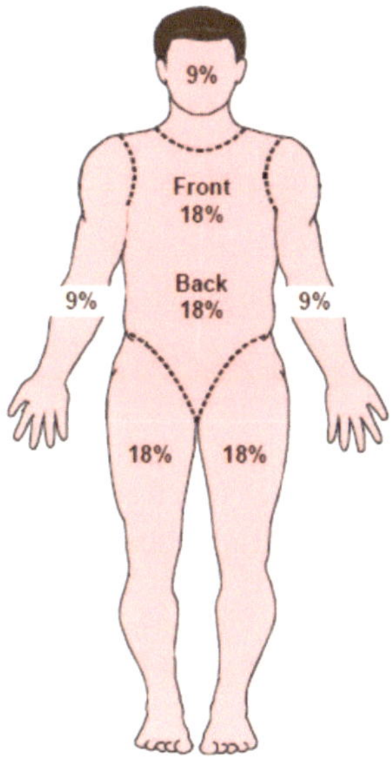

Adult body	BSA
Perineum	1%
Arm	9%
Head (front and back)	9%
Leg	18%
Chest	18%
Back	18%

Figure 5. Estimating body surface area (BSA: body surface area) (From: Hezode C. Boceprevir and telaprevir for the treatment of chronic hepatitis C: safety management in clinical practice. Liver Int 2012 Feb;32 Suppl 1:32-38)

Fatigue, nausea, dysgeusia, chills, insomnia, alopecia, diarrhoea, decreased appetite, irritability, vomiting, arthralgia, dizziness, dry skin rash, asthenia, dyspnoea on exertion are more common during boceprevir [21]. In particular, dysgeusia affects almost 50% of patients. Telaprevir induces hyperuricemia, fatigue, pruritus, diarrhoea, vomiting, haemorrhoids, anorectal discomfort, dysgeusia and anal pruritus relative to patients on standard of care. Cutaneous rash is the less tolerated side effect of telaprevir. Fortunately, more than 90% of such events is mild or moderate and does not progress. Discontinuation occurs only in 6% of cases [22]. Oral antihistamines or a topical steroid is effective in controlling symptoms. Moderate rash may associate with pruritus or mucosal involvement. When more than 50% of the body surface is involved or vesicles, bullae or ulceration develop, rash is considered severe and telaprevir should be stopped; peg-interferon and ribavirin can be continued for additional 6-7 days. If the rash does not improve, all drugs should be stopped and hospitalization and appropriate therapy is required [23].

Haemorrhoids, anal pruritus, anorectal discomfort and anal burning observed during telaprevir may be managed with topic steroid or local lidocaine.

Life threatening or systemic reaction (Steven-Johnson syndrome, drug reaction with eosinophilia and systemic symptoms – DRESS, erythema multiforme-EM) are rarely observed (refer to the specific chapter for details).

8. Drug interactions

Boceprevir and telaprevir are metabolized *via* the cytochrome P4503A pathway. They are potent inhibitors of CYP3A4 and also substrates and inhibitors of the drug transporter P-glycoprotein (P-gp).

Boceprevir and telaprevir availability depends on Child-Pugh but not on renal function.

Concentration of boceprevir in serum increases of 30% and 45-60% in patients with Child Pugh B and C, respectively.

Telaprevir is reduced of about 10-15% and 50% in Child Pugh B and C, respectively. Protease inhibitors greatly impact the metabolism of HMG-CoA reductase inhibitors.

Simvastatin and lovastatin are not recommended in patients treated with boceprevir or telaprevir. Atorvastatin should be avoided when telaprevir is administered and a lowest dose should be selected in boceprevir treated patients. Pravastatin is metabolized by other pathway and the risk of interaction is not completely defined. Rosuvastatin may be safely administered, even if it has not been specifically addressed in the trials.

STATINS	Use during Boceprevir	Use during Telaprevir
Simvastatin	NO	NO
Atorvastatin	POSSIBLE (USE THE LOWEST DOSE)	NO
Lovastatin	NO	NO
Pravastatin	YES	NO DATA
Rosuvastatin	POSSIBLE	POSSIBLE

Table 5. Potential association between protease inhibitors and statins.

Both boceprevir and telaprevir may reduce contraceptive efficacy of ethinyl estradiol. Moreover, boceprevir can increase plasmatic level of drosperidone while telaprevir reduces norethindrone.

Benzodiazepines (triazolam, alprazolam, flurazepam) may be greatly affected by protease inhibitors and should be avoided until new data are available.

Both boceprevir and telaprevir increase metabolism of escitalopram and its effect may be reduced.

Zolpidem concentration is reduced by of 42% in patients treated with telaprevir as well as trazodone.

Boceprevir and telaprevir reduce the clearance of cyclosporine and tacrolimus. The exposure to cyclosporine increases 4-fold with telaprevir and 3-fold with boceprevir, while tacrolimus plasmatic concentration increases 70-fold after telaprevir administration and 17-fold after boceprevir. On the other hands, immunosuppressive drugs seen not change boceprevir and telaprevir metabolism.

DRUGS	TO BE AVOIDED	INCREASED CONCENTRATION OF CONCOMITANT MED OR HCV PI	REDUCED CONCENTRATION OF CONCOMITANT MED OR HCV PI
Alpha-1 adrenoreceptor antagonist	Alfuzosin	Doxazosin Terazosin Tamsulosin Silodosin	
Anticonvulsant	Carbamazepime Phenobarbital Phenytoin		
Antifungals		Ketoconazole Itraconazole Posaconazole Voriconazole	
Antimicrobials		Clarithromycine Erythromycin	
Antimycobacterials	Rifampin Rifapentine	Rifabutin	
Antiretroviral drugs	Lopinavir (TPV) Darunavir (TPV) Fosamprenavir (TPV) Efavirenz (BOC)		Efavirenz (TPV)*
Benzodiazepines and sleep aids	Flurazepam Quazepam Triazolam Oral midazolam	Alprazolam Trazodone	
Cardiovascular	Amiodarone Bosentan Dofetilide Flecainide Lidocaine Propafenone Quinidine sildenafil and tadalafil for pulmonary arterial hypertension	Calcium-channel blockers Digoxin Carvedilol Nabivolol Irbesartan Losartan	

DRUGS	TO BE AVOIDED	INCREASED CONCENTRATION OF CONCOMITANT MED OR HCV PI	REDUCED CONCENTRATION OF CONCOMITANT MED OR HCV PI
Ergot derivatives	Dihydroergotamine Ergonovine Ergotamine Methylergonovine		
Herbal products	St. John's wort		
HMG-CoA reductase inhibitors	Lovastatin Simvastatin Atorvastatin (TPV)	Atorvastatin (BOC) Pravastatin Rosuvastatin	
Immunosuppressant	Tacrolimus Sirolimus	Cyclosporine	
Oral contraceptives		Drosperinone (BOC)	Ethynil estradiol
Respiratory		Fluticasone salmeterol	
Second-generation antipsycotic	Quetiapine	Iloperidone aripiprazole	

Interaction unique to one of the HCV protease inhibitors are indicated in parentheses (e.g. TPV or BOC).

Abbreviation: Med, medication; PI, protease inhibitor; HMG-CoA, 3-hydroxy-3-methyl-glutaryl-coenzyme A.

*A higher dose of TPV [1,120 mg every 8 hours) has been studied with efavirenz with promising preliminary rates of SVR.

(From: Kiser JJ, Burton JR, Anderson PL, Everson GT. Review and management of drug interactions with boceprevir and telaprevir. Hepatology 2012 May;55[5]:1620-1628]

Table 6. Summary of drugs to avoid and drugs to use with caution in combination with boceprevir (BOC) and telaprevir (TPV).

9. Triple therapy in cirrhotic and liver transplant patients

Cirrhosis increases morbidity and mortality and reduces SVR [24].

Clinical efficacy in cirrhosis has been investigated in phase 3 trials (ADVANCE, ILLUMINATE, REALIZE, RESPOND-2, SPRINT-2).

SVR is reached in 33% - 46% after 48 weeks of peg-interferon and ribavirin. [25, 26]

The addiction of a protease inhibitor improves the SVR to 50% [26]. In these cases, 48 weeks of treatment are commonly required.

In relapsers, the addition of a protease inhibitor increases SVR to 87%.

In partial responders SVR rate is lower (34% with triple therapy and 20% in peg-interferon and ribavirin schedule)

There are no benefits in cirrhotic null responders with by using telaprevir (14% vs 10%) [27].

The relapse rate remains high and side effects are too frequently observed in cirrhotic patients [24].

Until now, protease inhibitors are not approved for patients with liver transplantation for the interactions with immunosuppressive drugs [12].

10. Genetics and triple therapy

Interleukin 28B (IL28B) polymorfisms impacts the response to peg-interferon and ribavirin.

TRIPLE THERAPY	rs 12979860		
Boceprevir SVR	*C/C*	*C/T*	*T/T*
	80-82%	65-71%	55-59%
Telaprevir SVR	*C/C*	*C/T*	*T/T*
	90%	71%	73%

(From: Thompson AJ. Genetic factors and hepatitis C virus infection. Gastroenterology 2012 May;142(6):1335-1339)

Table 7. Response rate according to IL28B genotype in treatment-naive G1 HCV patients receiving triple therapy

Peg-interferon plus ribavirin	Polymorphism		
CAUCASIAN (n=1171)		rs 12979860	
SVR	C/C	C/T	T/T
	69%	33%	27%
AFROAMERICANS (n=300)		rs 12979860	
SVR	C/C	C/T	T/T
	48%	15%	13%

T/T genotype is associated with poor response.

The response is lower in Afro-Americans.

SVR, sustained virological response.

(From: Thompson AJ. Genetic factors and hepatitis C virus infection. Gastroenterology 2012 May;142(6):1335-1339)

Table 8. Response rate according to IL28B genotype (rs12979860) in treatment-naive North American G1 HCV patients receiving 48 week peg-interferon alpha plus ribavirin. Genotype C/C achieves SVR in 69% (good response).

The rs12979860 polymorphism has three possible genotypes (C/C, C/T, T/T), with C/C showing 2.5 or grater rate of SVR during therapy with peg-interferon and ribavirin.

The rs 8099917 polymorphisms has G/G, G/T, T/T genotypes. T/T genotype associates with higher SVR.

In G1 infected naive-patients eligible for antiviral therapy, the response after the "lead-in" phase and IL28B genotype are the most powerful predictors of response. In selective cases, when the benefit versus risk ratio is difficult to define IL28 may support the final decision.

Author details

R. Villani, F. Bellanti and G. Serviddio

C.U.R.E. (Centro Universitario per la Ricerca e la cura delle Epatopatie), Institute of Internal Medicine, Department of Medical and Surgical Sciences, University of Foggia, Italy

References

[1] Seeff, L. B, Hollinger, F. B, Alter, H. J, Wright, E. C, Cain, C. M, Buskell, Z. J, et al. Long-term mortality and morbidity of transfusion-associated non-A, non-B, and type C hepatitis: A National Heart, Lung, and Blood Institute collaborative study. Hepatology (2001). Feb;, 33(2), 455-463.

[2] Wasley, A, & Alter, M. J. Epidemiology of hepatitis C: geographic differences and temporal trends. Semin Liver Dis (2000). , 20(1), 1-16.

[3] Marcellin, P, Cheinquer, H, Curescu, M, Dusheiko, G. M, Ferenci, P, Horban, A, et al. High sustained virologic response rates in rapid virologic response patients in the large real-world PROPHESYS cohort confirm results from randomized clinical trials. Hepatology (2012). Jun 18.

[4] Bellanti, F, Vendemiale, G, Altomare, E, & Serviddio, G. The Impact of Interferon lambda 3 gene polymorfism on natural course and treatment of hepatitis C, Clinical and developmental Immunology. Clin Develop Immunol (2012).

[5] Hadziyannis, S. J, & Sette, H. Jr., Morgan TR, Balan V, Diago M, Marcellin P, et al. Peginterferon-alpha2a and ribavirin combination therapy in chronic hepatitis C: a randomized study of treatment duration and ribavirin dose. Ann Intern Med (2004). Mar 2;, 140(5), 346-355.

[6] Food and drug administrationChronic hepatitic C infection: developing direct acting antiviral agents for treatment. Guidance for Industry (2010).

[7] Dammacco, F, Sansonno, D, Piccoli, C, Racanelli, V, D'Amore, F. P, & Lauletta, G. The lymphoid system in hepatitis C virus infection: autoimmunity, mixed cryoglobulinemia, and Overt B-cell malignancy. Semin Liver Dis (2000). , 20(2), 143-157.

[8] Michielsen, P, Ho, E, & Francque, S. Does antiviral therapy reduce the risk of hepatocellular carcinoma in patients with chronic hepatitis C? Minerva Gastroenterol Dietol (2012). Mar;, 58(1), 65-79.

[9] Rosen, H. R. Clinical practice. Chronic hepatitis C infection. N Engl J Med (2011). Jun 23;, 364(25), 2429-2438.

[10] Tan, S. L. HCV genome and Life cycle. In: Horizon Bioscience, ed. Hepatitis C Viruses: Genomes and Molecular Biology. (2006).

[11] Brett, D, et al. Unravelling hepatitis C virus replication from genome to function. Nature (2005). , 436, 933-938.

[12] Barritt, A. S, & Fried, M. W. Maximizing opportunities and avoiding mistakes in triple therapy for hepatitis C virus. Gastroenterology (2012). May;, 142(6), 1314-1323.

[13] Hezode, C, Forestier, N, Dusheiko, G, Ferenci, P, Pol, S, Goeser, T, et al. Telaprevir and peginterferon with or without ribavirin for chronic HCV infection. N Engl J Med (2009). Apr 30;, 360(18), 1839-1850.

[14] Jacobson, I. M, Mchutchison, J. G, & Dusheiko, G. Di Bisceglie AM, Reddy KR, Bzowej NH, et al. Telaprevir for previously untreated chronic hepatitis C virus infection. N Engl J Med (2011). Jun 23;, 364(25), 2405-2416.

[15] Manns, M. P, Markova, A. A, Calle, S. B, & Cornberg, M. Phase III results of Boceprevir in treatment naive patients with chronic hepatitis C genotype 1. Liver Int (2012). Feb;32 Suppl , 1, 27-31.

[16] Marcellin, P, Reau, N, Ferenci, P, Hadziyannis, S, Messinger, D, Tatsch, F, et al. Refined prediction of week 12 response and SVR based on week 4 response in HCV genotype 1 patients treated with peginterferon alfa-2a (40KD) and ribavirin. J Hepatol (2012). Jun;, 56(6), 1276-1282.

[17] Zeuzem, S, Andreone, P, Pol, S, Lawitz, E, Diago, M, Roberts, S, et al. Telaprevir for retreatment of HCV infection. N Engl J Med (2011). Jun 23;, 364(25), 2417-2428.

[18] Bacon, B. R, Gordon, S. C, Lawitz, E, Marcellin, P, Vierling, J. M, Zeuzem, S, et al. Boceprevir for previously treated chronic HCV genotype 1 infection. N Engl J Med (2011). Mar 31;, 364(13), 1207-1217.

[19] Hezode, C. Boceprevir and telaprevir for the treatment of chronic hepatitis C: safety management in clinical practice. Liver Int (2012). Feb;32 Suppl , 1, 32-38.

[20] Barritt, A. S, & Fried, M. W. Maximizing opportunities and avoiding mistakes in triple therapy for hepatitis C virus. Gastroenterology (2012). May;, 142(6), 1314-1323.

[21] Kiser, J. J, Burton, J. R, Anderson, P. L, & Everson, G. T. Review and management of drug interactions with boceprevir and telaprevir. Hepatology (2012). May;, 55(5), 1620-1628.

[22] Cacoub, P, Bourliere, M, Lubbe, J, Dupin, N, Buggisch, P, Dusheiko, G, et al. Dermatological side effects of hepatitis C and its treatment: patient management in the era of direct-acting antivirals. J Hepatol (2012). Feb;, 56(2), 455-463.

[23] Incivek package. (2012).

[24] Bourliere, M, Khaloun, A, Wartelle-bladou, C, Oules, V, Portal, I, Benali, S, et al. Future treatment of patients with HCV cirrhosis. Liver Int (2012). Feb;32 Suppl , 1, 113-119.

[25] Poordad, F, & Mccone, J. Jr., Bacon BR, Bruno S, Manns MP, Sulkowski MS, et al. Boceprevir for untreated chronic HCV genotype 1 infection. N Engl J Med (2011). Mar 31;, 364(13), 1195-1206.

[26] Jacobson, I. M, Mchutchison, J. G, & Dusheiko, G. Di Bisceglie AM, Reddy KR, Bzowej NH, et al. Telaprevir for previously untreated chronic hepatitis C virus infection. N Engl J Med (2011). Jun 23;, 364(25), 2405-2416.

[27] Ahn, J. FS. Boceprevir versus telaprevir: a new era of directly acting antiviral therapy. Curr Hepatitis Rep (2012). , 11, 23-33.

Chapter 8

Management of HCV Infection in the Elderly

Antonino D. Romano and Gianluigi Vendemiale

Additional information is available at the end of the chapter

http://dx.doi.org/10.5772/55314

1. Introduction

During the past decade, the knowledge of clinical course and management of hepatitis C virus (HCV) infection has increased enormously, but there are few data on the course of the disease and its treatment in the elderly population (age > 60 years). According to its epidemiology, we are now facing HCV infection from the 20th century. We must take into account that in contrast to a younger population, old people who will develop Chronic C Hepatitis will be mainly women with genotype 1 and more severe fibrosis as clinical presentation pattern.

Thus, chronic infection is prevalent and may be severe in older population. Moreover, aging is an adverse factor for liver disease progression and treatment outcome.

2. Hepatitis C in elderly

Among younger people HCV infection declines [1]. HCV infections are common worldwide. It is estimated that about 3% of the world's population have HCV. There are about 4 million carriers in Europe alone. The prevalence of HCV in the general population varies widely across European countries, with ranges from 0.4% in Sweden, Germany and the Netherlands to over 20% in one region of Italy. According to an American National Health survey, the prevalence of HCV infection in elderly population varies from 0,9 % to 1.0% in subjects who were, respectively, in the age groups of 60-69 years and 70 years and more [2]. In general, countries in the southern part of Europe have a higher HCV prevalence compared to countries in the north or west of the EU. Italy in particular has a high general population prevalence of HCV, much higher than the country's estimated HBV prevalence [3]. In a large Italian study conducted among 1646 subjects, seroprevalence of HCV antibodies were found between 5% and 2% in patient ranging respectively, 58 to 67 years and 68 to 77 years [4].

Epidemiologic and phylogenetic assessments suggest this is caused by a period of increased iatrogenic transmission that took place around the 1960s due to the exposure to blood or blood products mainly deriving from using of non-disposable syringe [3, 5]. Subsequently, HCV infection is mainly due to risky behaviour, including tattooing, piercing, and sharing contaminated syringes among drug users. Finally, the rate of new infections decreased in the 1990s with the introduction of anti-HCV blood testing.

Hence, because chronic liver disease may develop many years after acute HCV infection, the past incidence of acute infections is a major determinant of the future burden of HCV-associated complications. Projections of the future prevalence of HCV-infected patients showed that, although the prevalence of HCV infection may be currently declining because of the decline in incidence in the 1990s, the number of persons infected for the next 20 years could increase substantially before peaking in 2015 [6].

If the incidence of new HCV infections does not increase in the future, persons born between 1940 and 1965 will be at highest lifetime risk of acquiring the infection [6]. To date, the true prevalence of HCV infection among elderly residing in nursing homes is largely underestimated; thus, data from a prospective study demonstrated a high seroprevalence (4,5%) in such population [7].

3. Natural history and age-related aspects

Given the statement above, we expect an increasing burden of decompensated cirrhosis and hepatocellular carcinoma (HCC) for the next two decades [1]. People who develop acute hepatitis C ignore this fact, so recognizing that disease onset is usually based on the potential circumstance of exposure. Progression into the chronic hepatitis is conventionally defined as persistence of increased levels of the aminotransferases for 6 months or, more appropriately, by the confirmation of HCV in the blood beyond that time period. The rate of persistence of HCV virus after an acute infection varies between several studies [8-11] but, in general, the HCV-RNA positivity is about 2,5-fold higher in old people than in person aged < 20 years [2]. Evolution from acute to chronic hepatitis mainly occurs in the absence of clinical manifestations that become clear only after the liver functions are significantly compromised. Decompensation of cirrhosis may occur soon or, more usually, several years after cirrhosis is recognized [12].

However it has been demonstrated in a cohort of patient with a known history of single blood transfusion in the past, that the period between the age at supposed infection and the development of cirrhosis was shorter if the infection was acquired at an older age [13]. The average period between the age of infection and the onset of cirrhosis was 33 years in patients who acquired the HCV infection at the age of 21 to 30, and was reported to decrease to 16 years in patients who acquired the infection after the age of 40 [13, 14]. Similar findings were demonstrated in a Japanese study: the mean time in developing cirrhosis in patients who had a blood transfusion at the age of 50 or older was reported to be 9.8 years, whereas were 23.6 years in patients who had a blood transfusion before 50 years [15]. The same study also demonstrated

http://dx.doi.org/10.5772/55314

that the mean time in developing HCC was 31.5 years against 14.7, depending from receiving blood transfusion respectively, before or after 50 years [15].

Moving from both findings, we can deduce that when HCV infection is acquired at an old age, it turns more rapidly into an advanced liver disease, including developing of HCC. Thus, it has been demonstrated that both patient with chronic HCV infection and HCV-related cirrhosis will develop an HCC in 1% to 2% of cases per year [3]. In contrast with younger people, acquiring HCV infection at older age means that complications of cirrhosis, such as ascitic decompensation, fibrosis and HCC, are often the initial manifestations of hepatitis.

Furthermore, the conjunction of old age at infection, long duration of infection, and aging, results in a higher risk of rapid fibrosis progression [16]. Liver fibrosis is more pronounced in elderly than in young people. A study conducted on 6865 patients older than 65 ys demonstrated a significant association with age and more intense fibrosis at liver biopsy, regardless of the duration of infection. Such results corroborate previous modelling, identifying the major role of aging as an accelerating factor for fibrosis progression after an age of 50 ys [16]. Authors raised several hypotheses to explain why HCV infection during aging is associated to enhanced liver fibrogenesis. Animal studies demonstrate in aging liver enhanced hepatic necrosis with a subsequent exacerbated free radical production and oxidative stress and enhanced susceptibility of senescent hepatic stellate cells to fibrogenetic stimuli.

Aging is undoubtedly associated with a higher susceptibility to environmental factors, reduction in the rate of hepatic blood flow and reduced mitochondrial capacity [17]. The association of Nonalcoholic fatty liver disease (NAFLD) and old age is also a factor that may contribute to the reduction of mitochondrial reserve, leading to liver deficiency in the presence of triggering events, such as HCV infection [18]. Taking into account the comorbidity and polypharmacology of the elderly patient, a good explanation might consider such conditions as contributor factors both in accelerating liver fibrosis and declining liver function.

Finally, it must also be outlined that immune system function declines with age [19, 20] and may be responsible for overreaction against HCV infection. With aging, virus T-cell immunomediated response is impaired due to both a decrease of T-cell function and the ability in recognizing new antigens [21]. Furthermore, memory subsets T-cell are reduced and cytokine profile is shifted from Th1 to Th2 leading to a pro-inflammatory response against the antigens [22, 23]. To sum up, such phenomena belong to the so-called immunosenescence that undoubtedly affects both the severity of liver inflammation and the efficacy of Interferon-based therapies.

4. HCV treatment in the elderly

The clinical course and management of liver disease in the elderly may differ in several aspects from those of younger adults. Comorbidities are the main culprits that render elderly patients more vulnerable to poor drug compliance. Therefore, physicians assign such patients to a lower priority treatment group, notwithstanding they need treatment since their infection advances rapidly. However, this issue is becoming of interest in countries such as Japan and Italy, where the average age of patients who receive antiviral therapy is about 10-15 years older than other countries [4, 24].

The efficacy and safety of treating elderly patients remain on debate. Mortality due to liver failure and HCC is expected to peak after 2030. One way to decrease mortality might be to extend access to current antiviral therapies and to develop more effective antiviral protocols. Despite the predictable epidemiological picture, a very limited number of studies have been dedicated to HCV treatment at old age and most of these have been conducted in the Japanese and Italian population.

Pegylated interferon (Peg-IFN) plus ribavirin combination therapy has led to a marked progress in the treatment of chronic C hepatitis [25-27]. However, in aged patients, the antiviral effect and tolerability to treatment are the main determinants in achieving results [25, 28]. As previously explained, with aging, development of both liver fibrosis and hepatocellular carcinoma has been shown to be faster. Accordingly the first goal of treatment of HCV-infected elderly patients should be HCV elimination [25]. Thus, a treatment strategy, aiming at the improvement of the antiviral efficacy, should be started as soon as possible.

4.1. Screening and initial assessment

According to the American Association for the Study of Liver Disease (AASLD), persons who received transfusion of blood or blood products before July 1992 should be checked for HCV infection [29]. Clinical statements about the opportunity of age-based HCV screening due to it's cost-effective are not clearly defined instead of current risk-based screening practices. However, it is conceivable that people older than 65 year with alterations in liver function might be screened for HCV infection even in the absence of known/suspected exposure to HCV.

The diagnosis of chronic hepatitis C is based on the detection of HCV infection (positive anti-HCV antibodies and HCV RNA) in a patient with signs of chronic hepatitis. Rarely, in immunosuppressed patients, anti-HCV antibodies are not detected and HCV RNA is present alone [30]. In order to determine the dose of Ribavirin and treatment decision, the HCV genotype [1-6] can be determined by various methods, including direct sequence analysis, reverse hybridization and genotype-specific real-time PCR [30]. Assessment of the severity of liver disease is recommended before beginning therapy. Liver biopsy, the gold standard and more recently, non-invasive methods, including serological markers and transient elastography (Fibroscan™, Echosens), have been extensively evaluated in patients with chronic HCV infection. The accuracy of non-invasive tests of liver fibrosis is good for identifying patients with mild fibrosis and cirrhosis, but is less reliable for discriminating moderate and severe fibrosis [31].

In any case, according to the geriatric medicine good practice, treatment decisions should be tailored on the basis of the severity of the liver disease and presence of comorbidity. Therapy is contraindicated for patients with decreased life expectancy (< 5 years) due to severe hypertension, heart failure, or coronary artery disease, poorly controlled diabetes or obstructive lung disease [29].

4.2. Individualised therapy for chronic hepatitis c and future perspectives

According to the European Association for the Study of the Liver (EASL), the primary goal of HCV therapy is to cure the infection, which results in eliminating detectable circulating HCV after cessation of treatment. Sustained virological response (SVR) is defined as an undetectable HCV RNA level (<50 IU/ml) 24 weeks after treatment withdrawal. SVR is generally associated with resolution of liver disease in patients without cirrhosis. The current standard of care (SOC) for the treatment of chronic hepatitis C and HCV-related compensated cirrhosis is the combination of a pegylated IFN and ribavirin.

On the basis of the evidence-based data produced by randomised clinical trials, current treatment guidelines recommend administering this therapy for 48 weeks to patients infected by HCV-1 (HCV-1a or HCV-1b) or HCV-4, and for 24 weeks to those infected by HCV-2 or HCV-3 [30, 32]. The same guidelines recommend stopping antiviral therapy after 12 weeks in HCV-1 or HCV-4 infected patients if their HCV-RNA levels have not decreased by at least 2 log 10 in comparison with baseline on the basis of solid evidence showing that such patients have little or no likelihood of achieving a sustained viral response (SVR) when treated for 48–52 weeks. No similar recommendations have been proposed for patients with HCV-2 and HCV-3 infection [30, 32].

Two pegylated IFN-α molecules can be used in combination with ribavirin (Peg-IFN α-2a or Peg-IFN α-2b). The pharmacokinetics of these compounds differs. A large-scale post-approval US trial comparing various schedules of administration of pegylated interferons with ribavirin in patients infected with HCV genotype 1 showed no significant difference between the tested strategies [30]. In contrast, two Italian trials in patients infected with HCV genotypes 1, 2, 3, and 4 showed some benefit, mostly in genotype 1 patients, in favor of pegylated IFN-α-2a in combination with ribavirin [30, 33, 34]. Although efficacy is still debated, there is currently no conclusive evidence that one pegylated IFN-α should be preferred to the other one as first-line therapy [30].

However, elderly patients with genotype 1 and high HCV loads have a lower SVR rate than younger patients because of higher dose reduction rates and discontinuation rates due to ribavirin-related anaemia and others side effects [35]. Reasons for discontinuation of therapy consisted mainly of anaemia, fatigue, anorexia and depression [35]. In clinical practice, < 15 % of adults treated with interferon and ribavirin discontinue therapy; however, discontinuation rates have been reported to be as high as 30 % and dose reductions are required in >70 % of individuals aged 60 years or older within the first 12 weeks of therapy [1, 36, 37].

The first-line treatment of chronic hepatitis C is based on the use of any of the two pegylated IFN-α available, administered weekly, subcutaneously, and daily oral ribavirin (evidence grading according to GRADE system: A1). Schedules and doses are the same as those recommended for younger patients (GRADE: B3). Pegylated IFN- α-2a should be used at a dose of 180 μg once per week, whereas pegylated IFN- α-2b should be used at a weight-based dose of

1.5 μg/kg per week. The ribavirin dose depends on the HCV genotype. Patients infected with HCV genotypes 1 and 4 should receive a weight-based dose of ribavirin: 15 mg/kg body weight per day. Patients infected with genotypes 2 and 3 can be treated with a flat dose of 800 mg of ribavirin daily, but those with a BMI beyond 25 or who have baseline factors suggesting low responsiveness (insulin resistance, metabolic syndrome, severe fibrosis or cirrhosis, older age) should receive a weight-based dose of ribavirin, similar to genotypes 1 and 4 [30].

Very recently, several progresses have been made in the development of new treatments, such as new specific inhibitors or direct antiviral agents that are active against hepatitis C virus. Many studies, mostly conducted in patients infected by HCV genotype 1 who were naïve to the treatment, showed an increase in the SVR rate of 27–31% [38]. Previous relapse patients show very high SVR rates of 75%–86%, while response rates are lower for partial responders (>2 log decline in HCV RNA at 12 weeks of prior therapy) [50–60%) and previous non-responder patients (33%, data only for telaprevir) [38-40]. Even though there are no data demonstrating the efficacy and toxicity of such drugs in elderly population, avoid antiviral therapy due to the advanced age is far from the good practice that should inspire clinicians. Using the antiviral agents in elderly patients undoubtedly requires special attention to co-morbid conditions and tolerance for potential side effects. In conclusion, waiting more clinical studies that will better characterize both the indicators of response and side-effects, we believe that antiviral therapy should be considered in elderly HCV patients with advanced fibrosis. It is important to take into account the life expectancy and co-morbidities in the decision of starting the treatment.

4.3. Treatment monitoring, side effects and stopping rules

According to the EASL Guidelines, patients treated with pegylated IFN-α and ribavirin should be seen at a minimum of weeks 4 and 12 after initiation of treatment, then, at a minimum of every 12 weeks until the end of treatment for both efficacy and side effects, and 24 weeks after the end of therapy to assess the SVR (GRADE: C2). Monitoring of treatment efficacy is based on repeated measurements of HCV RNA levels. A sensitive, accurate assay with a broad dynamic range of quantification, ideally a real-time PCR based assay, should be used. The same assay, ideally from the same laboratory, should be used in each patient to measure HCV RNA at different time points, in order to assure consistency of results [30].

Before considering typical side effect related to antiviral therapy some consideration are needed. Elderly have both lower haemoglobin levels and creatinine clearance. Because of a substantial amount of ribavirin is excreted by kidney, elderly with impaired renal function may be carefully followed-up. Ribavirin should not be administrated to patients with a creatinine clearance of < 50 mL/min. Ribavirin should be administered to elderly patients cautiously, starting at lower dosage, with renal function monitored and dosage adjustments made accordingly. Note that, in this population, the serum creatinine level might remain normal as the glomerular filtration rate decreases. Therefore, estimation of creatinine clearance should be done using equations incorporating age as a variable, such as the Cockroft-Gault equation [41].

Furthermore, if Elder have a history of neurological and psychiatric disorders, may be at risk of neurological side-effects of IFN, such as confusion, lethargy, cognitive changes and depression [41]. The most frequent side effect developing after 4–6 weeks of therapy due to the pegylated IFN-α injection, are a flu-like symptoms, which might be easily treated by paracetamol and paying attention to hydration. Severe fatigue, sleeping disorders, skin reactions, depression, irritability and dyspnoea may also be related to IFN therapy. Hematological and biochemical side effects of pegylated IFN-α and ribavirin include neutropenia, anaemia, thrombocytopenia, and ALT flares (Tab. 1). These parameters should be assessed at weeks 1, 2, and 4 of therapy and at 4–8 week intervals thereafter [30].

Frequency	IFN-α	Ribavirin
Common	Flu-like symptoms	Haemolysis, dyspepsia
Mild-Uncommon	Depression (mild to severe)	Anaemia
	Anorexia	Myocardial infarction
	Thyroid dysfunction	Angina
	Diabetes	Gastrointestinal symptoms
	Neuropathy	Cough and respiratory symptoms
	Leukocytopenia	Bacterial infections
	Thrombocytopenia	Bone marrow aplasia

Table 1. Most frequent side effect of anti viral therapy.

Most studies report a statistically significant higher ribavirin dose reduction and discontinuation rate in older patients. Based on these data, it would be very interesting knowing whether a close follow-up of the haemoglobin level could allow a better adjustment of the ribavirin dose. This strategy should decrease the discontinuation rate observed in the elderly population and improve the SVR rate. Such approach would take into account the reduction in renal function and the relative lower level of hemoglobin found in elderly, chronic HCV patients, making it possible to adapt the dose in relation to the clinical situation of each patient [42].

The pegylated IFN-α dose should be reduced in case of severe side effects, such as clinical symptoms of severe depression, and if the absolute neutrophil count falls below 750/mm^3, or the platelet count falls below 50,000/mm^3. In individual cases, clinicians may choose to maintain or reduce dosing in these situations but cautious monitoring is advised. When using pegylated IFN-α-2a, the dose can be reduced from 180 to 135 μg/week and then to 90 μg/week. When using pegylated IFN-α-2b, the dose can be reduced from 1.5 to 1.0 μg/kg/week and then to 0.5 μg/ kg/week. Pegylated IFN-α should be stopped in case of marked depression, if the neutrophil count falls below 500/mm^3 or the platelet count falls below 25.000/mm^3. If neutrophil or platelet counts go up, treatment can be re-started, but at a reduced pegylated IFN-α dose. If significant anaemia occurs (haemoglobin <10 g/dl), the dose of ribavirin should be adjusted downward by 200 mg at a time. Ribavirin administration should be stopped if the haemoglobin level falls below 8.5 g/dl. Furthermore, treatment should be promptly stopped in case of a hepatitis flare (ALT levels above 10 times normal, if not already present at the time of starting treatment) or if a severe bacterial infection occurs at any body site, regardless of neutrophil counts [30, 43, 44].

Recombinant erythropoietin (EPO) and erythropoiesis-stimulating agents (ESAs) can be administered when the haemoglobin level falls below 10 g/dl in order to avoid ribavirin dose reduction or discontinuation (GRADE: C2]. In selected population, such as neoplastic and diabetic patients, ESAs have been linked to increased risk of serious cardiovascular events, tumor progression, thrombosis, and death [45]. Nevertheless, using such drugs may help in managing ribavirin-associated anemia. It is conceivable that clinicians should attend to traditional thrombosis risk factors in patients prescribed ESAs.

Furthermore, it should be noted that there is no evidence that neutropenia during pegylated IFN-α and ribavirin therapy is associated with more frequent infection episodes (GRADE: C1), or that the use of granulocyte colony-stimulating factor (G-CSF) reduces the rate of infections and/or improves SVR rates (GRADE: B1) [30].

Moreover, patients with a history and/or signs of depression should be seen by a psychiatrist before therapy and should be treated with antidepressants (GRADE: C2) [30].

In studies using PEG-IFN plus ribavirin the SVR rate is always significantly lower in older patients than in younger [28, 35, 46]. However SVR depends mainly from HCV genotype. The study of Antonucci confirmed the effect of age in reducing SVR rate in patients infected by HCV 1 or 4 genotypes. Furthermore, such study demonstrated that hepatitis due to HCV genotypes 2 or 3 should be considered for treatment regardless patient's age suggesting that optimal treatment with peginterferon α plus ribavirin may be successfully and safely extended to elderly patients with no major contraindications which should be also included in clinical trials [28].

5. Risk of evolution

Several studies have clearly shown that risk of developing an HCC in those who are untreated is significantly higher than in IFN-treated groups hence, antiviral therapy is an effective way of reducing such risk and improving survival [47-49]. Interestingly, such observations are observed, both, from patients in whom SVR has been observed and a biochemical response obtained.

A retrospective study by Ikeda and colleagues considered the effect of antiviral therapy in a large cohort of elderly patients with HCV hepatitis. Stratifying patients according to their platelet count before therapy (high (> 150.000/mm^3), intermediate (100.000 – 149.000/mm^3) or low (< 100.000/mm^3), authors assessed survival and the risk of hepatocarcinogenesis. The study demonstrated that hepatocarcinogenesis was significantly and inversely correlated with platelet count, reflecting the degree of fibrosis. Interferon treatment for a subgroup of elderly patients with an intermediate or low platelet count conferred substantial advantages with regard to both hepatocarcinogenesis and survival [47, 50]. Furthermore, the study by Ikeda and colleagues demonstrates that platelet count can be used as a simple indicator of the risk of hepatitis progression. Imai and colleagues, using a conventional interferon-based regimen, found a significantly lower liver-related mortality rate in elderly patients when compared with their untreated counterparts [49].

6. Conclusion

There was no rigorous definition of old age and the upper limit for patient age allowed for interferon-based therapy. Moreover, several aspects should be taken into account; better stratifying elderly population might help physicians in managing HCV infection, regarding life expectancy, cost, side effects, and risks caused by interferon-based therapies (Table 2).

Managing chronic HCV infection in elderly
Identify and treat HCV patients before 60 years or as soon as possible
Carefully assess liver health and weigh the benefits-to-risk ratio of antiviral therapy
Treat HCV 2-3 patients more aggressively because of good response of treatment
Tailor the treatment to each patient
Manage side effect more aggressively

Table 2. Recommendation for managing HCV infection in elderly patients.

Furthermore, current guidelines endorse not to suspend antiviral therapy based exclusively on old age but suggest that special care should be paid to co-morbid conditions and tolerance for potential side effects [31]. Hence, treatment should be initiated under monitoring if there are no major contraindications or severe co-morbidities that would compromise the patient's life expectancy. Moreover, adverse effects typically resolve spontaneously within 2 – 3 weeks of discontinuing therapy.

In any case, treatment for the elderly should be individualized. In conclusion, a reduction in HCC incidence and liver-related deaths are the most desirable endpoints that could be achieved.

Author details

Antonino D. Romano and Gianluigi Vendemiale*

*Address all correspondence to: g.vendemiale@unifg.it

Institute of Geriatrics, Department of Medical and Surgical Sciences, University of Foggia, Foggia, Italy

References

[1] Carrion, A. F, & Martin, P. Viral hepatitis in the elderly. Am J Gastroenterol (2012).

[2] Alter, M. J, Kruszon-moran, D, Nainan, O. V, Mcquillan, G. M, Gao, F, Moyer, L. A, et al. The prevalence of hepatitis C virus infection in the United States, 1988 through 1994. N Engl J Med (1999).

[3] Mchutchison, J. G. Understanding hepatitis C. Am J Manag Care (2004). S, 21-29.

[4] Mazzeo, C, Azzaroli, F, Giovanelli, S, Dormi, A, Festi, D, Colecchia, A, et al. Ten year incidence of HCV infection in northern Italy and frequency of spontaneous viral clearance. Gut (2003).

[5] Chiaramonte, M, Stroffolini, T, Vian, A, Stazi, M. A, Floreani, A, Lorenzoni, U, et al. Rate of incidence of hepatocellular carcinoma in patients with compensated viral cirrhosis. Cancer (1999).

[6] Armstrong, G. L, Alter, M. J, Mcquillan, G. M, & Margolis, H. S. The past incidence of hepatitis C virus infection: implications for the future burden of chronic liver disease in the United States. Hepatology (2000).

[7] Chien, N. T, Dundoo, G, Horani, M. H, Osmack, P, & Morley, J. H. and Di Bisceglie AM. Seroprevalence of viral hepatitis in an older nursing home population. J Am Geriatr Soc (1999).

[8] Rodger, A. J, Roberts, S, Lanigan, A, Bowden, S, Brown, T, & Crofts, N. Assessment of long-term outcomes of community-acquired hepatitis C infection in a cohort with sera stored from 1971 to 1975. Hepatology (2000).

[9] Alter, M. J, Margolis, H. S, Krawczynski, K, Judson, F. N, Mares, A, Alexander, W. J, et al. The natural history of community-acquired hepatitis C in the United States. The Sentinel Counties Chronic non-A, non-B Hepatitis Study Team. N Engl J Med (1992).

[10] Alter, H. J, Conry-cantilena, C, Melpolder, J, Tan, D, Van Raden, M, Herion, D, et al. Hepatitis C in asymptomatic blood donors. Hepatology (1997). S-33S

[11] Yano, M, Kumada, H, Kage, M, Ikeda, K, Shimamatsu, K, Inoue, O, et al. The long-term pathological evolution of chronic hepatitis C. Hepatology (1996).

[12] Seeff, L. B. Natural history of chronic hepatitis C. Hepatology (2002). S, 35-46.

[13] Mindikoglu, A. L, & Miller, R. R. Hepatitis C in the elderly: epidemiology, natural history, and treatment. Clin Gastroenterol Hepatol (2009). quiz 124

[14] Minola, E, Prati, D, Suter, F, Maggiolo, F, Caprioli, F, Sonzogni, A, et al. Age at infection affects the long-term outcome of transfusion-associated chronic hepatitis C. Blood (2002).

[15] Tong, M. J, Farra, N. S, Reikes, A. R, & Co, R. L. Clinical outcomes after transfusion-associated hepatitis C. N Engl J Med (1995).

[16] Thabut, D. Le Calvez S, Thibault V, Massard J, Munteanu M, Di Martino V, et al. Hepatitis C in 6,865 patients 65 yr or older: a severe and neglected curable disease? Am J Gastroenterol (2006).

[17] Poynard, T, Ratziu, V, Charlotte, F, Goodman, Z, Mchutchison, J, & Albrecht, J. Rates and risk factors of liver fibrosis progression in patients with chronic hepatitis c. J Hepatol (2001).

[18] Serviddio, G, Bellanti, F, Tamborra, R, Rollo, T, Capitanio, N, Romano, A. D, et al. Uncoupling protein-2 (UCP2) induces mitochondrial proton leak and increases susceptibility of non-alcoholic steatohepatitis (NASH) liver to ischaemia-reperfusion injury. Gut (2008).

[19] Solana, R, & Pawelec, G. Molecular and cellular basis of immunosenescence. Mech Ageing Dev (1998).

[20] Linton, P. J, & Dorshkind, K. Age-related changes in lymphocyte development and function. Nat Immunol (2004).

[21] Pawelec, G, Barnett, Y, Forsey, R, Frasca, D, Globerson, A, Mcleod, J, et al. T cells and aging, January 2002 update. Front Biosci (2002). d, 1056-1183.

[22] Zanni, F, Vescovini, R, Biasini, C, Fagnoni, F, Zanlari, L, Telera, A, et al. Marked increase with age of type 1 cytokines within memory and effector/cytotoxic CD8+ T cells in humans: a contribution to understand the relationship between inflammation and immunosenescence. Exp Gerontol (2003).

[23] Ershler, W. B, & Keller, E. T. Age-associated increased interleukin-6 gene expression, late-life diseases, and frailty. Annu Rev Med (2000).

[24] Iwasaki, Y, Takaguchi, K, Ikeda, H, Makino, Y, Araki, Y, Ando, M, et al. Risk factors for hepatocellular carcinoma in Hepatitis C patients with sustained virologic response to interferon therapy. Liver Int (2004).

[25] Oze, T, Hiramatsu, N, Yakushijin, T, Mochizuki, K, Oshita, M, Hagiwara, H, et al. Indications and limitations for aged patients with chronic hepatitis C in pegylated interferon alfa-2b plus ribavirin combination therapy. J Hepatol (2011).

[26] Ghany, M. G, Strader, D. B, Thomas, D. L, & Seeff, L. B. and American Association for the Study of Liver D. Diagnosis, management, and treatment of hepatitis C: an update. Hepatology (2009).

[27] Manns, M. P, Mchutchison, J. G, Gordon, S. C, Rustgi, V. K, Shiffman, M, Reindollar, R, et al. Peginterferon alfa-2b plus ribavirin compared with interferon alfa-2b plus ribavirin for initial treatment of chronic hepatitis C: a randomised trial. Lancet (2001).

[28] Antonucci, G, Longo, M. A, Angeletti, C, Vairo, F, Oliva, A, Comandini, U. V, et al. The effect of age on response to therapy with peginterferon alpha plus ribavirin in a

cohort of patients with chronic HCV hepatitis including subjects older than 65 yr. Am J Gastroenterol (2007).

[29] Strader, D. B, Wright, T, Thomas, D. L, & Seeff, L. B. and American Association for the Study of Liver D. Diagnosis, management, and treatment of hepatitis C. Hepatology (2004).

[30] European Association for the Study of the LEASL Clinical Practice Guidelines: management of hepatitis C virus infection. J Hepatol (2011).

[31] European Association of the Study of the LEuropean Association of the Study of the Liver hepatitis C virus clinical practice guidelines. Liver Int (2012). Suppl , 1, 2-8.

[32] Italian Association for the Study of the LItalian Society of Infectious TD, and Italian Society for the Study of Sexually Transmitted D. Practice guidelines for the treatment of hepatitis C: recommendations from an AISF/SIMIT/SIMAST Expert Opinion Meeting. Dig Liver Dis (2010).

[33] Ascione, A, De Luca, M, Tartaglione, M. T, & Lampasi, F. Di Costanzo GG, Lanza AG, et al. Peginterferon alfa-2a plus ribavirin is more effective than peginterferon alfa-2b plus ribavirin for treating chronic hepatitis C virus infection. Gastroenterology (2010).

[34] Rumi, M. G, Aghemo, A, Prati, G. M, Ambrosio, D, Donato, R, & Soffredini, M. F. R. et al. Randomized study of peginterferon-alpha2a plus ribavirin vs peginterferon-alpha2b plus ribavirin in chronic hepatitis C. Gastroenterology (2010).

[35] Honda, T, Katano, Y, Shimizu, J, Ishizu, Y, Doizaki, M, Hayashi, K, et al. Efficacy of peginterferon-alpha-2b plus ribavirin in patients aged 65 years and older with chronic hepatitis C. Liver Int (2010).

[36] Iwasaki, Y, Ikeda, H, Araki, Y, Osawa, T, Kita, K, Ando, M, et al. Limitation of combination therapy of interferon and ribavirin for older patients with chronic hepatitis C. Hepatology (2006).

[37] Tsui, J. I, Currie, S, Shen, H, Bini, E. J, Brau, N, Wright, T. L, et al. Treatment eligibility and outcomes in elderly patients with chronic hepatitis C: results from the VA HCV-001 Study. Dig Dis Sci (2008).

[38] Flisiak, R, & Parfieniuk, A. Investigational drugs for hepatitis C. Expert Opin Investig Drugs (2010).

[39] Poordad, F, & Mccone, J. Jr., Bacon BR, Bruno S, Manns MP, Sulkowski MS, et al. Boceprevir for untreated chronic HCV genotype 1 infection. N Engl J Med (2011).

[40] Jacobson, I. M, Mchutchison, J. G, & Dusheiko, G. Di Bisceglie AM, Reddy KR, Bzowej NH, et al. Telaprevir for previously untreated chronic hepatitis C virus infection. N Engl J Med (2011).

[41] Marcus, E. L, & Tur-kaspa, R. Viral hepatitis in older adults. J Am Geriatr Soc (1997).

[42] Horsmans, Y. Treatment of chronic hepatitis C in elderly patients. Expert Opin Pharmacother (2010).

[43] Hadziyannis, S. J, & Sette, H. Jr., Morgan TR, Balan V, Diago M, Marcellin P, et al. Peginterferon-alpha2a and ribavirin combination therapy in chronic hepatitis C: a randomized study of treatment duration and ribavirin dose. Ann Intern Med (2004).

[44] Fried, M. W, Shiffman, M. L, Reddy, K. R, Smith, C, Marinos, G, Goncales, F. L, et al. Peginterferon alfa-2a plus ribavirin for chronic hepatitis C virus infection. N Engl J Med (2002).

[45] Sulkowski, M. S, Shiffman, M. L, Afdhal, N. H, Reddy, K. R, Mccone, J, Lee, W. M, et al. Hepatitis C virus treatment-related anemia is associated with higher sustained virologic response rate. Gastroenterology (2010). e1601

[46] Floreani, A, Minola, E, Carderi, I, Ferrara, F, Rizzotto, E. R, & Baldo, V. Are elderly patients poor candidates for pegylated interferon plus ribavirin in the treatment of chronic hepatitis C? J Am Geriatr Soc (2006).

[47] Ikeda, K, Arase, Y, Kawamura, Y, Yatsuji, H, Sezaki, H, Hosaka, T, et al. Necessities of interferon therapy in elderly patients with chronic hepatitis C. Am J Med (2009).

[48] Arase, Y, Ikeda, K, Suzuki, F, Suzuki, Y, Saitoh, S, Kobayashi, M, et al. Long-term outcome after interferon therapy in elderly patients with chronic hepatitis C. Intervirology (2007).

[49] Imai, Y, Kasahara, A, Tanaka, H, Okanoue, T, Hiramatsu, N, Tsubouchi, H, et al. Interferon therapy for aged patients with chronic hepatitis C: improved survival in patients exhibiting a biochemical response. J Gastroenterol (2004).

[50] Floreani, A. Hepatitis C: Should antiviral therapy be offered to elderly patients? Nat Rev Gastroenterol Hepatol (2009).

Chapter 9

Hepatitis E

Scotto Gaetano and Fazio Vicenzina

Additional information is available at the end of the chapter

http://dx.doi.org/10.5772/55568

1. Introduction

Hepatitis E virus (HEV) represents the major aetiological agent of enteric non-A hepatitis and it is the only member of a new virus, *Hepevirus*, belonging to the family of *Hepeviridae* [1-2]. HEV is often responsible of acute clinical hepatitis in developing world, specifically the Indian subcontinent and Southeast Asia, the Middle East and North Africa [3-5], where it is a common cause of sporadic and epidemic waterborne outbreaks and determines an important rate of morbidity and mortality, especially in pregnant women. In these countries, where the disease is endemic, antibodies HEV-IgG, which are indicative of past infections, have been detected in 5-60% of the general population. Once thought as an infection confined to developing countries, it is now recognized as a disease with a widespread geographic distribution. In industrialized countries this infection occurs sporadically; most cases are diagnosed in individuals who travel to regions where HEV is endemic [6], even though a growing number of infections have been identified also in patients with no history of recent travels to endemic countries [7-8]. However, in the last years, it has been shown that the host range, geographical distribution and ways of transmission of HEV and clinical features of this infection are much broader than it was previously believed.

2. The history

The existence of a different enteric transmitted hepatitis virus was suspected from epidemiological evidences already many years before the discovery of HEV. However, HEV Infection was first documented in 1955 during an outbreak in New Delhi and only two decades later some researchers have demonstrated the existence of a new non-A virus [3]. During the winter of 1955-56, a significant monsoon flooding in New Delhi caused the Jamuna River to change its direction. The waters ran through the city sewage and then into uptake pipes feeding a treatment plant that supplied water to most of New Delhi. The treatment facility broke down and contaminated water ran through the city's water supply. Over 30,000 cases of hepatitis were reported, representing 2.3% of the population residing in the affected areas. The epidemic peak was reached in 2 weeks and was reduced in about 7 weeks. The incidence of HEV infection is highest in young adults. Acute hepatitis is preceded by a brief prodromal period. The disease generally had a self-limited course, but pregnant women often had *fulminant hepatic failure* (FHF) with a high mortality rate [2]. It has been hypothesized this epidemic so great could be caused by the same old enteric hepatitis, as hepatitis A virus (HAV), overwhelming any previous immunity of individuals to this infection [3, 9-10]. In the early 1970s, with electron microscopy, were identified the hepatitis A virus and, the hepatitis B virus [11]. This led to the discovery of the serological tests for hepatitis A and B and to the recognition that many cases of post-transfusion hepatitis were not related to either of these agents; such cases were provisionally labeled as non-A, non-B post-transfusion hepatitis [3,5]. During an outbreak of acute viral hepatitis in the Kashmir Valley, India, in 1980, Khuroo was the first to suspect an enterically transmitted non-A, non-B hepatitis virus [12]. Among 16,620 inhabitants of the affected areas, there were 275 clinical cases; most of them were 11–40 years old, and occurred in villages with a common water source. Of the patients, 12 (4.4%) had fulminant hepatic failure, and 10 died; the outbreak was characterized by a high disease attack rate and mortality among pregnant women. With the availability of serological tests for hepatitis A and B, 31 patients were tested for these viruses; only one presented immunoglobulin M (IgM) anti-HAV antibodies and none had hepatitis B surface antigen (HBsAg); in fact, most subjects had evidence of prior immunity against HAV infection (IgG) [12]. After some months, *Wong et al* reported the results of retrospective serological testing on sample sera which had been collected and stored from the 1955–56 hepatitis outbreak in New Delhi; they proved that the outbreak victims at the time had not been infected with hepatitis A or B. Specimens from none of the outbreaks showed evidence of acute hepatitis A and only a few had markers of acute hepatitis B [3]. These findings suggested the existence of a water-transmissible agent distinct from HAV and HBV, and clearly a new virus was responsible for the outbreak. The name "enterically transmitted non-A, non-B hepatitis virus" was coined for this virus.

During the Soviet occupation of Afghanistan in the 1980s, after an outbreak of unexplained hepatitis at a military camp, a pooled aqueous faecal extract of faecal matter from nine patients with epidemic non-A, non-B hepatitis, was ingested by a member of the research team (*Dr. Balayan*), who was immune to HAV. The volunteer developed, on day 36, typical acute hepatitis, which lasted for about 3 weeks. Stool specimens were collected on days 28–45 and showed 27- to 30-nm spherical virus-like particles (VLPs); these VLPs presented aggregation with convalescent sera of patients with enteric non-A, non-B hepatitis, but not with those from patients with HAV virus hepatitis, hepatitis B or post transfusion non-A, non-B hepatitis. The volunteer showed seroconversion against VLPs, but no detectable HBsAg or boosting of anti-HAV antibodies [13].

About ten years after the discovery of a new virus, *Reyes et al.* isolated, from bile obtained from an experimentally-infected animal, a nucleic acid clone representing a part of its genome. They also identified similar genomic sequences in clinical specimens obtained from

http://dx.doi.org/10.5772/55568

several geographical regions at different time-points; the agent was christened as hepatitis E virus (HEV) [14]

The appearance of IgM anti- HEV antibodies was associated with the beginning of HEV virus hepatitis in most patients, while the IgG anti-HEV are detected shortly thereafter. The new-found molecular and serological tests for the diagnosis of HEV infection are actually used in different geographical areas to determine the frequency of HEV infection in patients with epidemic and sporadic hepatitis, and in different population groups. [15]

3. The virus

HEV is the single virus that belongs to the genus *Hepevirus* in the *Hepeviridae* family [1,2]. It can infect human and animal beings, as domestic pigs, wild boars, deer, rodents [2, 16-17]. The HEV virions are small, icosahedral, non-enveloped, spherical particles of 27-34 nm, with a single capsid protein and a linear, positive-sense RNA genome of approximately 7.2 kb [18]. The HEV genome contains three open reading frames (ORF). ORF1 non-structural polyprotein encodes a protein of 1693 amino acids, and contains domains with methyl-transferase, putative papain-like cysteine protease, RNA helicase, and RNA-dependent RNA polymerase activities, which are important for viral replication [19-20]. The ORF2 encodes the viral capsid protein of 660 amino acids protein, consists of three linear domains and is responsible for virion assembly, interaction with target cells, and immunogenicity [21-22]. ORF3, which overlaps with ORF2 and encodes a small protein of 114 amino acids, is required for HEV replication in the host; moreover, it has pleiotropic effects on host cell pathways and plays a role in viral egress from infected cells [23-24]. In HEV capsid organisation, three domains have been defined: the shell domain (S; amino acids 129–319), the middle domain (M; amino acids 320–455), and the protruding domain (P; amino acids 456–606). These studies placed the neutralising epitope(s) in the P domain of ORF2 [25-26]. At present, are recognized four different HEV genotypes, whose genotype 1-2 are found in human species [19, 27], genotype 1 and 2 strains are transmitted via contaminated water in developing countries, HEV1 occurs mainly in Asia [28-29], and HEV2 in Africa [30] and Mexico [31]. Genotypes 3 and 4 have a broader host range and are also *zoonotic* viruses; in fact they infect human beings, pigs, and other mammalian species and are responsible for sporadic cases of autochthonous hepatitis E in both developing and developed countries [2,16]. Interspecies transmission has been demonstrated for HEV genotypes 3 and 4. HEV3 has a worldwide distribution [32-33]; by contrast, HEV4 mostly occurs in southeast Asia [28-29], but has recently been isolated also in European pigs [33]. On the basis of full-length genome-sequence analyses, HEV genotypes have recently been characterized in rats in Germany [34], wild boars in Japan [35], and farmed rabbits in China [36]. HEV1 can be classified into five sub-genotypes, HEV2 into two, HEV3 into three, and HEV4 into seven. *Phylogenetic analyses show that HEV sub-genotypes, circulating in human beings and animals in the same area are closely related, supporting zoonotic transmission* [27].

The cellular receptor and the mode of entry of HEV into the cell are not known, but heparin sulphate proteoglycans are required for HEV attachment and infection of target cells [37].

It appears that HEV is not directly cytopathic, and liver injury results from the host immune response; this response is marked by an initial increase in anti-HEV immunoglobulin (Ig)M, followed closely by an IgG response; whereas IgM titers wane off in 4- 6 months, IgG persists for longer periods. [38]. Viremia begins 1-2 weeks before and last 2-4 weeks after the onset of symptoms. In experimentally infected nonhuman primates, HEV RNA is observed in serum, bile, and faeces before the elevation of aminotransferases [28]. The HEV antigens first appear in hepatocytes about 7 days post-infection, followed by rapid spread to 70%-90% of hepatocytes [39].

4. The epidemiology

HEV infection can cause both epidemic and acute sporadic hepatitis in developing world. However, the true incidence of this infection is unknown because it is most often a self-limited hepatitis, except for HEV infection during in pregnancy characterized by high mortality, and often for the lack of available serological tests in these areas of the world. Seroprevalence studies have led to establish that HEV can infect about one-third of worldwide population [40].

Anti-HEV IgG antibodies represent evidence of past exposure to HEV; furthermore, the duration of persistence of circulating IgG anti-HEV antibodies remains unclear, varying from some months to several years after acute disease, though its titers declined over time. Anti-HEV antibodies have been found worldwide also in healthy subjects; prevalence rates are higher in developing countries where HEV hepatitis is common, than in countries where clinical cases due to hepatitis E are sporadic [32].

The mode of transmission or risk factors for sporadic HEV transmission is not yet understood. HEV infection is mainly transmitted through contaminated water, perhaps during outbreaks [41], that can last from a few-week to prolonged time, [42]. Other routes of transmission are possible: food-borne, zoonotic, infected-blood products, needle sharing, and vertical (materno-fetal) transmission [9, 11]. Person-to-person spread occurs in only 0.7% to 2.2% of cases compared to 50% to 75% for hepatitis A; even when multiple cases occur in a family, the time interval between cases is usually short, indicating a shared primary water-borne infection rather than person-to-person spread [43-44]. However, person-to person transmission could become efficient perhaps in a peak of HEV infection and, in addition, promiscuity and poor hygienic practices could contribute to HEV infection in households [45]. It is not yet clear if protracted viremia or prolonged fecal shedding of HEV, with endless pollution of sewage, could be the reservoir of HEV, responsible for maintaining the infection in hyperendemic populations. Persons affected with subclinical infection could contribute to maintain HEV infection through fecal dissemination of the virus contaminating water supplies [28,46].

The existence of an animal reservoir in hyper-endemic regions is suggested by the high prevalence of anti-HEV antibodies in several animal species, and by the isolation of HEV genomic sequences from pigs in these regions. above all in genotype 4 [47-48]. On the contrary, genotype 1 has never been isolated from pigs and other domestic and wild animals [49] and so it is not responsible of zoonotic transmission. The way of transmission of HEV infection not always can be identified, especially in low-endemic regions and sporadic cases in highly endemic areas.

In epidemics, the incubation period varied from 2 to 10 (with an average of 6-7) weeks. Two distinct epidemiological patterns have been observed: endemic and non-endemic, characterized by different routes of transmission and the disease characteristics [4,32].

In high-endemic areas, a large proportion of HEV infections manifest itself as acute sporadic hepatitis in all age groups; the clinical characteristics of these patients are similar to those of epidemic hepatitis E. Main routes of transmission might be the contamination of water or food and this is confirmed by the identification of the HEV genomic sequences in sewage from high-endemic regions [34]. Route of transmission is unclear in such patients, but is likely to be through contamination of water or food; identification of the HEV genomic sequences in sewage from high-endemic regions around the year suggests nearly ubiquitous circulation of HEV in these populations; this could act as a reservoir of infection responsible for sporadic cases [34].

4.1. Epidemiology of hepatitis E in developing countries

The first, retrospectively identified outbreak of hepatitis E caused about 30,000 cases in India in 1955–56 [3]. Other large outbreaks of this disease, subsequently, have been reported frequently in the Indian subcontinent [12], China [5], Southeast and Central Asia [52], the Middle East, and northern and western parts of Africa (Somalia, Uganda) [53-54], affecting up from several hundred to several thousand people. Two small outbreaks occurred in North America (Mexico) during 1986–1987, but none has been reported thereafter [31]. Epidemics of hepatitis E occur periodically throughout the developing world, and are mainly caused by HEV genotype 1 in Asia and HEV genotype 2 in Africa [53] and Mexico [31]. Most infections are due to HEV1 but also to HEV4, although HEV3 has recently been isolated in endemic regions. In the last years, hepatitis E in China has occurred mainly as sporadic cases and occasional food-borne outbreaks. The predominant circulating genotype is HEV4, with only occasional HEV1 cases; this might reflect improvements in water supply and in the sanitary infrastructure in China over the past few decades, allowing zoonotically transmitted HEV4 to predominate in the human population [27]. Sporadic HEV4 cases are more common in elderly men.

Seroprevalence studies conducted in various endemic countries have demonstrated that the rate of HEV seropositivity seldom exceeds 40% of population, and in some countries, such as India, Algeria, and in some parts of China, there is a higher prevalence of anti-HEV [50]. A study in rural areas of southern China demonstrated a prevalence of anti-HEV that ranged from 25% to 63%, particularly in young males [51]. Moreover, a higher incidence of hepatitis E outbreaks occurs during pregnancy, especially, greater incidence is often associated with prematurity, low birth weight and a major risk of perinatal mortality.

Instead, children have lower HEV infection rates, probably because in children there are frequently asymptomatic infections.

In fact in the children, asymptomatic infections are usually more frequent by two to four times in waterborne outbreaks and sporadic cases.

Mortality rates of HEV infection in epidemics range from 0.2% to 4.0% and they are higher in infants under 2 years of age and in pregnant women (10% to 25% of cases).

Mortality in pregnancy occurs largely in the third trimester, and is caused by *fulminant hepatic failure* and obstetric complications such as eclampsia or hemorrhage. [55] Moreover, pregnant cases more often (22.2%) developed FHF than the cases who were non-pregnant women (0%) or men (2.8%). These associations were first noted during the Kashmir and the Delhi outbreaks. The exact cause of this specific predilection for occurrence of the worsening of the disease among pregnant women remains unknown; immunological or hormonal factors have been suspected [56].

4.2. Epidemiology of hepatitis E in developed countries

Previous seroprevalence studies in industrialized countries reported the discovery of locally-acquired cases of HEV hepatitis, determining a substantial change in epidemiological pattern of this infection in regions where HEV is infrequent. Variable rates of anti-HEV antibodies were observed in healthy populations: 2.5% in the USA [57] and 0.4-3% in Western Europe, mainly in Mediterranean European Countries [58-60] (Italy, Spain, France and Greece), where there is a high prevalence of immigrants. However also in other developed countries (Japan, Denmark), high anti-HEV antibodies prevalence (up to above 20%) have been reported; these appear to be markedly higher than those expected from the low rate of hepatitis E disease diagnosed in these areas [61-62]. In the last years, isolated cases or small case series related to autochthonous (locally-acquired) acute hepatitis E have been described in the US, Europe, and in developed countries of Asia-Pacific (Japan, Taiwan, Hong Kong, Australia)). In a recent Italian long-term prospective study, the prevalence of acute hepatitis E was 20.6% in a cohort of 651 patients with acute viral non A-non C hepatitis [69]. A prospective study (unpublished data) was conducted by our group in Southern Italy, in 2010-2011, to evaluate the seropreva-lence of HEV in a cohort of 1,217 subjects, 412(34%) of whom were immigrants who had recently arrived in Italy, and 805 were from four different Italian populations (blood donors, general population, HIV-positive patients, haemodialysis patients). A total of 107 (8.8%) of the 1,217 serum samples examined were reactive to anti-HEV IgG and confirmed by Western Blot. The prevalence in immigrants was 19.7%, in Italians was 3.9% (blood donors 1.3%, general population 2.7%, HIV-positive patients 2.0%, haemodialysis patients 9.6%). In our study, we found 38/107 (35.5%) patients with anti-HEV IgM positive. Most of them (34 cases) were immigrants. Several of these cases can be traced to traveling to developing countries and/or immigration, but others occurred among autochthonous individuals reporting no trips abroad or at-risk contacts (travelers and/or immigrants). While the HEV genotypes in immigrant and/or travelers are mainly 1-2, autochthonous acute hepatitis E was determined by genotypes 3-4 [63].The reason for this high anti-HEV seroprevalence is unclair, and might reflect past subclinical HEV infection due to travel in endemic countries or a cohort effect due to recent past HEV infections imported by immigrants. Sporadic cases of the infection are owed to faecal contamination of drinking water. Autochthonous HEV, in industrialized countries, is due mainly exposure to animals; people with occupational exposure to swine or wild animals in these regions often show a high seroprevalence of anti-HEV antibodies. The genotypes (3-4) also widely circulate in swine populations; these findings reinforce that some cases of autochthonous hepatitis E in developed countries could strengthen zoonotic transmission. Inadequately-cooked deer meat could represent a possible source of HEV infection, as it has been reported in some Japanese cases. The genomic sequences of HEV isolated from these cases were identical to those from the left-over frozen meat, establishing food-borne transmission. A proportion of commercial packets of pig liver sold in Japanese and US grocery stores have been shown to contain genotype 3 or 4 HEV [64]. Contaminated shellfish has also been proposed as a potential vehicle in developed countries. To-day this finding suggests that at least some autochthonous cases are related to consumption of contaminated foods, but the extent of zoonotic transmission is not fully understood. Other routes of transmission, in developed countries, were described:

1. Higher rates of hepatitis E antibodies were found in drug users in Denmark [62] and Sweden [65]: this might indicate parenteral transmission by needle sharing within the group.

2. Furthermore, HEV was found in sewage samples collected in some western countries (France, Spain, USA), with evidence of autochthonous HEV infection in these areas; in southwest France, HEV is hyper-endemic [66].

3. Moreover, several studies unexpectedly showed a high prevalence of antibodies to HEV in haemodialysis patients, and blood donors in developed countries; the mode of exposure and clinical significance of these infections are not well understood [67-68].

Acute HEV-3 and HEV-4 infections in developed countries are usually self-limiting illnesses that last 4–6 weeks; symptomatic HEV infection is much more common in middle-aged and elderly men. The high pregnancy-associated mortality in HEV-1 has not been reported with HEV-3 or HEV-4. In developed countries the mortality rates can to be up to 10%, especially in individuals with several comorbidities in symptomatic cases of HEV infection [8, 33]. Excessive alcohol consumption could contribute to the onset of HEV infection, because these individuals are characterized by major risk of hepatic steatosis or hepatic fibrosis and so by a more severe host response to HEV infection [70-71].

4.3. Epidemiology in travelers

The incidence of HEV in travelers is not well known, but it is very low, on the order of *1 case per 1 million travelers* [6]. This supports the hypothesis that the fecal–oral route is the most important transmission route of HEV infection and it is highly endemic in several countries, particularly the Indian subcontinent, which is a popular travel destination of over 4 million people traveling annually, as reported by World Tourism Organization, and Southeast Asia. Despite the low number of reported HEV cases in travelers, many cases of HEV in travelers are underdiagnosed, perhaps because of the lack of awareness of HEV infection among physicians and the lack of commercial diagnostic tools preventing the confirmation of HEV infection diagnosis in many industrialized countries. Moreover, travelers are not immune to the disease. A thorough review of the literature from 1989 to 1999 identified 161 reported cases of acute HEV in travelers and military personnel coming mainly from the Indian subcontinent and Southeast Asia [6]. Recent Geo-Sentinel surveillance data from returning travelers during the period 1999-2005 report 33 cases of acute HEV [72]; almost all of these cases were in travelers visiting the Indian subcontinent. Between 1994 and 2003, there were 30 cases of documented Hepatitis E among travelers, expatriates, and Peace Corps volunteers in Nepal who asked for medical treatment at three local clinics in Kathmandu (unpublished data). During a world cruise in 2008, seven UK citizens contracted acute HEV infection during their 12-week voyage, which included visiting several Asian port cities [73]. In a recent long-term prospective study in Italy, a total of 134 out of 651 patients tested had acute hepatitis E, and 109 (81.3%) of them developed hepatitis E traveling to endemic areas [69].

Seroconversion studies among travelers might help to sustain the evidence of HEV risk to travelers from a low to a highly endemic region of the world, but only few data of HEV antibody seroconversion in travelers have been reported. A prospective seroconversion study was conducted in 1993 among 356 American short-term travelers to developing countries: of the 236 initially seronegative patients, 4 (1.7%) seroconverted to HEV IgG positive after 6 months; all were asymptomatic [74]. A 1995 retrospective study of 328 North American missionaries serving in Africa, Asia, and Central and South America between 1967 and 1984 showed no seroconversion [75]. Another seroconversion study was conducted in Nepal from June 1997 to December 1998 and it showed the seroprevalence of anti-HEV among foreigners living in Nepal and it has determined seroconversion rates over a 12-month period. This study conclused that among the 373 persons seronegative for anti-HEV, there was one case of acute HEV infection, for a seroconversion rate of 0.3%; there were no cases of asymptomatic seroconversion.

According to these seroconversion studies, a HEV infection is not widespread among travelers [76]. The acute HEV infection associated with travel is observed mainly in patients of mean age 30 (range 6–65) and 52% female. Most of these individuals (53/69-77%) had traveled to the Indian subcontinent (India, Nepal, Pakistan, and Sri Lanka). The mean duration of travel was about 3 months, but there was a report of HEV infection after only 1 day in an endemic area (range 1 day to 12 months) [77].

5. Clinical course

After the infection there is an incubation period of 15 to 60 days, with an average of 40 days, then the infected patients develop symptoms and clinical signs similar to those of other forms of acute viral hepatitis. The most prominent feature is jaundice accompanied by malaise, anorexia, abdominal pain, nausea, vomiting, fever and hepatomegaly; diarrhea, pruritus, arthralgia and rash can also be present. Serum levels of liver enzymes (AST-ALT) can be elevated and there can be bilirubinemia. These markers usually return to normal values within 6 weeks of onset. Hepatitis E is typically a self-limited disease, lasting 1–4 weeks; most patients recover completely within a few months. However, in about half the cases, HEV infection may occur with protracted coagulopathy and cholestasis in more than half of patients [78].

Liver histology in a study of eleven patients with sporadic acute hepatitis E showed acute lesions in all cases: necro-inflammatory activity and confluent necrosis in nine and five samples, respectively. Moreover, there were also siderosis and cholestasis in eleven and nine patients, respectively [79]. The clinical significance of the genotypes in determining the severity of the diseases is still unknown; a study from Japan compared the clinical features of patients infected with genotypes 3 and 4 and showed that genotype 4 tends to have more severe clinical manifestations than genotype 3 with a significantly higher ALT peak levels and a lower trough prothrombin time [80]. The severity of infections can range from subclinical disease to fulminant hepatitis. Overall mortality ranges from 0.1% to 4%. The mortality rate among pregnant women infected with HEV during their third trimester is as high as 25%. Pathogenetic events leading to increased mortality after HEV infection during pregnancy are not fully understood; endotoxin-mediated hepatocyte injury and elevated T-helper type 2 responses may have some role [81].

Fulminant hepatitis is often associated with patients with chronic liver disease; some patients, however, progress to fulminant hepatitis without any apparent precipitating factors [82]. In 2004 in Dhaka, 23 patients, without other diseases, presented fulminant hepatitis, more than half (13/23) of those were HEV IgM positive; the mortality rate was 87% [83].

The seroepidemiology of hepatitis E suggests a long-term post-infection immunity against subsequent HEV infections during epidemics of the diseases, but lifelong immunity has not been confirmed.

5.1. Clinical course in developing countries

In these regions the disease usually lasts for a few weeks and improves spontaneously; only a few patients have a prolonged illness with cholestatic manifestations, though the outcome is usually good. Some patients, as above said, have a particularly severe illness, presenting as FHF, particularly common in pregnant women. During hepatitis E outbreaks, some patients presented anicteric hepatitis (elevated liver enzymes with normal serum bilirubin) and HEV infection (HEV viremia and seroconversion), and later only the detection of anti-HEV antibodies indicate a prior acute hepatitis [78,82].

In these areas, HEV super-infection can occur in patients with pre-existing chronic liver disease of viral or non-viral etiology, leading to superimposed acute liver injury and clinical presentation with acute on chronic liver disease, determining a higher risk of a poor outcome. In some patients, chronic liver disease had been clinically silent till the time of HEV super-infection [84]. Case-fatality rates of hepatitis E have been reported as 0.5% to 4%. For unknown reasons, mortality is higher in infants <2 years of age, and in pregnant women [54, 85]. However, these data derive from hospitalized cases with more severe disease. In population surveys at the time of disease outbreaks, much lower mortality rates of 0.07% to 0.6% have been observed [3]. The highest rates of mortality are reported in patients affected with acute HEV infection and other chronic liver diseases; studies from the Indian subcontinent showed a 12-month mortality up to 70% in patients with HEV genotype 1 and prior chronic liver disease [86].

5.2. Clinical course in developed countries

Hepatitis E is a neglected disease in Western countries, and many physicians do not consider the diagnosis when there is no history of travel to endemic countries. In these areas the diagnosis is most often recognized when all the markers for other hepatitis are negative and HEV test is undertaken in patients with unexplained liver injury; several studies report anti-HEV seroprevalence rates of less than 5% [87-88]. Clinical features in these patients are generally similar to those in high-endemic regions, except that most patients are *middle aged or elderly men* and often have another coexistent disease, thus patients in developed countries have a more severe disease than those in high-endemic areas [33, 40]. Moreover, some cases were initially suspected to have drug-induced liver injury.

The very high fatality rate among pregnant women in endemic areas cannot be evaluated in the traveler population or in industrialized countries because cases are very rare. Reports of "severe hepatitis" in two pregnant women from the UK in their third trimesters were noted [6]. Another case of liver transplantation due to fulminant HEV occurred in an Israeli woman a few days after an uneventful delivery, and she had no history of travel [83].

Most deaths from HEV genotype 3 is determined by acute or subacute liver failure in patients with prior hepatic disease. Indeed, the mortality and morbidity of this disease in patients in developed countries with pre-existing liver disease is not well-established, since these patients are not routinely tested for HEV infection. Two studies have shown an association between pork consumption (HEV genotype 3 has been detected in pork destined for human food in several countries) and mortality from chronic liver disease [88-90].

5.3. Clinical course in travelers

The incubation period and clinical course in travelers are identical to those observed in inhabitants of HEV-endemic areas affected from acute HEV hepatitis. A study on travelers with HEV infection showed that 96% (155/161) completely recovered without sequelae; only 2.5% (4/161) developed fulminant hepatitis and two of them died [6]. One of these was a 65-year-old man with chronic hepatitis C and the other was a woman with no reported underlying liver disease. The case fatality in this review was 1.2% (2/161), similar to the value of those with autochthonous hepatitis.

In the already mentioned Italian study, in all 109 patients who developed hepatitis E traveling to endemic areas, the acute disease had a self-limited course with ALT normalization within 3-6 weeks. Phylogenetic analysis on 39/109 isolated patients showed that they belonged to genotype 1 [69]. Also our study on patients with a travel-related disease presented similar results both in regards to the genotype of virus and the outcome of the disease.

5.4. Clinical extra-hepatic manifestations

In the last years some reports described HEV-associated neurological syndromes, mainly in developing countries; most cases originate from the Indian subcontinent and the cause is HEV genotype 1. These complications include Guillain-Barre syndrome [91], Bell's palsy [92],

http://dx.doi.org/10.5772/55568

neuralgic amyotrophy [93], and acute meningo-encephalitis [94], and seem to be related to the viral load of HEV. The diagnosis is not sure, it is only serologic, because most of these studies did not use molecular techniques to confirm the presence of the virus and/or the genotype.

Recently, neurological complications were described in seven (6%) of 126 patients with acute and chronic HEV genotype 3 infection; HEV RNA was detected in the in the cerebrospinal fluid (CSF) of all four patients with chronic HEV infection. A complete resolution of neurological symptoms or a significant improvement was observed in patients who achieved viral clearance [95]. Two further cases of HEV-associated Guillain-Barre syndrome (presence of anti-ganglioside GM1 antibodies) and one case of meningoencephalitis have been described in Belgium [96] and France [97]. The patients with Guillain-Barre syndrome responded well to treatment with intravenous immunoglobulin [96].

Other extra-hepatic HEV-related manifestations can be represented by membrano-proliferative glomerulonephritis and membranous glomerulonephritis; some cases have been reported in India in patients with acute HEV genotype 1 infection [97], and in France in patients with chronic HEV genotype 3 infection [98]. Further complications were observed during acute HEV infection as acute pancreatitis [99] and severe thrombocitemia [100].

5.5. Chronic HEV infection

Hepatitis E is considered a self-limited disease, evolving rarely into chronic disease. However, some patients, undergoing organ transplants and subsequent immunosuppressive therapy, may have developed chronic HEV infection. HEV chronic infection is defined by persisting HEV RNA in serum or stools for 6 months or more, in immunosuppressed patients. For the first time in 2008, a French study described a group of 14 solid-organ transplant recipients (liver, kidney, and pancreas) that were diagnosed with acute HEV, who were receiving immunosuppressive drugs. Consumption of game meat, pork products and mussels were associated with viral infections in these patients. About 60% (8 patients) of organ-transplants recipients failed to clear the virus and developed chronic hepatitis, as confirmed by a recent onset, the persistently presence of transaminase elevation (7 asymptomatic, 7 with non-specific symptoms), and persistent HEV viremia. All patients had genotype 3 HEV [101]. Sequential liver biopsies in some of the patients with chronic HEV infection showed portal hepatitis with dense lymphocytic infiltrate, and variable degrees of piecemeal necrosis, with rapid progression in fibrosis, and 10% of patients showed progress to cirrhosis. In this study no correlation between serum HEV RNA load and liver fibrosis progression has been reported [102]. Death occurred in few of these patients due to decompensated chronic liver disease. The patients with persistent infection had a significantly shorter time from organ transplantation to the development of HEV infection, and thus had lower total, and CD2, CD3, and CD4 lymphocyte counts than those with resolving HEV infection [81]. Another study reported two cases of chronic HEV infection in liver transplant recipients leading to cirrhosis and graft-failure. The same study found a prevalence of HEV infection acquired after liver transplantation in only 1% of 274 patients. [103]. Chronic HEV hepatitis was later reported also in HIV positive patients and in immunosuppressed patients for chemotherapy or hematological diseases [82].

The most of chronic hepatitis E cases have been reported among immunosuppressed subjects with genotype 3.

6. Diagnosis

For the diagnosis of acute hepatitis E, the detection of antibodies to HEV or detection of HEV RNA in serum or faeces are essential tests.

6.1. Serology

After the incubation period, the immune response to HEV follows the usual pattern: an initial specific IgM response that remains positive for months followed by IgG antibodies that can be detectable as early as in the second week of clinical symptoms [104]. In the beginning we notice the presence of the low avidity IgG antibodies, and when response matures they are replaced by antibodies with higher avidity [105]. Although four genotypes of HEV are recognized, they elicit very similar antibody responses and appear to represent a single serotype [106]. Confirmation of HEV acute hepatitis diagnosed in this way is either by molecular techniques, detecting rising reactivity in a specific IgG assay, or by positivity in immunoblot IgM assays [107]. The determination of immunity or previous exposure to HEV infection, by serological diagnosis, would be very important but it is difficult because available enzyme immunoassays use different antigens and present various effectiveness. A concentration of anti-HEV antibodies that reliably prevent infection has not been defined, but a vaccine study suggests that antibodies concentrations of 20 Walter Reed units/mL (2,5 WHO units/mL) are protective [104].

Commercial ELISA tests for antibody detection are available in Europe, Canada, and parts of Asia. In the USA, however, these tests are not commercially available. In research settings, there are tests for detecting hepatitis E virus antigen (HEVAg) in the serum. Diagnosing HEV remains a challenge given the lack of available diagnostic methods. PCR is not available in many areas of the world and serology cannot be relied upon.

6.2. Molecular techniques

HEV RNA detection using amplification techniques is a key test for the diagnosis, confirmation, and monitoring of HEV infections. In addition, recently, emerging data on the use of antiviral treatment in patients with chronic hepatitis E have emphasized the role for HEV RNA detection and quantification for monitoring therapeutic responses [100-1071].

In patients with an acute HEV infection, viral RNA occurs during the incubation period and the early phase of disease, it can be detected just before the onset of clinical symptoms in both blood and stool samples. HEV RNA usually becomes undetectable in blood and stool within one to six weeks after the onset of symptoms [108]. The window of detectable RNA is close and so if the detection has been searched later, an undetectable HEV RNA result does not exclude a recent infection. Detection of HEV RNA is very important in the diagnosis of patients with chronic HEV infection because, in immunosuppressed individuals, a specific serological response (IgM-IgG) might be absent and there are no markers for HEV infection [78].

7. HEV prevention

Currently, there are two strategies preventing HEV infections in healthy population: decreasing exposure to the virus and inducing immunity through vaccination. Individuals with prior exposure to HEV, demonstrated by pre-existing anti-HEV antibodies, appear to be protected when subsequently exposed to the virus [109]. The reduction of exposure to HEV, in developing countries, is obtained by the provision of safe drinking water, by improving the sanitary infrastructure, and by education about personal hygiene. In developed countries, prevention is more complicated for many transmission routes of infection. Sanitary handling, proper cooking of pork meat and ensuring the proper disposal of pig faeces is recommended in areas with zoonotic transmission.

The use of immune-globulins prepared in HEV-endemic regions of the world does not appear to provide significant protection. This may be because there are relatively low titers of anti-HEV antibody in the general population. There have, however, been studies of the protective efficacy of anti- HEV when immuno-globulins from patients in the convalescent period of natural infection are pooled [110].

Vaccination is, at present, the most important way to prevent HEV infection, two hepatitis E vaccines have undergone clinical testing. The first, a recombinant HEV vaccine, has been developed and a phase 2/phase 3 trial of the vaccine was carried out in seronegative members in the Nepalese army. The soldiers were randomized in two groups to receive either three doses of vaccine (898 participants) or placebo (896 participants) at 0, 1, and 6 months, and were followed for an average of 804 days. The vaccine was well tolerated and was proven highly efficacious, with protective rates of 95.5% in subjects who received all three doses. Administration of two doses was associated with a somewhat lower efficacy rate of 86%. The duration of protection is not known, but the vaccine appeared to render significant protection for at least 2 years after vaccination. The vaccine's safety and efficacy in women has not been established [111]. The second vaccine consisted of a truncated ORF2 protein, p239, which is expressed in Escherichia Coli and occurs as virus-like particles, 23 nm in diameter. In phase 3, in a large clinical trial, in 11 townships in south-eastern China, participants were randomly assigned to receive either three doses of vaccine at 0, 1, and 6 months (56,302 participants) or hepatitis B vaccine as a placebo (56,302 participants), and were followed for a 13-month period. This study enrolled participants aged 16-65 and from both genders, irrespective of their anti-HEV antibody status. The vaccine was well tolerated and showed a protective efficacy of 100% during the following one year; even after two doses of vaccine, 100% protection was noted, though these data are more limited [112]. This vaccine has recently been licensed in China, but it is uncertain whether and when it will be licensed for marketing in other developing and developed countries, possibly because the industry is not assured of a sufficient market. But, due to the zoonotic factor in transmission, there may be an overall increase in HEV infection worldwide; therefore, in developed countries vaccination might be useful in immune-suppressed patients, in those with a chronic liver disease, and in travelers to endemic areas. However, the studied vaccine regimens of three doses is difficult for travelers, but the need for HEV vaccine remains uncertain in that the attack rate in travelers remains low. On the other hand, with very effective vaccines now available for both hepatitis A and hepatitis B virus, the prevalence of these viruses may decline significantly and HEV may become the dominant hepatitis among travelers.

There are still no comparative data on the safety and immunogenicity of the two vaccines. The results of vaccinations are very promising but many questions about vaccines are still unanswered: 1) whether these vaccines can reduce transmission of infection in community; 2) the duration of protection determined by the vaccines; 3) the protective efficacy when the vaccines are administered post-exposure; 4) whether the vaccines can prevent asymptomatic HEV infection (important reservoir of HEV); 5) if the vaccines could also bring benefits to people at high risk of severe complications following HEV infection; 6) whether the vaccines may reduce the incidence of hepatitis E outbreaks in high endemic areas.

Only when we will obtain the response to these questions, there will be a complete knowledge of these vaccines, thus the exact role for HEV vaccines currently remains unclear. As said above, no vaccine has reached the market at the time of writing this chapter.

8. Treatment of HEV infection

8.1. Acute HEV

Currently, there is not a specific treatment for hepatitis E infection and often some specific interventions are not required. Physician can only monitor this disease, that, in most cases, is self-limiting and is followed by complete recovery, without chronic sequelae. However, patients with acute severe HEV genotype 3 infection have been treated successfully with ribavirin monotherapy [113-114]. Patients with hepatic failure should be transferred to a centre capable of performing liver transplants. In developing countries, the treatment of pregnant women with HEV genotype 1 infection would be necessary, but teratogenicity of ribavirin may pose a problem for use during pregnancy. Taking into account the rapid downhill course of such patients and the high risk of untreated HEV to the mother and foetus, in some cases it is needed to start the treatment with ribavirin, because the temporal window of opportunity for the drug to act and alter the outcome of disease in such patients may also be limited.

8.2. Chronic HEV

In organ-transplant recipients in immunosuppressive treatment, who are affected by chronic HEV infection, viral clearance is needed to avoid the risk of rapid progressive liver injury. Withdrawal or reduction in dose of immunosuppressive therapy (especially drugs that target T cells), if possible, should be tried before considering antiviral treatment. Reduction of immunosuppression results in viral clearance in 30% of patients [116]. Antiviral therapy is

http://dx.doi.org/10.5772/55568

needed for patients for whom it is impossible to reduce immunosuppressive treatment and for those without clearance of HEV RNA after reducing immunosuppression. Pegylated interferon [117] and ribavirin [116] as mono-therapy or in combination for 3-12 months have been tried in subjects with chronic HEV infection, with moderate success in achieving an absence of detectable serum HEV RNA for 3-6 months after stopping the administration of drugs [116,117]. In kidney-transplant recipients it is better not to use the interferon-α, because it increases the risk of acute rejection. HEV infection seems, in these patients, to respond to ribavirin monotherapy, achieving viral clearance within a few weeks. This treatment (duration of 3 months) is now the antiviral agent of choice in kidney-transplants recipients.

In other immunosuppressed patients, treatment options are less well established. Ribavirin and interferon-α have been successfully used in monotherapy and in combination only in a short case series and controlled trials with longer follow-ups are needed [118-119].

9. Concluding remarks

In the last 30 years the landscape of hepatitis HEV has changed enormously. Once thought as an infection confined to developing countries, deriving from a waterborn infection, it is now recognized as a widespread geographic distribution disease, with different ways of transmission, causing an acute and/or chronic hepatic disease. This new knowledge has led to an increasing research activity to better understand the virology and the clinical features of HEV infection. Recent studies deal the treatment and the prevention: the therapy of the chronic disease, at the moment, is represented mainly by ribavirin; the only prevention possible is the use of HEV vaccines, particularly in some high-risk groups or certain situations (e.g. populations displaced due to floods, war or conflicts). At the moment HEV infection is not a major problem in Western European countries, but the increasing number of travelers to endemic regions for HEV, the high number of immigrants arriving in Italy and the new zoonotic aspect of the infection could change this epidemiologic situation in the future. The new epidemiological spreading of HEV infection and the emerging clinical features of the disease require constant surveillance for a better control and prevention of this disease.

Author details

Scotto Gaetano[1*] and Fazio Vicenzina[2]

*Address all correspondence to: g.scotto@medicina.unifg.it

1 Clinical of Infectious Diseases, University of Foggia, Italy

2 Department of laboratory, Unit of virology, Hospital of Foggia, Italy

References

[1] Meng XJ, Anderson DA, Arankalle VA, et al. Hepeviridae. In:King AMQ, Adams MJ,Carstens EB, Lefkowitz EJ, eds. Virus taxonomy: classification and nomenclature of viruses: Ninth Report of the International Committee on Taxonomy of Viruses. San Diego, CA: Elsevier; 2011: In press

[2] Purcell RH, Emerson SU. Hepatitis E: an emerging awareness of an old disease. J Hepatol 2008;48:494–503.

[3] Wong DC, Purcell RH, Sreenivasan MA, Prasad SR, Pavri KM. Epidemic and endemic hepatitis in India: evidence for a non-A, non-B hepatitis etiology. Lancet 1980; 2: 876–9.

[4] Wierzba TF, Panzner U. Report on the International Symposium on Hepatitis E, Seoul, South Korea, 2010. Emerg Infect Dis. 2012 May;18(5). doi: 10.3201/eid1805.111916.

[5] Aggarwal R Hepatitis E: historical, contemporary and future perspectives. J Gastroenterol Hepatol. 2011;26(Suppl 1):72–82.

[6] Piper Jenks N, Horowitz H, Schwartz E. The risk of hepatitis E infection to travelers. J Travel Med 2000; 7:194-9

[7] Kwo PY, Schlauder GG, Carpenter HA, Murphy PJ, Rosenblatt JE, Dawson GJ et al. Acute hepatitis E by a new isolate acquired in the United States. Mayo Clin Proc 1997;72:1133-1136.

[8] Dalton HR, Stableforth W, Thurairajah P, Hazeldine S, Remnarace R, Usama W, et al. Autochthonous hepatitis E in Southwest England: natural history, complications and seasonal variation, and hepatitis E virus IgG seroprevalence in blood donors, the elderly and patients with chronic liver disease. Eur J Gastroenterol Hepatol 2008;20: 784-790.

[9] Vishwanathan R. Infectious hepatitis in Delhi (1955–1956): a critical study: epidemiology. Indian J. Med. Res. 1957; 45 (Suppl.1): 1–29.

[10] Vishwanathan R, Sidhu AS. Infectious hepatitis: clinical findings Indian J. Med. Res. 1957; 45 (Suppl.): 49–58.

[11] Dane DS, Cameron CH, Briggs NM. Virus-like particles in serum of patients with Australia antigen-associated hepatitis. Lancet 1970;1:695–98.

[12] Khuroo MS. Study of an epidemic of non-A, non-B hepatitis: possibility of another human hepatitis virus distinct from post-transfusion non- A, non-B type. Am. J. Med. 1980; 68:818–23.

[13] Balayan MS, Andjaparidze AG, Savinskaya SS et al. Evidence for a virus in non-A, non-B hepatitis transmitted via the fecal-oral route. Intervirology 1983; 20: 23–31

[14] Reyes GR, Purdy MA, Kim JP et al. Isolation of a cDNA from the virus responsible for enterically transmitted non-A, non-B hepatitis. Science 1990; 247: 1335–9.

[15] Dawson GJ, Chau KH, Cabal CM, Yarbough PO, Reyes GR, Mushahwar IK. Solid-phase enzyme-linked immunosorbent assay for hepatitis E virus IgG and IgM antibodies utilizing recombinant antigens and synthetic peptides. J. Virol. Methods 1992; 38: 175–86.

[16] Meng XJ. Hepatitis E virus: animal reservoirs and zoonotic risk. Vet Microbiol 2010; 140: 256–65.

[17] Payne CJ, Ellis TM, Plant SL, Gregory AR, Wilcox GE. Sequence data suggests big liver and spleen disease virus (BLSV) is genetically related to hepatitis E virus. Vet Microbiol 1999; 68: 119–25.

[18] Kalia M, Chandra V, Rahman SA, et al. Heparan sulfate proteoglycans are required for cellular binding of the hepatitis E virus ORF2 capsid protein and for viral infection. J Virol 2009;83:12714–12724.

[19] Wedemeyer H, Pischke S, Manns MP. Pathogenesis and treatment of hepatitis e virus infection. Gastroenterology. 2012 May;142(6):1388-1397

[20] . Mushahwar IK. Hepatitis E virus: molecular virology, clinical features, diagnosis, transmission, epidemiology, and prevention. J Med Virol 2008;80:646–658.

[21] Li TC, Yamakawa Y, Suzuki K, et al. Expression and self-assembly of empty virus-like particles of hepatitis E virus. J Virol 1997;71: 7207–13.

[22] Xing L, Wang JC, Li TC, et al. Spatial configuration of hepatitis E virus antigenic domain. J Virol 2011; 85: 1117–24.

[23] Yamada K, Takahashi M, Hoshino Y, et al. ORF3 protein of hepatitis E virus is essential for virion release from infected cells. J Gen Virol 2009; 90: 1880–91.

[24] Emerson SU, Nguyen HT, Torian U, Burke D, Engle R,Purcell RH. Release of genotype 1 hepatitis E virus from cultured hepatoma and polarized intestinal cells depends on open reading frame 3 protein and requires an intact PXXP motif. J Virol 2010; 84: 9059–69.

[25] Tang X, Yang C, Gu Y, et al. Structural basis for the neutralization and genotype specifi city of hepatitis E virus. Proc Natl Acad Sci USA 2011; 108: 10266–71.

[26] Takahashi M, Tanaka T, Takahashi H, et al. Hepatitis E Virus (HEV)strains in serum samples can replicate efficiently in cultured cells despite the coexistence of HEV antibodies: characterization of HEV virions in blood circulation. J Clin Microbiol 2010; 48: 1112–25

[27] Lu L, Li C, Hagedorn CH. Phylogenetic analysis of global hepatitis E virus sequences: genetic diversity, subtypes and zoonosis. Rev.Med. Virol. 2006; 16: 5–36.

[28] Ippagunta SK, Naik S,Sharma B, Aggarwal R. Presence of hepatitis E virus in sewage in northern India. Frequency and seasonal pattern. Journal of Medical Virology.2007; 79, 1827-1831.

[29] Labrique AB, Zaman K, Hossain Z. Epidemiology and risk factors of incident hepatitis E virus infection in rural Bangladesh. American Journal of Epidemiology.2010; 172(8), 952-961

[30] Goumba AI, Konamna X, Komas NP. Clinical and epidemiological aspects of a hepatitis E outbreak in Bangui, Central African Repubblic. BMC Infectious Diseases.2011; 11, 93-99

[31] Huang CC, Nguyen D, Fernandez J et al. Molecular cloning and sequencing of the Mexico isolate of hepatitis E virus (HEV).Virology 1992; 191: 550–8.

[32] Aggarwal R, Naiks S. Epidemiology of hepatitis E: current status. J Gastroenterol Hepatol 2009; 24:1484-1493

[33] Dalton HR, Bendal L, Ijaz S,Banks M. Hepatitis E: an emerging infection in developed countries. Lancet Infect Dis 2008; 8: 698-709

[34] Johne R, Plenge-Bonig A, Hess M, Ulrich RG, Reetz J, Schielke A. Detection of a novel hepatitis E-like virus in faeces of wild rats using a nested broad-spectrum RT-PCR. J Gen Virol 2010; 91: 750–58.

[35] Takahashi M, Nishizawa T, Sato H, et al. Analysis of the full-length genome of a hepatitis E virus isolate obtained from a wild boar in Japan that is classifi able into a novel genotype. J Gen Virol 2011; 92: 902–08.

[36] Zhao C, Ma Z, Harrison TJ, et al. A novel genotype of hepatitis Evirus prevalent among farmed rabbits in China. J Med Virol 2009; 81: 1371–79.

[37] Kalia M, Chandra V, Rahman SA, Sehgal D, Jameel S. Heparan sulfate proteoglycans are required for cellular binding of the hepatitis E virus ORF2 capsid protein and for viral infection. J Virol 2009;83:12714-12724.

[38] Khuroo MS, Kamili S, Dar MY, Moecklii R, Jameel S. Hepatitis E and long-term antibody status. Lancet 1993;341:1355.

[39] .Purcell RH, Emerson SU, Prevention. In : Thomas HC, Lemon S, Zuckerman AJ, editors. Viral Hepatitis. Malder, MA: Blackwell Publishing; 2005, p. 635–45.

[40] Yamashita T, Mori Y, Miyazaki N, Cheng RH, Yoshimura M, Unno H, et al. Biological and immunological characteristics of hepatitis E virus-like particles based on the crystal structure. Proc Natl Acad Sci U S A 2009;106:12986-12991.

[41] Naik SR, Aggarwal R, Salunke PN, Mehrotra NN. A large waterborne viral hepatitis E epidemic in Kanpur, India. Bull World Health Organ 1992;70:597-604.

http://dx.doi.org/10.5772/55568

[42] Aggarwal R, Naik SR. Hepatitis E: does person-to-person spread occur? Indian J Gastroenterol 1992, 11:109-112.

[43] Somani SK, Aggarwal R, Naik SR et al. A serological study of intra-familial spread from patients with sporadic hepatitis E virus infection. J Viral Hepat 2003; 10: 446-449

[44] Teshale EH, Grytdal SP, Howard C, Barry V, Kamili S, Drobeniuc J, Hill Vr, Okware, S, Hu DJ, Holmberg SD. Evidence of person-to-person transmission of hepatitis E virus during a large outbreak in Northern Uganda. Clin Infect Diseas 2010; 50:1006-1010

[45] Aggarwal R, Kini D, Sofat S, Naik SR, Krawczynski K. Duration of viraemia and faecal viral excretion in acute hepatitis E. Lancet 2000;356:1081-1082.

[46] Shukla P, Chauhan UK, Naik S, Anderson D, Aggarwal R. Hepatitis E virus infection among animals in northern India: an unlikely source of human disease. J Viral Hepat 2007;14:310-317.

[47] Arankalle VA, Chobe LP, Joshi MV, Chadha MS, Kundu B, Walimbe AM. Human and swine hepatitis E viruses from Western India belong to different genotypes. J Hepatol 2002;36:417-425.

[48] Meng XJ, Halbur PG, Haynes JS, Tsavera TS, Bruna JD, Royer RL, et al. Experimental infection of pigs with the newly identified swine hepatitis E virus (swine HEV), but not with human strains of HEV.Arch Virol 1998;143:1405-1415.

[49] Fix AD, Abdel-Hamid M, Purcell RH, Shehata MH, Abdel-Aziz F, Mikhail N, et al. Prevalence of antibodies to hepatitis E in two rural Egyptian communities. Am J Trop Med Hyg 2000;62:519–23.

[50] Li RC, Ge SX, Li YP, Zheng YJ, Nong Y, Guo QS, et al. Seroprevalence of hepatitis E virus infectrion, rural southern People's Republic of China. Emerg Infect Dis 2006;12(11):1682–8.

[51] Labrique AB, Zaman K, Hossain Z (2010) Epidemiology and risk factors of incident hepatitis E virus infection in rural Bangladesh. American Journal of Epidemiology. 2010; 172(8), 952-961

[52] Bile K, Isse A, Mohamud O, et al. Contrasting roles of rivers and wells as sources of drinking water on attack and fatality rates in a hepatitis E epidemic in Somalia. Am J Trop Med Hyg 1994; 51: 466–74.

[53] Teshale EH, Howard CM, Grytdal SP, et al. Hepatitis E epidemic,Uganda. Emerg Infect Dis 2010; 16: 126–29.

[54] Khuroo MS, Teli MR, Skidmore S, Sofi MA, Khuroo MI. Incidence and severity of viral hepatitis in pregnancy. Am J Med 1981;70: 252-255.

[55] Bhatia V, Singhal A, Panda SK, Acharya SK. A 20-year single-center experience with acute liver failure during pregnancy: is the prognosis really worse? Hepatology 2008;48:1577-1585.

[56] Tsang TH, Denison EK, Williams HV, Venczel LV, Ginsberg MM, Vugia DJ Acute hepatitis E infection acquired in California. Clin Infect Dis 2000; 30:618-619

[57] Mansuy JM, Peron JM, Abravanel F, Poirson H, Dubois M, Miedouge M, Vischi F, Alric L, Vinel JP, Izopet J. Hepatitis E in the south west of France in individuals who have never visited an endemic area. J Med Virol 2004; 74:419-424

[58] Scotto G, Saracino A, Pempinello R, El Hamad I, Geraci S, Panunzio M, Palumbo E, Cibelli DC, Angarano G; Italian Study Group for Infectious Diseases in Immigrants. et al. SIMIT epidemiological multicentric study on hospitalized immigrants in Italy during 2002. J Immigr. Health 2005; 7: 55-60.

[59] Clemente-Casares P, Pina S, Buti M, Jardi R, MartIn M, Bofill-Mas S, Girones R. Hepatitis E virus epidemiology in industrialized countries. Emerg Infect Dis. 2003 Apr; 9:448-54.

[60] Mitsui T, Tsukamoto Y, Hirose A, et al. Distinct changing profi les of hepatitis A and E virus infection among patients with acute hepatitis, patients on maintenance hemodialysis and healthy individuals in Japan. J Med Virol 2006; 78: 1015–24.

[61] Christensen PB, Engle RE, Jacobsen SE, Krarup HB, Georgsen J, Purcell RH. High prevalence of hepatitis E antibodies among Danish prisoners and drug users. J Med Virol. 2002 Jan; 66:49-55

[62] Reuter G, Fofor D, Forgach P, Katai A, Szucs G. Characterization and zoonotic potential of endemic hepatitis E virus (HEV) strains i humans and animals in Hungary. J Clin Virol 2009; 44: 277-281

[63] Christensen PB, Engle RE, Hjort C, Homburg KM, Vach W, Georgsen j, Purcell RH Time trend of the prevalence of hepatitis E antibodies among farmers and blood donors: a potential zoonosis in Denmark Clin. Inf. Diseases 2008; 47:1026-1031

[64] Sylvan SP. The high rate of antibodies to hepatitis E virus in young, intravenous drug-abusers with acute hepatitis B-virus infection in a Swedish community: a study of hepatitis markers in individuals with intravenously or sexually acquired hepatitis B-virus infection Scand J Infect Dis. 1998; 30:429-30.

[65] Mansuy JM, Bendall R, Legrand-Abravanel F, et al. Hepatitis E virus antibodies in blood donors, France. Emerg Infect Dis 2011;17: 2309–12.

[66] Stefanidis I, Zervou EK, Rizos C, Syrganis C, Patsidis E, Kyriakopoulos G, Sdrakas L, Tsianas N, Rigopoulou EI, Liakopoulos V, Dalekos GN. Hepatitis E virus antibodies in hemodialysis patients: an epidemiological survey in central Greece. Int J Artif Organs. 2004 Oct; 27:842-847.

http://dx.doi.org/10.5772/55568

[67] Boutrouille A, Bakkali-Kassimi L, Crucière C, Pavio N Prevalence of anti-hepatitis E virus antibodies in French blood donors J. Clin. Microbiol. 2007, 45:2009-2010

[68] Romanò L, Paladini S, Tagliacarne C, Canuti M, Bianchi S, Zanetti AR Hepatitis E in Italy. A long-term prospective study. J Hepatol 2011; 54: 34-40

[69] Said B, Ijaz S, Kafatos G, et al, and the Hepatitis E Incident Investigation Team. Hepatitis E outbreak on cruise ship. Emerg Infect Dis 2009; 15: 1738–44.

[70] Dalton HR, Bendall RP, Rashid M, et al. Host risk factors and autochthonous hepatitis E infection. Eur J Gastroenterol Hepatol 2011; 23: 1200–05.

[71] Reed C, Freedman DO, Castelli F,Chen L, Pandy P, Parola P et al. Increase in hepatitis E among travelers reported to the GeoSentinel surveillance system [Abstract]. 43rd Annual Meeting of the Infectious Diseases Society of America. San Francisco; October 2005.

[72] Potasman I, Koren L, Peterman M, Srugo I. Lack of hepatitis E infection among backpackers to tropical countries. J Travel Med 2000;7:208–10.

[73] Ooi W, Gawoki J, Yarbough P, Pankey G. Hepatitis E Seroconversion in United States travelers abroad. Am J Trop Med Hyg 1999;61(5):822–24.

[74] Smalligan R, LangeW, Frame J, et al. The rik of viral hepatitis A,B, C and E among North American missionaries. Am J Trop Med Hyg 1995;53:233–6.

[75] Shlim DR, Pandey P, Scott R, Vaughn DW. Risk of Hepatitis E infection among foreigners living in Nepal [Abstract FC 1.4]. In: Proceedings of the 6th Conference of the International Society of Travel Medicine, Montreal; 1999.

[76] Cowie B, Adamopoulos J, Carter K, Kellly H. Hepatitis E infections, Victoria Australia. Emerg Infect Dis 2005;11(3): 482–4.

[77] Aggarwal R, Jameel S. Hepatitis E. Hepatology. 2012 Dec;54(6):2218-26.

[78] Peron JM, Danjoux M, Kamar N, Missoury R, Poirson H, Vinel JP, Mansuy JM, Bureau C, Izopet J, Brousset P, Selves J. Liver histology in patients with sporadic acute hepatitis E: a study of 11 patients from South-West France. Virchows Arch. 2007 Apr; 450(4):405-10

[79] Ohnishi S, Kang JH, Maekubo H, Arakawa T, Karino Y, Toyota J, Takahashi K, Mishiro S. Comparison of clinical features of acute hepatitis caused by hepatitis E virus (HEV) genotypes 3 and 4 in Sapporo, Japan Hepatol Res. 2006 Dec;36(4):301-7.

[80] Pal R, Aggarwal R, Naik SR, Das V, Das S, Naik S. Immunological alterations in pregnant women with acute hepatitis E. J Gastroenterol Hepatol 2005;20:1094-1101

[81] Aggarwal R.Hepatitis E: Historical, contemporary and future perspectives. J Gastroenterol Hepatol. 2011 Jan;26 Suppl 1:72-82.

[82] Mantab MA, Rahman S, Khan M, Marmum AA, Afroz S. Etiology of fulminant hepatic failure: experience from a tertiary hospital in Bangladesh. Hepatobilary Pancreat Dis Int 2008;7(2):161–2.

[83] Kamar N, Bendall R, Legrand-Abravanel F, Xia NS, Ijaz S, Izopet J, Dalton HR. Hepatitis E. Lancet. 2012 Jun 30;379(9835):2477-88.

[84] Sharapov MB, Favorov MO, Yashina TL, et al. Acute viral hepatitis morbidity and mortality associated with hepatitis E virus infection: Uzbekistan surveillance data. BMC Infect Dis 2009; 9: 35-42.

[85] Kumar Acharya S, Kumar Sharma P, Singh R, et al. Hepatitis E virus (HEV) infection in patients with cirrhosis is associated with rapid decompensation and death. J Hepatol 2007; 46: 387–94.

[86] Boutrouille A, Bakkali-Kassimi L, Cruciere C, Pavio N. Prevalence of anti-hepatitis E virus antibodies in French blood donors. J Clin Microbiol 2007; 45: 2009–10.

[87] Bouwknegt M, Engel B, Herremans MM, et al. Bayesian estimation of hepatitis E virus seroprevalence for populations with diff erent exposure levels to swine in The Netherlands. Epidemiol Infect 2008; 136: 567–76.

[88] Tei S, Kitajima N, Takahashi K, Mishiro S. Zoonotic transmission of hepatitis E virus from deer to human beings. Lancet 2003;362: 371-373.

[89] Takahashi K, Kitajima N, Abe N, Mishiro S. Complete or near-complete nucleotide sequences of hepatitis E virus genome recovered from a wild boar, a deer, and four patients who ate the deer. Virology 2004; 330:501-505.

[90] Sood A, Midha V, Sood N. Guillain-Barre syndrome with acute hepatitis E. Am J Gastroenterol 2000; 95: 3667–68.

[91] Dixit VK, Abhilash VB, Kate MP, Jain AK. Hepatitis E infection with Bell's palsy. J Assoc Physicians India 2006; 54:418

[92] Fong F, Illahi M. Neuralgic amyotrophy associated with hepatitis E virus. Clin Neurol Neurosurg 2009; 111: 193–95

[93] Kejariwal D, Roy S, Sarkar N. Seizure associated with acute hepatitis E. Neurology 2001; 57: 1935.

[94] Kamar N, Bendall RP, Peron JM, et al. Hepatitis E virus and neurologic disorders. Emerg Infect Dis 2011; 17: 173–79.

[95] Maurissen I, Jeurissen A, Strauven T, Sprengers D, De Schepper B. First case of anti-ganglioside GM1-positive Guillain-Barre syndrome due to hepatitis E virus infection. Infection 2011; 7:341-9

[96] Despierres LA, Kaphan E, Attarian S, et al. Neurologic disorders and hepatitis E, France, 2010. Emerg Infect Dis 2011; 17: 1510–12.

http://dx.doi.org/10.5772/55568

[97] Ali G, Kumar M, Bali S, Wadhwa W. Heptitis E associated immune thrombocytopenia and membranous glomerulonephritis. Indian J Nephrol 2001; 11: 70–72

[98] Kamar N, Weclawiack H, Guilbeaud-Frugier C, et al. Hepatitis E virus and the kidney in solid organ transplant patients. Transplantation 2012; published online Jan 31. DOI:10.1097/ TP.0b013e318245f14c

[99] Deniel C, Coton T, Brardjanian S, Guisset M, Nicand E, Simon F. Acute pancreatitis: a rare complication of acute hepatitis E. J Clin Virol 2011; 51: 202–04.

[100] Fourquet E, Mansuy JM, Bureau C, et al. Severe thrombocytopenia associated with acute autochthonous hepatitis E. JClin Virol 2010;48: 73–74.

[101] Kamar N, Selves J, Mansuy JM, Ouezzani L, Peron JM, Guitard J, et al. Hepatitis E virus and chronic hepatitis in organ-transplant recipients. N Engl J Med 2008;358:811-817.

[102] Gerolami R, Moal V, Colson P. Chronic hepatitis E with cirrhosis in a kidney-transplant recipient. N Engl J Med 2008;358:859-860.

[103] Haagsma EB, van den Berg AP, Porte RJ, Benne CA, Vennema H, Reimerink JH, Koopmans MP. Chronic hepatitis E virus infection in liver transplant recipients. Liver Transpl. 2008 Apr;14(4):547-53.

[104] Huang S, Zhang X, Jiang H, et al. Profile of acute infectious markers in sporadic hepatitis E. PLoS One 2010; 5: e13560.

[105] Bendall R, Ellis V, Ijaz S, Thurairajah P, Dalton HR. Serological response to hepatitis E virus genotype 3 infection: IgG quantitation, avidity, and IgM response. J Med Virol 2008; 80: 95–101.

[106] Engle RE, Yu C, Emerson SU, Meng XJ, Purcell RH. Hepatitis E virus (HEV) capsid antigens derived from viruses of human and swine origin are equally efficient for detecting anti-HEV by enzyme immunoassay. J Clin Microbiol 2002; 40: 4576–80.

[107] Herremans M, Bakker J, Duizer E, Vennema H, Koopmans MP. Use of serological assays for diagnosis of hepatitis E virus genotype 1 and 3 infections in a setting of low endemicity.Clin Vaccine Immunol 2007; 14: 562–68.

[108] Takahashi M, Kusakai S, Mizuo H, Suzuki K, Fujimura K, Masuko K, Sugai Y, Aikawa T, Nishizawa T, Okamoto H. Simultaneous detection of immunoglobulin A (IgA) and IgM antibodies against hepatitis E virus (HEV) Is highly specific for diagnosis of acute HEV infection. J Clin Microbiol. 2005 Jan;43(1):49-56

[109] Bryan JP, Tsarev SA, Iqbal M, Ticehurst J, Emerson S, Ahmed A, et al. Epidemic hepatitis E in Pakistan: patterns of serologic response and evidence that antibody to hepatitis E virus protects against disease. J Infect Dis 1994;170:517–21.

[110] Pillot J, Turkoglu S, Dubreuil P, Cosson A, Lemaigre G,Meng J, et al. Cross-reactive immunity against different strains of the hepatitis E virus transferable by simian and human sera. C R Acad Sci III 1995;318:1059–64.

[111] Shresta MP, Scott RM, Joshi DM, Mammen MP Jr, Thapa GB, Thapa N, et al. Safety and efficacy of a recombinant hepatitis E vaccine. N Engl J Med 2007;365:895–903.

[112] Zhu FC, Zhang J, Zhang XF, et al. Effi cacy and safety of a recombinant hepatitis E vaccine in healthy adults: a large-scale, randomised, double-blind placebo-controlled, phase 3 trial. Lancet 2010; 376: 895–902.

[113] Peron JM, Dalton H, Izopet J, Kamar N. Acute autochthonous hepatitis E in western patients with underlying chronic liver disease: a role for ribavirin? J Hepatol 2011; 54: 1323–24, author reply 1324–25.

[114] Gerolami R, Borentain P, Raissouni F, Motte A, Solas C, Colson P. Treatment of severe acute hepatitis E by ribavirin. J Clin Virol 2011; 52: 60–62.

[115] Mallet V, Nicand E, Sultanik P, et al. Brief communication: case reports of ribavirin treatment for chronic hepatitis E. Ann Intern Med 2010; 153: 85–89.

[116] Kamar N, Rostaing L, Abravanel F, et al. Ribavirin therapy inhibits viral replication on patients with chronic hepatitis E virus infection. Gastroenterology 2010; 139: 1612–18.

[117] Kamar N, Rostaing L, Abravanel F, Garrousta C, Esposito L, Cardeau-Desangles I, et al. Pegylated interferon-alpha for treating chronic hepatitis E virus infection after liver transplantation. Clin Infect Dis 2010; 50:e30-e33.

[118] Alric L, Bonnet D, Laurent G, Kamar N, Izopet J. Chronic hepatitis E virus infection: successful virologic response to pegylated interferon-alpha therapy. Ann Intern Med 2010; 153: 135–36.

[119] Alric L, Bonnet D, Beynes-Rauzy O, Izopet J, Kamar N. Definitive clearance of a chronic hepatitis E virus infection with ribavirin treatment. Am J Gastroenterol 2011; 106: 1562–63.

Chapter 10

The Skin and Viral Liver Disease

Mastrolonardo M.

Additional information is available at the end of the chapter

http://dx.doi.org/10.5772/56140

1. Introduction

It is undisputable that a multifaceted biological interplay exists between the skin and the liver.

The integument can firstly be viewed as a 'gate' through which hepatotropic viruses may access the blood stream. In this respect, one may think of the huge number of B and C virus hepatites that must have been acquired in a more or less distant past due to either intravenous drug consumption, use of contaminated equipment in beauty and health care-related procedures, or even dermal tattooing. Moreover, one may consider that some cases of herpes simplex virus hepatitis have been reported in the literature which are not unlikely ascribable to systemic dissemination from primary muco-cutaneous lesional *foci*.

Yet, the skin may also be viewed as a 'mirror' capable of projecting on the body surface more or less specific *echoes* of disease conditions involving the liver. A recent review of the issue by Hazin and coworkers [1] is introduced by the following simple but just as brilliant statement: "Dysfunction in the body's second largest organ, the liver, often yields changes in the body's largest organ, the skin". The most trivial paradigm sustaining such an obvious assumption is *jaundice* when it is sustained by primary failure of hepatocytes to perform one of their main functions, that is to conjugate bilirubin into a secretable form. However, further and less obvious paradigms, such as cutaneous manifestations of mixed cryoglobulinemia in HCV infected patients, will also be discussed.

Since the issue that will be specifically reviewed in this chapter is all the many possible links between skin and virus-induced liver disease, this introductory framework is to be completed by mentioning the not unusual circumstances in which neither the skin nor the liver disease in itself, but treatments undertaken to cure a disease of one of the two organs may have undesired consequences on the other one. This seems obviously true thinking of some double-edged risky circumstances in which either worsening of psoriasis in patients undergoing interferon plus ribavirin therapy, or reactivation of latent viral infections under immunosuppressive treatment of the skin disease, is observed.

2. The skin as a 'gate' for hepatotropic virus infections

2.1. Tatooing as risk factor for viral liver disease

Tatooing has been practiced for many centuries worldwide, and is a well-established risk factor for transfusion-transmitted diseases, including HBV and HCV [2]. A recent meta-analysis highlights that the above menace is still currently far from being remote, especially in certain at-risk categories (such as prison inmates and subjects undergoing home-made procedures without proper aseptic techniques) [3].

2.2. Rare forms of viral hepatitis caused by agents which usually involve only the skin

After primary infection, in the absence of any severe immune deficiency condition, *herpesviruses* like Herpes Simplex Viruses (HSV) type 1 or 2, and Varicella-Zoster virus (VZV) establish latency by remaining dormant in the dorsal root nerve ganglia. Viral reactivation results in cutaneous or muco-cutaneous manifestations that usually run an overall benign course (Figg 1, 2, 3), with an inflamed vesicular and/or bullous rash which is customarily restricted to a limited district of the body surface. Though in some patients rather impressive clinical *scenarios* may be observed (Figg. 4, 5 and 6), herpetic lesions tend to heal within few weeks, with no or only minor scarring and dyschromic sequelae. As for VZV, post-herpetic neuralgia develops quite rarely, and is the worst occurrence reported after skin manifestations have faded.

In otherwise healthy subjects, disseminated herpes simplex virus hepatitis have been reported very exceptionally. In one case described by Miyazaki and coworkers in 1991 [4], the possibility that patient's mucosal herpetic lesions might have behaved as a 'gate' for a large virus *inoculum* leading to visceral involvement either directly or after having overwhelmed local immune defenses has been considered.

By contrast, HSV and VZV hepatitis are possible in patients whose cell-mediated immunity is severely impaired, for instance in malignancy or organ transplanted patients [5]. In these cases, the skin rash may either be absent, coincide with, or supervene after visceral involvement. When cutaneous lesions are present, severity of skin involvement is often significantly increased compared to standard clinical pictures both in terms of number of lesions, diffusion over the body surface, and severity of tissue impairment. Notably, in a recent review of 74 cases of herpes simplex hepatitis [6], Sharma and Mosunjac highlighted that proper diagnosis was delayed in more than two-third of cases, despite a herpetic muco-cutaneous involvement was present in at least 70% of patients. Conversely, the occurrence of an unexplained impairment of liver function tests in an immunocompromised patient exhibiting skin herpetic lesions should always arouse a high degree of suspicion of visceral dissemination [7]. Fulminating herpetic hepatitis is a life-threatening occurrence, but it can be treated effectively if therapy is

http://dx.doi.org/10.5772/56140

started early. Inclusion of herpes virus in the differential diagnosis procedures is thus mandatory.

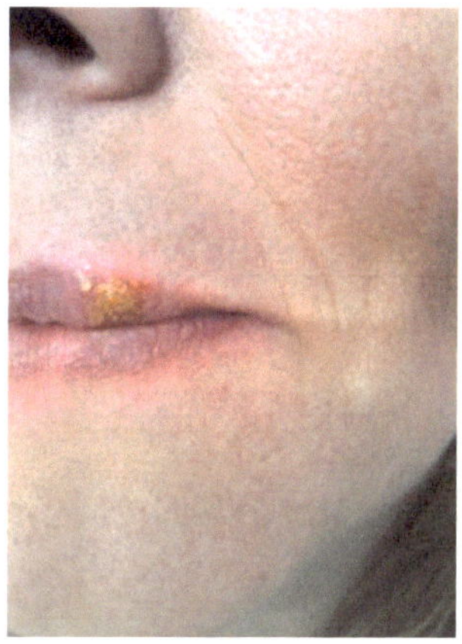

Figure 1. Herpes simplex labialis

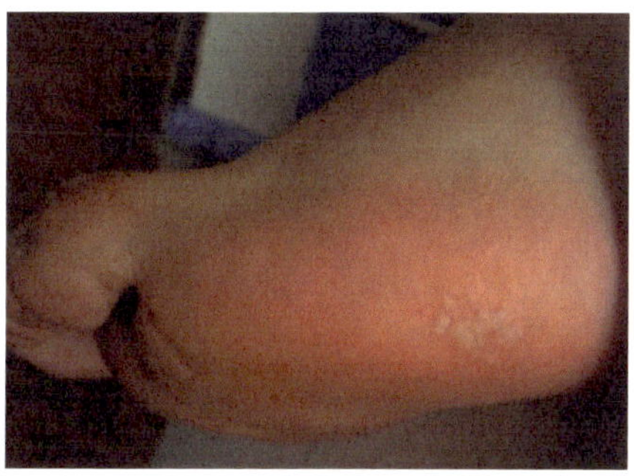

Figure 2. Herpes simplex on the foot: an unusual localization

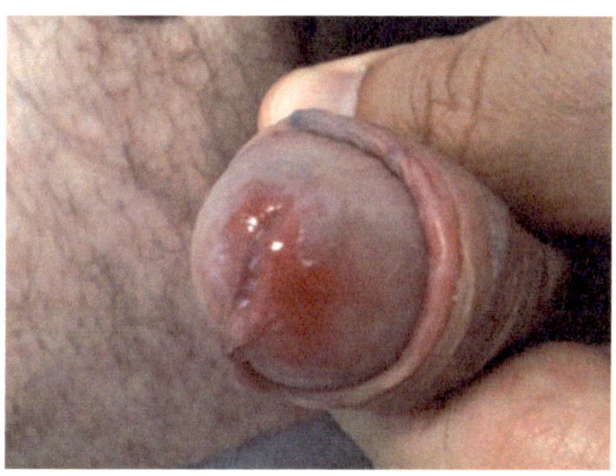

Figure 3. Herpes simplex progenitalis

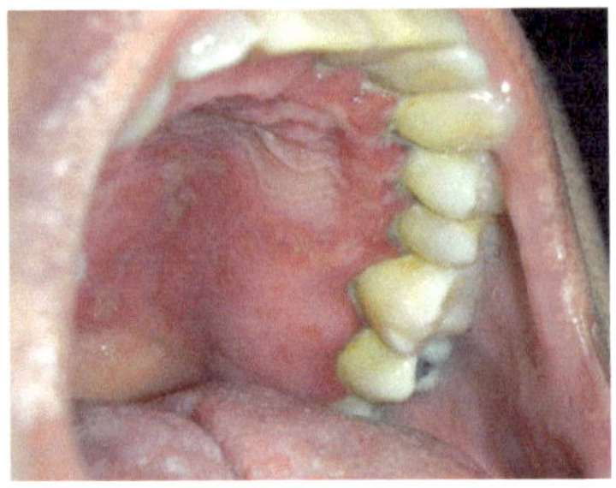

Figure 4. Severe herpetic gingivostomatitis

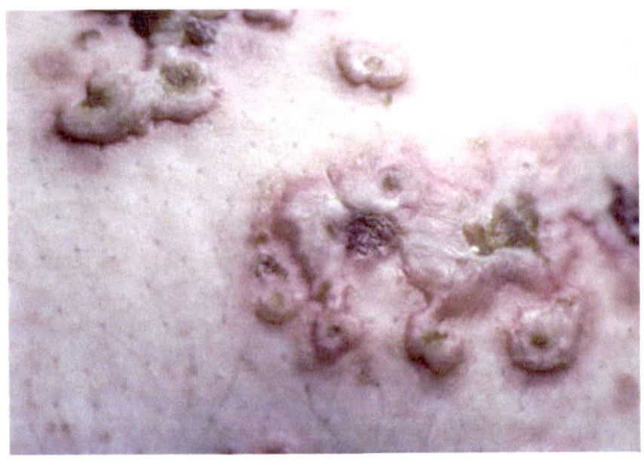

Figure 5. Severe cutaneous herpes simplex with extensive vesico-bullous elements

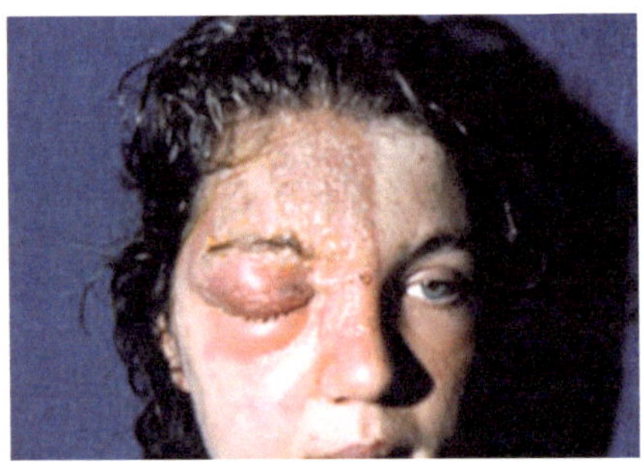

Figure 6. Severe, necrotic and hemorrhagic herpes zoster

3. Skin manifestations occurring in viral liver disease

3.1. Skin manifestations related to HCV

Cutaneous manifestations of *acute* infection are sporadic and show no substantial specificity, ranging from urticaria, erythema multiforme, leukocytoclastic vasculitis to erythema nodosum. On the contrary, there exists a wide panel of skin conditions linked, to a varying degree, with *chronic* HCV infection [8, 9]. The occurrence of skin disorders of any type has been in fact reported in up to 17% of HCV patients (Table 1) [10]. In this context, the association with the 'big three' i.e. mixed cryoglobulinemic vasculitis, porphyria cutanea tarda and lichen planus show the highest robustness on both biological and epidemiological ground. On the other hand, the clinical alliance between HCV and a broad list of other skin conditions has not yet received sufficient support [9, 11]. In this context, anecdotal reports have mostly been made in the literature of associations with pityriasis rubra pilaris [12], sarcoidosis [13], vitiligo [8], cholestatic and non-cholestatic pruritus [14, 15], prurigo nodularis [16], cutaneous polyarteritis nodosa [17], pyoderma gangrenosum [18], subacute cutaneous lupus erythematosus [19], primary localized cutaneous amyloidosis [20], pigmented purpuric dermatosis [21], actinic porokeratosis [22], pityriasis lichenoide [23], generalized granuloma annulare [24], disseminated Kaposi's sarcoma [25] and necrolytic acral erythema [26]. Of note, in most of the above circumstances it seems quite difficult to sift consistently the direct contribution of HCV infection *per se* from that attributable to antiviral treatment. A data set which is therefore of the outmost relevance in this regard is that provided by an U.S. nationwide hospital-based case-control study in which El-Serag and coworkers [8] surveyed comorbidity in as many as 34,204 HCV-infected subjects, the vast majority of whom (notably, >95%) were naïve to antiviral therapy. In this study, the aforementioned strong association with cryoglobulinemia, porphyria cutanea tarda and lichen planus found an authoritative confirmation. However, a statistically significant link was also observed with vitiligo, but this finding did not receive further comparable support from the rest of the literature, and remains rather inexplicable.

3.1.1. Mixed cryoglobulinemic vasculitis

Cryoglobulins are a family of anomalous proteins which tend to precipitate at low temperatures (<37°C), such as those currently found in the extremities (namely hands, feet, ear and nose). The prototype of cryoglobulinaemic diseases in HCV infected patients is 'mixed cryoglobulinemia' (MC). Of note, up to more than a half of HCV-infected patients show circulating cryoglobulins, and rates of 30 to 100% of HCV positive serologies have been reported in carriers of circulating cryoglobulins, with an unexplained predominance in the Mediterranean basin.

In MC tissue damage results from deposition of immune complexes containing rheumatoid factor, polyclonal IgG, complement and HCV RNA on endothelial surfaces of small- to medium-sized vessels, which in turn leads to vascular inflammation. The prevalent histological pattern of MC is neutrophilic 'leukocytoclastic' vasculitis; however, 'necrotizing' vasculitis, with intimal fibrinoid necrosis and infiltration of the entire vessel wall and perivascular space, may also be observed [27].

The skin is one of the most commonly affected organs, along with kidneys and peripheral nerves. Thus, the dermatologist may play a helpful role in early detection of previously unrecognized HCV infections. In fact, the appearance of cutaneous lesions on extremities, particularly in cooler weather, must always raise clinical suspicion. The spectrum of skin involvement in MC ranges widely from 'palpable purpura' (which is the absolutely prevalent

Disorders with an obvious linkage with HCV
-mixed cryoglobulinemic vasculitis
-porphyria cutanea tarda
-lichen planus
Other skin diseases described in association with HCV
-pityriasis rubra pilaris
-sarcoidosis
-vitiligo
-cholestatic and non-cholestatic pruritus
-prurigo nodularis
-cutaneous polyarteritis nodosa
-pyoderma gangrenosum
-subacute cuteneous lupus erythematosus
-primary localized cutaneous amyloidosis
-pigmented purpuric dermatosis
-actinic porokeratosis
-pityriasis lichenoide
-generalized granuloma annulare
-disseminated Kaposi's sarcoma
-necrolytic acral erythema

Table 1. Skin manifestations in hepatitis C infection

clinical scenario) [9] to urticarial vasculitis, necrotizing vasculitis, isolated necrotic ulcers, acral ischemias, acrocyanosis, and livedo reticularis (Figure 7 and 8). Of note, even in cases characterized by the highest clinical severity, the skin behaves very often like a sort of 'emuntory system', with poor or absent signs of internal organ involvement. Systemic vasculitis, involving the kidneys, the heart, the central nervous system and other viscera, is in fact unusual. First-line treatment of MC diseases consists of associated pegylated INF-α and ribavirin. In patients who are intolerant to antivirals, or those with severe systemic disease, or those who have failed to reach SVR after antiviral therapy, symptomatic treatment with plasmapheresis, steroids or rituximab should be considered [27].

3.1.2. *Porphyria cutanea tarda*

Porphyria cutanea tarda (PCT) is related to a deficient activity of the heme synthetic enzyme uroporphyrinogen decarboxylase (UROD), which may in turn be sustained by either UROD gene mutations or acquired liver insufficiency [28]. A strong association has been reported between acquired PCT and HCV infection. HCV prevalence in PCT sufferers is significantly higher than that reported in the general population. Prevalence rates range from 17 to 65%, the latter having been reported in Southern Europe [29, 30]. However, HCV alone is not likely to cause the disease, but it is thought to be a strong trigger for the development of deranged porphyrin metabolism in subjects with other known predisposing factors (such as, alcohol abuse or iron overload) [31].

Laboratory diagnosis is based on detection of increased levels of uro-carboxyl porphyrins and heptacarboxyporphyrins in the urine, and on the presence of isocoproporphyrin in the feces. Due to its porphyrin content, the urine of PCT patients is discoloured (chiefly after air and light exposure), while all 'iron tests' are negative. On clinical ground, diagnosis derives from an array of dermatological findings, as follows: vesicular or vesico-bullous swellings on skin sites subjected to even minor actinic and/or mechanic traumas; ensuing eroded areas that take weeks or months to heal; scarred and/or melasma-like hyperpigmented patches; keratin-filled milial cysts; lilac erythematous rash of periorbital areas; hypertrichosis on the lateral aspects of the face; chloracne; skin dystrophic calcifications with ulceration; alopecia; and onycholysis.

3.1.3. Lichen planus

Lichen planus (LP) [32] is an inflammatory immune mediated disease of the skin and/or mucous membranes most commonly affecting middle-aged adults of both sexes, the etiology of which has not yet been fully clarified. The occurrence of the disease in the general population is rare. Prevalence rates of 0.1 to 0.3 have been calculated for cutaneous LP, and of 1.15 to 2.3 for mucous (oral) LP. However, the persisting lack of aim-oriented studies based on standardized methods and criteria results in some uncertainty [33].

Clinically, cutaneous LP is characterized by flat, polygonal, lilac red papules which may remain isolated, or merge into larger plaques (Figure 9 and 10). The rash has an unpredictable duration, from few weeks to several months or years. Lesions may resolve with atrophy, scarring or brownish hyperpigmentation. The flexor aspects of the limbs, the upper back, and the lumbar region are frequently involved, but the disease can spread over the entire body surface. Hair and nails may also be affected. Severe, recalcitrant itch is very common. Mucous LP chiefly affects the mouth and, less frequently, genitalia, conjunctiva, and esophagus. The mucosal lesions consist of erosive erythematous patches (Figure 11), or horny micro-papules arranged in a reticular pattern recalling a lace network (or a sprinkle of lime) (Figures 12 and 13), or a combination of both (Figure 14). The erosive variant is usually accompanied by intense burning sensations.

LP histology is the prototype of a morphological scenario that has traditionally been referred to as "lichenoid tissue reaction/interface dermatitis", in which a band-like mononuclear cell inflammatory infiltrate in the papillary dermis obscuring the dermal-epidermal junction (DEJ) is seen, coupled with more or less pronounced epithelial changes, as follows: hydropic/vacuolar degeneration in the basal cell layer, scanty 'ghost' epithelial cells (*'colloid bodies'*), spongiosis and clefting at the DEJ (*'Max Joseph spaces'*), irregular acanthosis and thickening of the granular layer, dense hyperkeratosis, disappearance of intra-epidermal melanocytes along with melanin 'leakage' into the dermis (*pigmentary incontinence*) (Figure 15).

The pathogenesis of LP has not yet been fully elucidated, however the disease is universally alleged to be an autoimmune disease. The prominence of certain HLA haplotypes (such as, HLA-DR1), or detection of cytokine gene polymorphisms in some case series [34], support a genetic predisposition to the disease. The basal epidermis injury observed in LP is attributed to cytotoxic T lymphocytes, which in fact predominate into the infiltrate along with minor subpopulations of macrophages and dendritic cells. In this context, a significant role of plasmacytoid dendritic cells has been also recognized. In fact, these cellular effectors are viewed as the driving force to the end-stage T cell-mediated epidermal damage, in that they would be able to give rise to an inflammatory type I interferon signaling pathway which, in turn, would amplify and maintain cytotoxic T cell attack to keratinocytes [35]. Cross-reactivity between endogenous and environmental antigens is widely suspected, but the exact nature of the triggering antigen is still obscure. Among the putative exogenous factors involved in LP, one of the most outstanding candidates appears to be HCV. An ample body of biological evidences supporting this view exists in the literature, and has been reviewed in recent years [36, 37]. However, the conclusive proof of the causal linkage between HCV and LP is still lacking. These circumstances have recently led Baccaglini and coworkers [37] to launch somewhat provocatively the subversive hypothesis of a fake association via a 'third factor' consisting of a still unidentified *confounder*.

However, at least on epidemiological grounds, the existence of a 'two-way' association between LP and HCV infection seems currently beyond question worldwide. On these regard, two well-designed meta-analyses have been recently carried out showing that LP sufferers have an odds ratio of being HCV seropositive up to 5.4 times higher compared to controls, and that the risk of having LP is up to 4.47 times higher in HCV patients than in seronegative controls [38, 39]. On the basis of these circumstances, screening for anti-HCV antibodies is substantially advisable in patients with LP, especially in countries with the highest seroprevalence rates. In this regard, it has been suggested that routine HCV testing would be cost-effective in geographical districts in which HCV prevalence is 7% or more [40]. Yet, in the absence of standardized criteria and guidelines, individual case-by-case screening strategies are more suitably recommended [37].

This section is to be concluded by underscoring that *true* cases of idiopathic LP need sometimes to be differentiated from so-called *lichenoid eruptions* (LE), which somehow resemble LP on both clinical and histological grounds [41]. LE are often caused by (and develop at sites of) contact with dental restorative amalgams or stomatological devices, due to their content of methacrylic acid esthers, nickel, mercury, copper and gold [32]. However, LE may be also induced by a huge array of systemic drugs whose number is in steady increase [42], ranging from angiotensin-converting enzyme inhibitors to non-steroidal anti-inflammatory drugs, antimalarials and proton pump inhibitors. The reader should be aware that the list includes the agents employed for treatment HCV infection, interferon and ribavirin [43]. In such occurrences, LE may either be exanthematic, or stay confined to oral mucosa, or just involve the site of interferon injection [43].

3.2. Skin manifestations related To HBV

Both range and frequency of extrahepatic manifestations in patients with HBV infection are considerably lower compared with those observed in HCV infected subjects [44, 45]. A French multicenter, retrospective, cross-sectional study of 190 patients with chronic hepatitis B has rated the overall incidence of clinical and biologic extrahepatic manifestations to be 16% and 15%, respectively [46]. As more specifically regards the skin, vasculitis, psoriasis and pruritus were found to occur in only 1% of cases each. Of note, in striking contrast with HCV populations, in HBV patients cryoglobulinemia and related disease manifestations have been reported in only 2% of cases. Many clinical and laboratory observations have long cast significant doubts on the actual biological relevance of this association. On this regard, literature yields rates up to 15% for cryoglobulin detection in HBV patients, although no signs or symptoms of related vasculitis are observed in the great majority of cases [47].

Both cutaneous and non-cutaneous extrahepatic manifestations of HBV infection have been largely attributed to deposition of circulating immune complexes (IC) containing HBs and/or possibly HBe antigens. Alternatively, induction of local IC formation by viral antigens, interaction between tissue antigens and virus-induced autoantibodies, or direct tissue damage by viral replication have also been invoked. However, this issue remains highly controversial [45, 48, 49].

Cutaneous manifestations of HBV infection (Table 2) are observed both in the incubation, prodromal phase and in chronic state of disease. In the former, a clinical scenario in which intermingled signs of either a mild 'flu-like' or a more serious 'serum sickness-like' syndrome have been described. In this phase, up to 30% of the patients may have fever, weakness, headaches, arthralgias/myalgias, and glomerulonephritis which not infrequently develop in association with varied dermatological manifestations, such as non-specific (toxic) erythema, urticaria, angio-oedema, erythema multiforme, erythema nodosom, Henoch-Schonlein (rheumatoid) purpura, or palpable purpura [44, 45, 50-53]. Other extrahepatic manifestations of HBV infection in which skin involvement is either a prominent feature or an ancillary finding include Gianotti-Crosti syndrome and polyarteritis nodosa, respectively.

3.2.1. Gianotti-crosti syndrome

Gianotti-Crosti syndrome (GCS) [54], also termed 'papular acrodermatitis of childhood', is a peculiar, self-limited and largely asymptomatic skin eruption featuring almost monomorphous papular or papulovesicular lesions located mainly on the face and distal aspects of the four limbs (Figure 16). Mucosal involvement is never described. Histology is noncontributory, with upper dermis perivascular round cellular infiltrates and endothelial swelling as the prevailing findings. Children aged from a few months to 15 years (with a peak between 1 and 6 years) are mostly involved, but adults (of note, only females) may be also affected. Spontaneous recovery usually occurs within 25 to 45 days. Systemic findings, which are observed rarely, include malaise, fever or diarrhea. Limited lymphadenopathy, splenomegaly and hepatomegaly are sometimes detected. When present, hepatitis is usually anicteric. Originally described as in strict conjunction with sole HBV infection, GCS has been subsequently linked to an array of infectious agents, including other viruses (such as, HAV, CMV and EBV) and bacteria (such as, Borrelia burgdorferi and β-hemolytic streptococci). Neither viral bodies nor viral antigens have ever been demonstrated in the context of skin lesions, and the pathogenesis of GCS remains largely unclear. Current views on the issue span from a role of immune complex deposition to occurrence of virus-related delayed hypersensitivity reactions. Furthermore, an association between immunization and GCS has long been outlined, with anti-HBV and anti-HAV vaccinations being included in the list of triggering factors [54-57]. Remarkably, it has been proposed that occurrence of GCS after the first vaccine administration does not contraindicate completion of the immunization protocol, as GCS does not recur after the subsequent boostering injections [55]. Finally, in addition to that with GCS, an association has also been reported between HBV infection and a much rarer, but equally peculiar skin eruption involving the extremities, i.e. so-called 'papular-purpuric gloves and socks syndrome', in which a triggering role of HBV (along with other infections such as measles, parvovirus B19, coxsakie B6 and cytomegalovirus) has been assumed [58].

3.2.2. Polyarteritis nodosa

Recognition of a strong linkage between HBV and polyarteritis nodosa (PAN) dates back to the 1970s. Rates of prevalence of positive HBV serologies have been estimated up to 50% among PAN patients. However, these figures have decreased significantly over the last four decades, and are currently less than 5% [45]. A major role in this respect must have been played by improved blood transfusion safety measures, other general hygiene precautions and extensive vaccination campaigns. The pathogenesis has largely been attributed to deposition of immune complexes containing HBsAg. Of note, unlike other forms of PAN, in HBV-related PAN serum antineutrophilic cytoplasmic antibodies (ANCA) are only exceptionally detected. Histologically, PAN is characterized by transmural, usually segmental, necrotizing infiltration of medium-to-small vessels resulting in ischaemia, infarcts and haemorrhage, which ultimately lead to end-organ damage. If untreated, the course of PAN is often protracted, and symptoms and signs of multi-organ involvement are generally observed. Organs more commonly affected are kidneys, heart, gut and peripheral nerves. Cutaneous PAN has also been reported in 10 to 50% of cases, depending on the case series examined. Livedo reticularis and painful subcutaneous nodules (usually along the arteries of the lower limbs) are commonly described. Nodules ulceration and distal gangrene are frequent findings as well [44, 59, 60].

Further anecdotal reports of skin disorders observed in conjunction with HBV infection include acanthosis nigricans [61] and generalized granuloma annulare [62]. Finally, the association with lichen planus (LP), which is now undisputed in HCV infection, is instead highly controversial in HBV carriers. A number of earlier studies have provided some support for this view, but such biological alliance has more recently received repeated confutations [63, 64] and is currently considered unfounded.

3.2.3. Skin unfavorable effects of HBV immunization

Hepatitis B vaccination may also be hazardous for the skin. In this respect, the following dermatological undesired manifestations have been reported: erythema nodosum [65], generalized granuloma annulare [66], Gianotti-Crosti syndrome [54, 56, 67], cutaneous

-urticaria
-angio-oedema
-non-specific (toxic) erythema
-erythema multiforme commonly observed in the prodromal phase of infection
-erythema nodosom
-Henoch-Schonlein purpura
-palpable purpura
-Gianotti-Crosti syndrome ('papular acrodermatitis of childhood')
-polyarteritis nodosa
-acanthosis nigricans
-generalized granuloma annulare
-lichen planus (highly controversial)

Table 2. Skin manifestations in hepatitis B infection

polyarteritis nodosa [68] and pityriasis rosea-like rash [68], lichen planus [69], lichenoid and pseudolymphomatous reactions confined to site of injection [70], and generalized pseudo-lymphomatous reactions [71].

3.3. Skin manifestations related to HAV

Apart from the 'paradigm' of jaundice, HAV infection is very occasionally linked to significant cutaneous side-events. Few reports have been made of urticaria, purpura or other exanthemas [72]. A case of Henoch-Schönlein purpura has been described after immunization [73].

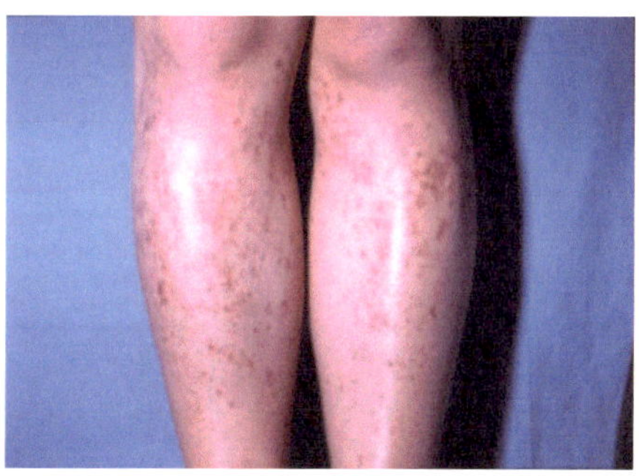

Figure 7. Palpable purpura

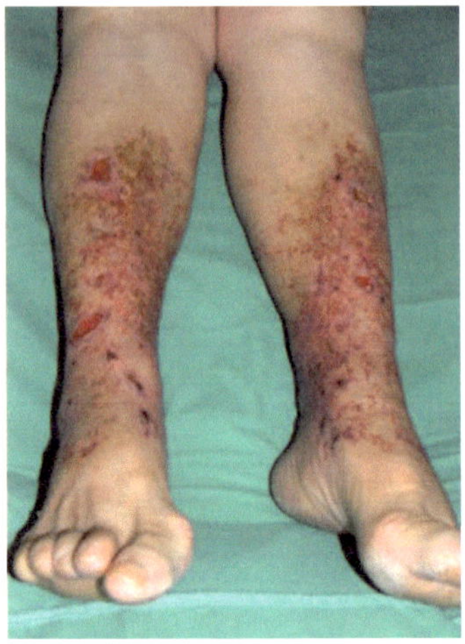

Figure 8. Nodular, necrotic vasculitis

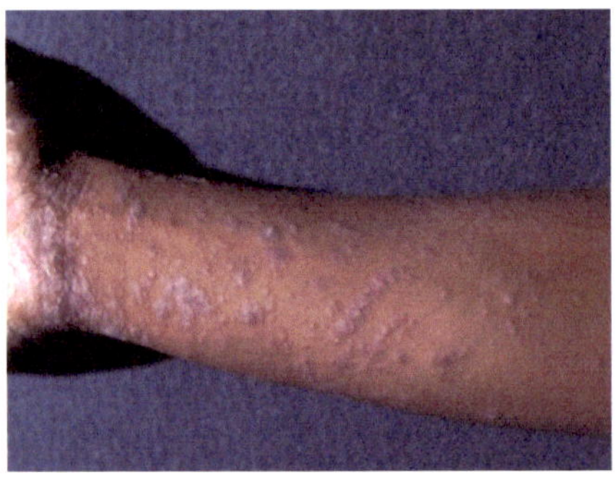

Figure 9. Cutaneous lichen planus (LP): flat, polygonal, lilac red-coloured pruritic papules (Courtesy of Professor M. Lomuto, Bari, Italy)

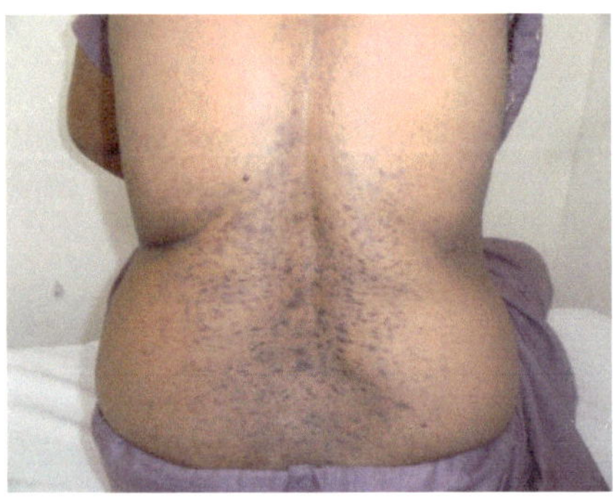

Figure 10. Cutaneous LP (Courtesy of Professor A. J. Kanwar, Chandigarh, India)

http://dx.doi.org/10.5772/56140

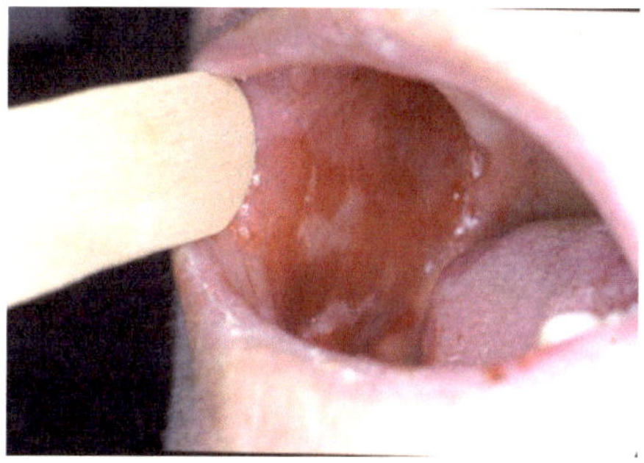

Figure 11. Mucous LP: erosive variant (Courtesy of Professor M. Lomuto, Bari, Italy)

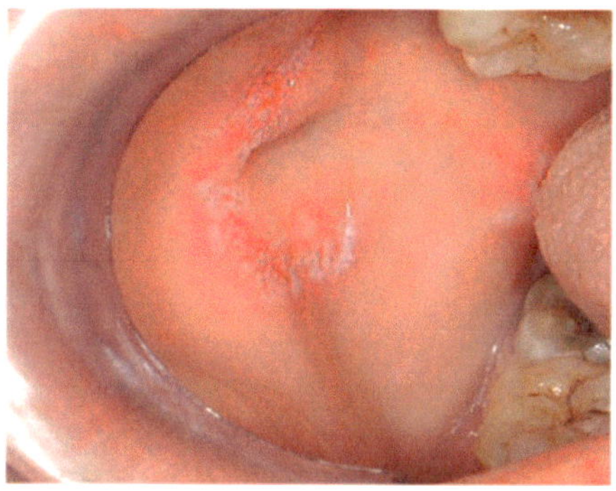

Figure 12. Mucous LP: papular, hyperkeratotic variant ('lace network' pattern) (Courtesy of Professor M. Lo Muzio, Foggia, Italy)

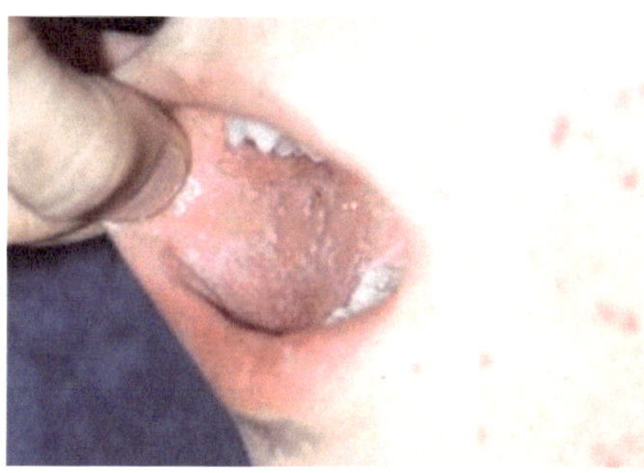

Figure 13. Mucous LP: papular, hyperkeratotic variant ('sprinkle of lime' pattern) (Courtesy of Professor E. Bonifazi, Bari, Italy)

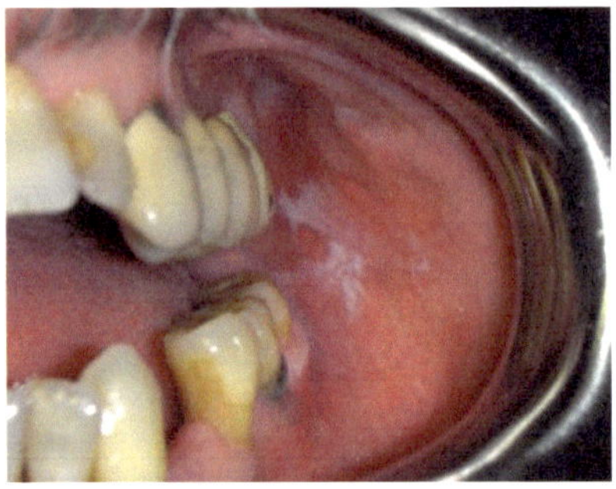

Figure 14. Mucous LP: mixed type, with a combination of erosive and hyperkeratotic lesions (Courtesy of Professor M. Lo Muzio, Foggia, Italy)

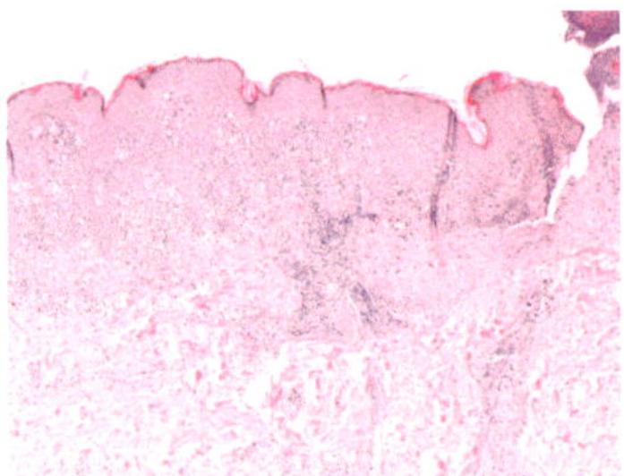

Figure 15. Histological picture of LP: a fully developed prototype of so-called "lichenoid tissue reaction/interface dermatitis" (Courtesy of Professor P. Bufo, Foggia, Italy)

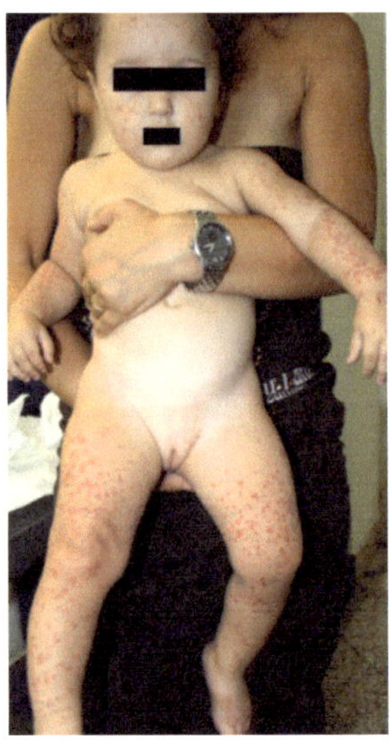

Figure 16. Gianotti-Crosti syndrome ('papular acrodermatitis of childhood') (Courtesy of Professor E. Bonifazi, Bari, Italy)

http://dx.doi.org/10.5772/56140

4. Skin manifestations associated with treatment of viral liver disease

4.1. Skin adverse effects related to 'standard of care' treatment of chronic HCV infection

The 'fingerprint detector' effect

The combination of pegylated interferon α (PEG-INF) and ribavirin (RBV), which is the current 'standard of care' (SOC) in the management of chronic HCV infection, has significantly improved the treatment outcome. Due to the side effect profile of both drugs, a considerable number of chronic hepatitis C patients are ineligible for PEG-INF/RBV-based treatment because of medical contraindications. Moreover, vast rates of patients are unable to tolerate antiviral therapy, and account for nearly 10% of premature treatment discontinuations [74, 75].

More specifically regarding skin adverse events (AEs), in a recent large-scale prospective study of 2871 Japanese patients, dermatologic undesired manifestations were the third most common reason for therapy withdrawal [75]. INF alone may give raise to a wide variety of cutaneous AEs, the frequency of which has been estimated from 13 to 23%, and the association with RBV has led to an increased incidence of skin AEs compared to those observed during INF monotherapy era [75-80]. Cutaneous AEs related to SOC treatment may be divided into three major groups: local reactions occurring at INF injection sites (Figure 17); non-local or generalized reactions; and signs of hypothyroidism caused by INF-induced autoimmune thyroiditis (Table 3). Local reactions are more consistently ascribable to the action of INF alone. By contrast, not local or generalized manifestations have to be linked to both agents, considering that the modes of action of INF and RBV are rather intermingled and their individual contribution seem thus quite undistinguishable. As shown in the table, a long array of cutaneous manifestations have been observed. Some reports are almost anecdotal, while the *triad* pruritus, skin xerosis and eczematous lesions are the principal hallmark of 'hepatitis C treatment-associated dermatitis' according to an in-depth review recently carried out by Lübbe and coworkers [81]. *Xerosis* is customarily spread over the entire body surface. *Pruritus* is also generalized, and is not rarely refractory to standard antihistamine agents. *Eczema*, which mainly affects the extensor aspects of limbs and sites exposed to friction (Figure 18 and 19), has been reported to sometimes take the appearance of so-called 'nummular' (discoid) eczema (Figure 20 and 21 or prurigo nodularis (Figure 22).

As regards 'eczema', an extensive discussion of the vast archipelago of disease conditions which are currently collected under such term in the dermatological literature [82] is beyond the scope of the present textbook. However, a brief digression on the matter will perhaps be useful to the reader. Clinically, along with variable degrees of itching and soreness, eczematous dermatoses display a variety of signs which range from acute to chronic forms as follow: erythema, vesiculation, exudation, excoriation, fissuring, dryness, scaling, hyperkeratosis, papulation and lichenification (Figure 23.A to -C). Accordingly, histological hallmarks vary from epidermal oedema ('spongiosis'), thickening of spinous and horny layers ('acanthosis' and 'hyperkeratosis', respectively) and more or less dense round cell infiltrates in the dermis. The simplest classification framework of eczemas implies division into two forms, i.e. exogenous and endogenous. Exogenous forms (also referred to as 'contact dermatitis') result from direct exposure of the skin surface to toxic agents ('irritant contact dermatitis') or allergens ('allergic contact dermatitis'). Cell-mediated (not humoral), 'delayed'-type hypersensitivity is involved in the latter. As a counterpart, in the endogenous forms all the other forms of eczema (ranging from atopic eczema to so-called *discoid* or *nummular* eczema) which are not attributable to any recognizable contact offender, and whose pathomechanisms still remain largely obscure are to be included.

Interferon-related injection site (local) reactions
-ill-defined, roundish, pruritic, self-recovering erythematous patches (Figure 17)
-vesico-bullous rashes
-Skin necrosis
-Dermal mucinosis
-Sarcoidosis
-Foreign body granulomatous reaction
-Lichen planus
-Patchy hypermelanosis
-Vasculitis
-Vitiligo
-Alopecia
Non local, or generalized reactions
-Generalized pruritus
-Skin xerosis
-Eczema
-Generalized nummular eczema
-Prurigo-like eruptions
-Meyerson's phenomenon ('halo dermatitis') around melanocytic naevi
-Fixed drug eruption
-Nonspecific erythematous or maculopapular exanthemas
-Nonspecific 'acantholytic dermatitis'
-Grover's disease
-Dry pulpitis and fissured fingers
-Vitiligo
-Sarcoidosis
-Tongue hyperpigmentation
-Psoriasiform drug eruptions
-Psoriasis (triggered or worsened)
-Lichen planus (triggered or worsened) and other lichenoid eruptions

-Cryoglobulinemic vasculitis (worsened)
-Leukocytoclastic vasculitis
-Pyoderma gangrenosum
-Polyarteritis nodosa
-Dermatitis herpetiformis and/or other gluten hypersensitivity states
-Rosacea fulminans
-Systemic lupus erythematosus
-Systemic sclerosis
-Alopecia areata and universalis
-Dystrophic alopecia and diffuse thinning of the hair
-Diffuse or localized hypertrichosis
-Hair curling
-Hair repigmentation
-Eyebrow and eyelash
Skin and hair signs of hypothyroidism caused by INF-induced autoimmune thyroiditis
-diffuse skin hyperkeratotic thickening
-scalp and body hair dryness and coarseness
-diffuse loss of scalp hair
-slow growth, dystrophy and atrophy of nails
-skin pallor
-carotenemia with skin yellowing (more prominently, on the palms, soles, and in the nasolabial folds)
-impaired wound healing
-petechial purpuric patches

References cited in this table are partly compiled from the works of Cacoub and coworkers [78], Mistry and coworkers [77], Lübbe and coworkers [81], and Jadali [89].

Table 3. Cutaneous adverse events reported under INF *plus* RBV treatment of patients with chronic HCV infection

The *'fingerprint detector'* effect - According to what has been said above, eczematous manifestations occurring during treatment for HCV infection may be classified as 'endogenous'. This seems appropriate also considering that no data are currently available in the literature concerning possible past history of delayed-type hypersensitivity conditions or present skin reactivity to standard contact allergen series in patients developing eczema under treatment for HCV infection. In this context, it might be hypothesized that the combination of INF and RBV acts as a sort of 'fingerprint detector' over the skin surface being able to unmask and trigger reactivation of clones of skin-resident T cells that could have been primed at any time in the past via indeterminable antigenic challenges, without ever exceeding the threshold which could have given rise to overt clinical manifestations. Indeed, the skin is the outermost barrier against a huge number of environmental threats, including chemical and infectious agents. So that the magnitude of immune host defense reactions taking place at any moment in the skin are immeasurable. Since its first description by Streiler in 1989 [83], the so-called 'skin-associated lymphoid tissue' has acquired an ever-increasing number of immunological prerogatives, including the capacity of keratinocytes (an ectodermal cell lineage), in concert with Langerhans cells and dermal dendritic cells, to play a role in antigen-presenting processes and, additionally, to prime naïve skin-reactive T cells directly [84]. Thus, some evidence has been provided to look at the skin as a true lymphoid organ in its ability to mount an immune response framework within its own milieu. Yet, there is still insufficient information on biological mechanisms driving leukocyte migration and homing to target tissues in immune responses and inflammation [85]. However, the hypothesis that memory CD8 T cells are able to persist as a stable, 'dormant' population in the skin after specific priming has taken place, has received authoritative confirmations from studies performed on both lichen planus (Figure 9 to 14) [86] and fixed drug eruption (Figure 24) [87], two prototypes of a vast group of skin conditions (comprehensively referred to as 'lichenoid tissue reaction/interface dermatitis') in which a common role of antigen presenting cell-mediated type I intereferon signaling has been assumed [35]. Taken as a whole, all these data might provide the key to at least theoretically closing the pathogenetic loop linking treatment and occurrence of the otherwise clinically 'no sense' eczematous rashes in patients with HCV infection. However, a body of evidence which is strict enough to fully clarify the exact mechanisms underlying eczema and each of the many other skin AEs (Table 3) attributed to PEG-INF/RBV is still lacking. Yet, one might consider that notwithstanding the specific clinical and histological characteristics exhibited by each of the skin unfavorable events observed, many of them show a mixed type III and IV hypersensitivity reaction pattern in which Th-1 shifted inflammatory clones are likely to drive the inflammatory process. In such an immunopathogenetic framework, both the well-known proinflammatory properties of interferon and the multifaceted immune enhancing effects exerted by ribavirin on Th-1 cell mediated processes [88], may well intervene by worsening the course of pre-existing conditions, or triggering the new onset of diseases in subjects who would otherwise be unaffected clinically.

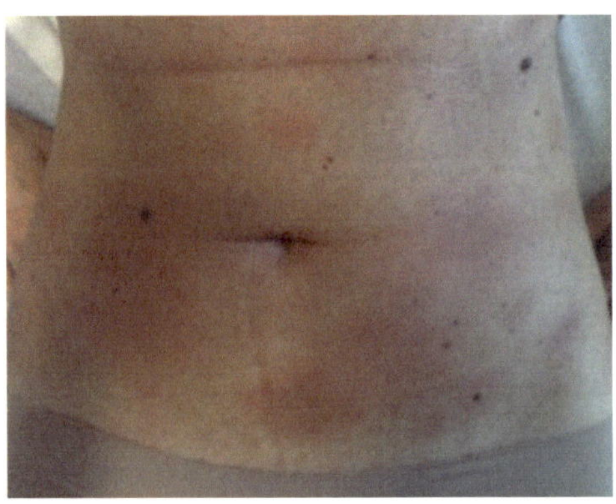

Figure 17. Erythematous patches at the site of injection of INF

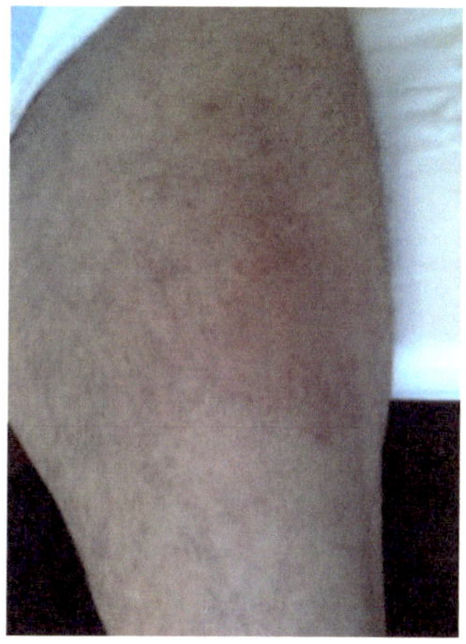

Figure 18. Vague eczematous patches on the extensor aspects of the limbs

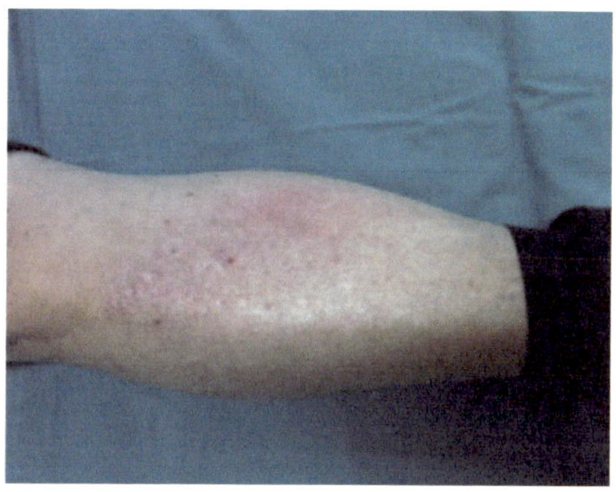

Figure 19. Eczema involving areas exposed to friction

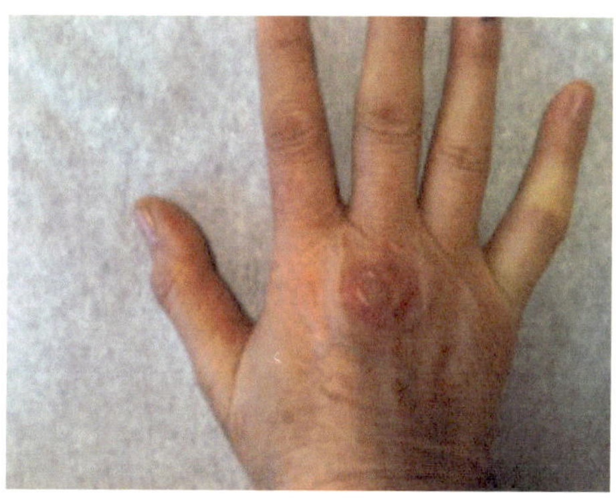

Figure 20. A 'coin' shaped, sharply demarcated eczematous lesion (*nummular eczema*)

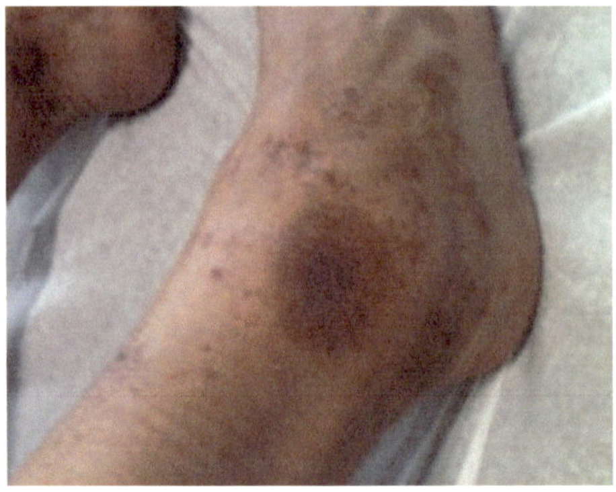

Figure 21. Nummular eczema: dyschromic sequelae

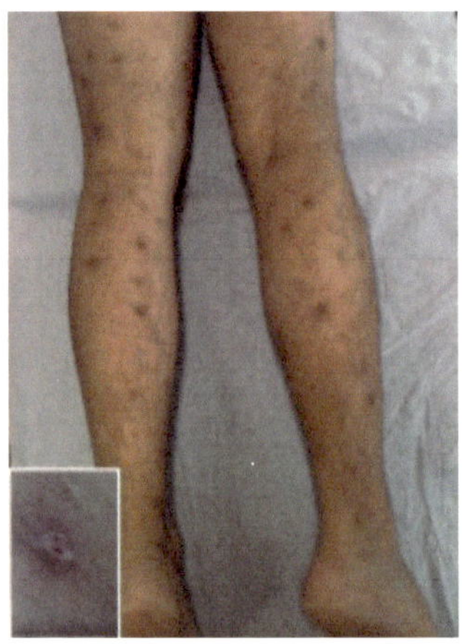

Figure 22. Prurigo nodularis - Bottom left corner: closeup of an excoriated nodule

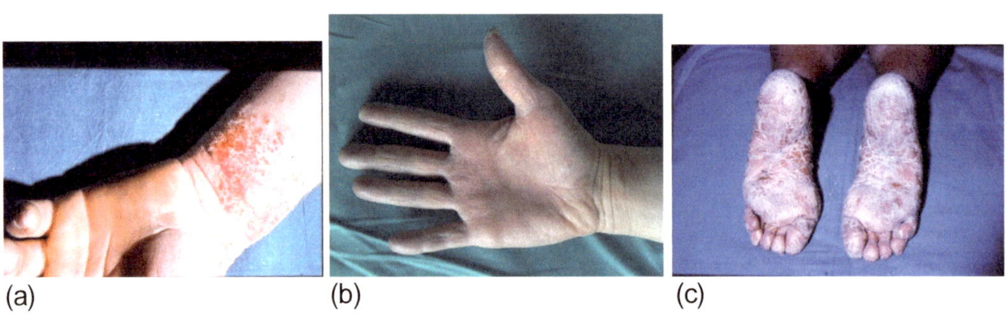

Figure 23. Clinical grading of eczema: A, acute; B, subacute; C, chronic

http://dx.doi.org/10.5772/56140

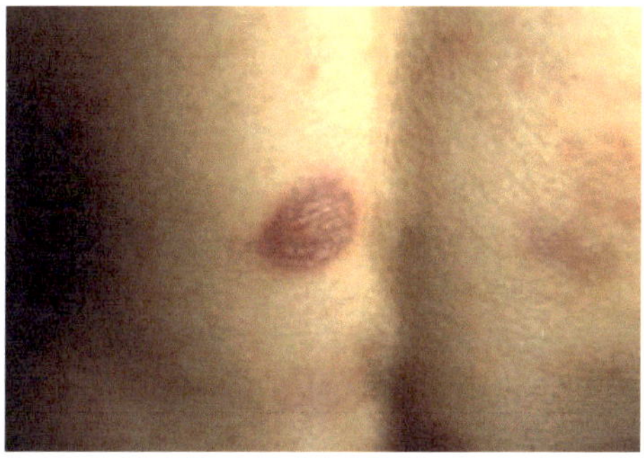

Figure 24. Fixed drug eruption (Courtesy of Doctor R. Pellicano, San Giovanni Rotondo, Italy)

4.2. Skin adverse effects related to newly developed agents for treatment of chronic HCV infection

'*Telaprevir dermatitis*': what are we dealing with?

The recent introduction of the NS3/4A protease inhibitors telaprevir and boceprevir, the first direct-acting antiviral agents (DAAs) approved for treatment of chronic infection with genotype 1 HCV in conjunction with PEG-INF and RBV, has led to increased viral response rates. Although PEG-INF plus RBV are still responsible for the majority of adverse effects related to 'triple therapy', DAA have been reported to induce exacerbation of traditional adverse events and development of new undesired occurrences.

As more specifically regards skin unfavorable manifestations, telaprevir seems to play a major role. Pruritus, independent of, or associated with skin manifestations are in fact the most significant cutaneous AEs [78, 90]. The analysis of the safety profile exhibited by telaprevir in the phase 1 to 3 studies available in the literature has yielded the almost invariable finding of consistently increased frequency rates of skin rashes appearing during telaprevir treatment phases compared with those occurring under SOC regimens. Rashes of any severity have been in fact reported in 36 to 82% of patients [90-93], and seemed to be virtually indistinguishable from the PEG-IFN/RBV-related rashes, having 'dry skin', 'pruritus' and 'eczema' as prominent features. It has also been noted that some rashes were of greater severity and occurred on a larger body surface area (BSA), but in the vast majority of cases the BSA 30% limit was not exceeded. Of note, these rashes have been reported to largely occur during the first weeks of treatment and recover after telaprevir withdrawal.

Some efforts have recently been made to conceive strategy protocols of early intervention to minimize treatment-linked AEs. As for skin AEs, in the trials carried out by Jacobson and coworkers [94] and Zeuzem and coworkers [95] a 'rash management plan' was established and the intensity of rash was accordingly graded as *grade 1* (mild, localized to one or several sites); *grade 2* (moderate, with a diffuse skin eruption involving up to 50% of the body surface); and *grade 3* (severe, involving more than 50% of the body surface, or rash with the appearance of substantial systemic signs or symptoms). In patients with a progressive grade 2 rash, or any grade 3 rash telaprevir administration was stopped, while continuing PEG-INF/RBV treatment. In case of worsening of the rash within the subsequent 7 days, RBV (and possibly PEG-INF) was to be discontinued as well (Table 4.A) [94, 95].

Severe rashes were observed in only 3-7% of patients, with some cases featuring Stevens-Johnson syndrome, toxic epidermal necrolysis, acute generalized exanthematous pustulosis, or 'drug rash with eosinophilia and systemic symptoms' (DRESS) syndromes. As a whole, however, only in 4-7% of subjects enrolled in clinical trials was telaprevir discontinued owing to skin rash. The absolute majority of skin rashes were instead *mild* to *moderate*, and were quite easily controlled through oral anti-histamines, topical emollients and/or high-to-mean potency steroid ointments [96].

There is a great number of reports concerning prevalence of and clinical warnings raised by telaprevir-induced dermatologic manifestations. However, to the best of my knowledge, no evidence is yet available in the literature giving '*telaprevir dermatitis*' some taxonomical profiling at least on morphological grounds. At the time of this writing, those of Cacoub and coworkers [78], Dupin and coworkers [97], Kumada and coworkers [93] and Awwad and coworkers [98] are the sole papers in the literature reporting some iconography of telaprevir-related dermatological AEs. Skin lesions are almost invariably and vaguely referred to as 'primarily eczematous' or 'maculopapular', and, as such, indeed appear to be rather indiscernible from those allegedly linked to PEG-INF/RBV. No or little information is available on cases that are 'not eczematous'. Could they be alternatively urticarial, dermographical, or polymorphic? When the rash is 'eczematous', are the skin lesions haphazard or symmetrical? Had any of these eczematous patients a history of delayed-type hypersensitivity and/or was he subsequently skin tested? Related to these circumstances, one should consider that the clinical grading of skin AEs (as described above), and thus the possibility of driving decision-making algorithms, currently lie on the need to assess severity of the skin rash through criteria that are not strict enough to prevent some unpredictable levels of intra- and inter-observer variability. In this respect, one may consider the rather significant differences existing in 'rash management strategies' conceived by different research groups (see Table 4.A and 4.B for comparison). Consequently, extensive dermatologist-oriented surveys are still warranted to better define the clinical edges (if any) of '*telaprevir dermatitis*' and possibly shed new light on the pathophysiology of such largely unexplained occurrences.

The same insufficiencies observed in morphological assessment of AEs related to telaprevir also involve studies carried out with other DAAs, which seem however to bear an overall lower potential of inducing dermatological unfavorable manifestations compared to the former. In this regard, in two recent phase 3 trials [99, 100] in which boceprevir was administered in combination with PEG-INF plus RBV for up to 44 weeks after a 4-week 'lead-in' phase with SOC agents, skin AEs (such as, 'rash' and 'dry skin') were observed in consistently lower rates of patients compared to telaprevir studies, and in no case were they the reason for pre-term discontinuation of treatment. Interestingly, in the trial involving naïve subjects [99], frequency of 'pruritus', 'rash' and 'dry skin' were found to be not significantly different between SOC and boceprevir groups. Instead, in the trial involving non-naïve subjects [100], 'rash' and 'dry skin' were reported in up to 17 and 22% of patients, respectively, and between-arm differences with respect to this were found to be significant. Reasons for the above discordances appear definitely obscure.

Concerning possible reasons for the striking differences observed between telaprevir and boceprevir in terms of cutaneous (and noncutaneous) pathogeneticy, the obviously different chemical structures of the two agents may well account for most of *intrinsic* differences in specific harmful potentials. However the different treatment protocols applied (telaprevir associated with SOC agents at the beginning of the trial period, while boceprevir started only after a lead-in phase of SOC alone) could also be taken into consideration as being able to influence type and severity of undesired complaints. Particularly regarding skin AEs, one might speculate that PEG-INF and RBV, being delivered in association with telaprevir from the beginning of the trial, act as 'proinflammatory boosters' by virtue of their multifarious immunomodulating actions which would be able to create a sort of synergy with telaprevir noxious capacity.

As for other developing DAAs, the protease inhibitor BI 201335 has also to be considered. A small trial enrolling 53 chronic HCV genotype-1 patients (34 treatment-naïve and 19 treatment-experienced subjects) evaluated efficacy and safety profiles of 'multiple rising dose' regimens of BI 201335 in the short-term (4 weeks) [101]. In this study, no skin AEs during therapy with BI 201335 alone were reported. 'Mild rash or photosensitivity' was observed only in four patients during combined treatment with SOC agents, but in no case did this cause pre-term treatment discontinuation. It should additionally be reported that, according to interim (12 weeks) outcome analyses of an earlier study of BI 201335 with PegIFN/RBV in 288 patients in the long-term (24 weeks) [102], 'mostly mild to moderate rash and photosensitivity reactions' were referred to as the most frequent adverse events, along with gastrointestinal disorders. 'Severe rash' was observed in 0.7-1.3% of subjects receiving daily BI 201335 doses of 240mg, while this rate increased up to 5.7% in patients undergoing daily doses of 480 mg. Finally, in a phase 1b open-label trial, 34 treatment-naïve patients with chronic HCV-1 infection were randomized to receive an association of the polymerase inhibitor BI 207127 (400 to 600 mg 3 times daily) and BI 201335 (120 mg once daily) plus RBV (1000 to 1200 mg per day) for 4 weeks [103]. In this study a 'rash management plan' was established and the intensity of skin AEs was accordingly graded as *mild* (localized), *moderate* (diffuse, 30% to 70% body surface area), or *severe* (diffuse generalized, mucous membrane involvement, organ dysfunction, signs of anaphylaxis, or life threatening). A part from mild gastrointestinal disorders (diarrhea, nausea, vomiting), a mild 'rash or photosensitivity reaction' was observed in 42% of subjects receiving the highest daily dosages. Yet, due to drug overlap within the treatment regimens, it was not possible to ascribe any of these AEs to an individual compound. Nevertheless, no *severe* AEs were observed, and no AE-related preterm discontinuation of treatment occurred throughout the study period.

Rash severity	Description	Early intervention strategy protocol
Grade 1	*mild*, localized to one or several sites	Stable *mild/moderate* rash → Medical management performed at the discretion of the investigator
Grade 2	*moderate*, with a diffuse skin eruption involving up to 50% of the body surface	
Grade 3	*severe*, involving more than 50% of the body surface, or rash with the appearance of substantial systemic signs or symptoms	Progressive *moderate* rash, or *severe* rash → telaprevir discontinued ↓ Rash not improving within 7 days → RBV ± PEG-INF discontinued (suggested)

Table 4.A Telaprevir - Skin AEs severity scale and rash management plan according with Jacobson et al [94] and Zeuzem et al [95]

Rash severity	Description	Early intervention strategy protocol
Grade 1	Localized skin lesions	Routine, non specific management
Grade 2	Diffuse or multiple skin lesions	
Grade 3	Skin lesions covering >50% of the body surface or rashes with some characteristics such as bullae, ulceration of mucous membrane, epidermal detachment detachment, target lesion or significant systemic signs	Telaprevir discontinued PEG-IFN and RBV reduced or discontinued, as required Dermatologists' consultation for diagnosis and specific cares
Grade 4	Stevens–Johnson syndrome and drug rashes with eosinophilia and systemic symptoms (DRESS)	

Table 4.B Telaprevir - Skin AEs severity scale and rash management plan according with Kumada et al [93]

4.3. Skin adverse effects related to treatment of HBV infection

Current mainstays of treatment for HBV infection are interferon (INF) and nucleotide/nucleoside analogues (NAs), which are used following standardized guidelines in both 'first line, definite duration' and 'long-term, indefinite duration' protocols [104]. Considering, on one hand, the high diffusion of HBV infection in the general population [105] and the significant amounts of these agents that must have been, and are delivered worldwide accordingly, and on the other hand, the vast arrays of skin unfavorable manifestations observed under treatment for HCV infection (see above paragraph), the substantial paucity in the literature of systematic reviews or clinical reports on cutaneous side effects occurring in association with HBV treatment is somewhat surprising. The difference will be evident at a glance by comparing

Table 3 and 5. One may confidently infer that NAs are overall biologically inert within the 'skin milieu', but interferon does remain a shared weapon in the treatment of both viral agents, and has been the backbone tool in the management of HBV infection for many years before the advent of NAs. Differences in the prevalence rates of HBV and HCV infection worldwide, or mere underreporting could be well invoked in this respect. Yet, a possible explanation of such striking divergence between INF impact on the skin of patients with HBV and HCV infection could also lie in the more faithful hepatotropism of HBV compared to HCV. The latter has indeed been found in many tissue other than liver [106, 107], skin included [108, 109]. These circumstances might suggest a possible (yet indeterminable) synergy in skin pathogenicity between INF and HCV, which could play some direct role in local promotion of INF-related skin untoward manifestations in HCV but not in HBV patients. Another explanatory hypothesis could lie on the unique capacity of HCV (not ascribed to HBV) to induce B cell lymphoproliferation and trigger a number of autoimmune processes.

4.3.1. Skin events related to INF

Apart from the almost invariable occurrence of an erythematous roundish plaque at the injection site (Figure 17), administration of INF in HBV patients has been implicated in the following undesired effects (Table 5): skin necrosis at the injection site [110], angioedema-urticaria syndrome [111], diffuse patchy erythematous rash [112], morbilliform exanthema [113], psoriasis [114, 115], vitiligo [115], lichen planus [116], ocular trichomegaly [117].

4.3.2. Skin events related to NAs

The potential exhibited by these agents to sustain any skin pathogenicity appears to be overall contained. Not better specified 'rash and/or anaphylaxis' have been recently assumed to be 'infrequent' [$1/10^3$ to $1/10^4$: tenofovir), 'common' [1/10 to $1/10^2$: lamivudine, telbivudine and adefovir) or 'with unknown frequency' (entecavir) [104]. Reports on NAs-related skin untoward effects are quite scanty in the literature. Lamivudine has been reported in relation with an ichthyosiform eruption in a patient with chronic HBV infection [118]. Clinical and histological iconography is also available of a severe, diffuse eczematous rash observed in an additional case of HBV infection in a Korean-language paper [119]. Reports of other skin AEs related to lamivudine refer to subject with HIV infection [120]. Entecavir has been reported to cause a diffuse maculopapular rash in one HBV patient [121] and an 'immediate allergy' erythematous eruption in an additional HBV patient [122]. Tenofovir has been implicated in development of a maculopapular rash on the face, extremities and trunk observed in HIV patients [123]. Adefovir has been found to trigger a case of Stevens-Johnson/toxic epidermal necrolysis overlap syndrome in a patient with HBV infection [124].

5. Virus-related liver hazards related to treatment of skin diseases

Treatment of a wide variety of skin inflammatory, immune mediated disorders poses a concrete risk for hepatic disease and toxicity. Possible undesired liver injuries are constantly a significant limitation in case management with a great number of pharmaceutical agents.

Injection site (local) reactions
-ill-defined, roundish, pruritic, self-recovering erythematous patches (figure 17)
-skin necrosis
Non local, or generalized reactions
-angioedema-urticaria syndrome
-diffuse patchy erythematous rash
-morbilliform exanthema
-psoriasis
-vitiligo
-lichen planus
-ocular trichomegaly
A – related to INF
Lamivudine:
-ichthyosiform eruption
-severe, diffuse eczematous rash
Entecavir:
-diffuse maculopapular rash
-erythematous eruption
Adefovir:
-Stevens-Johnson/toxic epidermal necrolysis overlap syndrome
B – related to NAs

Table 5. Skin adverse effects under treatment of HBV infection

Hepatotoxicity can derive directly from many drugs used in the treatment of psoriasis, such as methotrexate, ciclosporin or retinoids. Potential hazards may also indirectly result from drugs used to contrast unfavorable complications of dermatological treatment regimens, such as reactivated tuberculosis necessitating isoniazid or rifampicin administration. Also, unsurveyed administration of immunomodulating/immunosuppressive agents, ranging from corticosteroids to TNF- α antagonists, may be also associated with exacerbation of an underlying chronic viral hepatitis [125-127].

An in-depth analysis of all skin disorders the treatment of which may result in liver injury is certainly beyond the scope of this chapter. Instead, I will only concisely focus on systemic therapy of moderate-to-severe psoriasis (Table 6), in view of the fact that psoriasis is the leading item in cutaneous immune mediated pathology affecting 1 to 3% of population in Western industrialized countries [128]. Notably, it has been estimated that more than 11 million people suffer from psoriasis in Europe [129, 130]. Severity of psoriasis is 'quantitatively' assessed through so-called 'psoriasis area-and-severity index' (PASI), whose score ranges from 0 to 72 (with higher scores indicating more severe disease). Overall, patients with PASI scores of 12 or higher are candidates to systemic treatment. Yet, the magnitude of disease severity is also to be evaluated 'qualitatively', considering that the skin condition may often lead to substantial burden in terms of disability and psychosocial stigmatization (I believe that the reader will readily agree on this view after taking a look at figures 25.A to -D). In this regard, it has been calculated that impairment of physical and mental functioning in psoriatic patients is not consistently different from that observed in subjects with major medical illnesses, such as cancer, heart disease, chronic respiratory disease or type 2 diabetes [131]. Also, it should be underlined that a striking discrepancy between the objective 'weight' of the disease on clinical ground and the patients' subjective appraisal of the skin problem 'dimension' often exists [132]. The degree of patient dissatisfaction with treatment outcome is frequently high, and significant levels of intentional noncompliance with prescribed regimens are not uncommon accordingly [133].

Huge numbers of patients with psoriasis undergo systemic treatment, and thus are subject to some risk of undesired liver injury. In this context, the possibility of reactivation of chronic hepatitis B and C is of significant concern. As for Europe, the recently audited 'European S3-Guidelines on the systemic treatment of psoriasis vulgaris' [134] reflect a high level of physician awareness about this risk. 'Active chronic hepatitis B' and 'hepatitis C', respectively, are listed as absolute and relative contraindications on use of many systemic treatments. Accordingly, pre-treatment necessary measures include HBV/HCV serology and liver function tests. Liver enzymes are also to be evaluated throughout the treatment period at regular intervals. Moreover, some caveats concerning the use of anti-TNFα biologic agents (such as infliximab, etanercept, alefacept, efalizumab) in chronic carriers of HBV and HCV have been explicitly expressed [134]. Pre-treatment or concomitant use of antiviral agents has been assumed to allow systemic treatment use in some trials involving non-dermatological (Crohn's disease) patients, with no reports of viral reactivation under high potency regimens [135]. Co-administration of lamivudine has also been considered in the management of HBsAg carrier psoriatic patients [136, 137]. However, concerns are raised by the recognized risk of viral resistance development and acute disease flare occurrence after prolonged use of lamivudine. Thus, more studies are warranted to reliably assess whether antiviral prophylaxis is a viable option in the management of chronic inflammatory conditions.

5.1. Safety profile of traditional ('nonbiologic') and anti-TNFα ('biologic') agents in viral hepatitis patients

First, it must be strongly emphasized that reliable assessment of the safety profile of systemic agents employed in the treatment of moderate-to-severe psoriasis is inherently biased by many factors. Available information from randomized trials is often poor owing to low sample size and insufficient power to ascertain safety outcome conclusively [138]. Furthermore, clinical trials typically involve healthy patients or, at least, not 'difficult-to-treat' cases. In this regard, an inadequate representation in case populations of subjects with some relevant covariates, such as pediatric or elderly age, pregnancy or breastfeeding, history of kidney or liver disease, cancer, HIV, HBV and HCV infection, has been consistently documented [139-141]. Taken as a whole, these circumstances dictate extreme caution in extrapolating results to the broader population of patients in day-to-day clinical practice.

5.1.1. HBV setting

Many papers can be found in the literature reporting TNFα inhibitors to worsen chronic HBV disease in subjects suffering from noncutaneous diseases, such as rheumatic conditions or Crohn's disease [142-144]. Instead, I found only one case concerning a patient with psoriasis vulgaris and psoriatic arthropathy caused by adalimumab [126]. An additional case, related to infliximab, was reported in the results of a questionnaire-based survey involving a nation-wide sample of physician members of the American Academy of Dermatology in 2011 [145]. As for nonbiologic treatment-related events, a retrospective study carried out on ninety-eight patients undergoing prolonged corticosteroid treatment for psoriasis-unrelated skin conditions (namely, pemphigus vulgaris and dermatomyositis) showed only four cases of HBV reactivation, two of whom had a fatal outcome [125].

Reasons for such low reporting rates remain to be fully clarified. A role of so-called 'Weber effect' [146], or other factors possibly affecting spontaneous reporting of adverse events, might be invoked. Alternatively, a consistently high level of alertness among dermatologists might be assumed. In this respect, it can incidentally be considered that since 2005 all Italian dermatologists involved in the management of psoriasis with 'biologic' and 'nonbiologic' systemic agents have to mandatorily adhere to the well-established pharmacovigilance roadmap dictated by the so-called 'Psocare' program.[1] Moreover, another independent aim-oriented dermatology registry network, the Psonet (http://www.psonet.eu) [129, 147], has more recently branched off from the Psocare program in order to merge data and strategy protocols from most European countries, along with Israel and Australia. Properly surveyed administration of anti-TNFα agents in HBV patients has been reported to be an overall safe treatment option in the setting of both noncutaneous inflammatory conditions [148, 149] as well as psoriasis [136, 150, 151]. However, the use of systemic ('biologic' or 'nonbiologic') agents in psoriatic patients who are chronic carriers of HBV is only an end-line tool in the ranking of therapeutic options, phototherapy and/or topical agents being more properly recommended (Table 7) [139].

5.1.2. HCV setting

Despite the wide range of noncutaneous inflammatory diseases in which TNFα inhibitors are now used as well-established therapeutic tools, literature yields only few papers in which these

1 Psocare is an Italian joint venture of psoriasis patients, dermatologists, epidemiologists and drug safety experts who are proactively involved since 2005 in a nationwide process linking drug prescription data to information on treatment outcome, such as effectiveness and long-term safety. Registration and participation to Psocare program, which is funded by the Italian Drug Administration Agency (AIFA), is mandatory to administer conventional treatments (including phototherapy) and new generation biologics. To date, Italian regional health authorities have appointed nearly 150 reference centers, in which patients' admission and follow-up visits are carried out, and demographic and lifestyle characteristics, disease severity, treatment exposure, treatment outcome, and any medical event (i.e. new diagnoses, hospitalizations, outpatient specialist visits) are registered. Before starting therapy, and throughout the treatment period, patients are rigidly evaluated according to standardized guidelines aimed at assuring the closest postmarketing surveillance of effectiveness and safety of systemic agents.

agents are reported to worsen HCV disease in subjects suffering from sole rheumatoid arthritis [141, 152-156]. TNFα inhibitors have also been assayed in HCV patients suffering from psoriasis. In this context, a number of small case series or anecdotal cases have been reported in which etanercept, efalizumab and alefacept do not induced HCV exacerbation. Of note, mild improvement in viral load and/or liver function tests were also observed in many of these cases [151, 157-170]. Only in one case, described by Ventura and coworkers [163], a significant increase of viral load (from 1.52×10^4 to 1.94×10^6 IU/mL), not coupled with increased liver enzymes, was observed after a 6-month therapy and led to treatment discontinuation. On the basis of such evidence, the overall harmful impact of anti-TNFα therapies in the setting of chronic HCV infection may appear to be lower than that exhibited in HBV infection. Indeed, the TNFα cascade has been consistently involved in the pathogenesis of liver damage, scar formation and fibrosis in chronic hepatitis C, and promising data have been reported suggesting a protective role of TNFα inhibitors against both INF-RBV-related undesired effects and virus-related hepatocyte injury [171]. Nevertheless, treatment of HCV infected psoriasis populations is subject to the same caution expressed by current guidelines for the management of patients who are chronic carriers of HBV [134]. Concerning this aspect, two different authority panels have recently audited all pros and cons, and drawn up a ranking list each of therapeutic options for treatment of moderate-to-severe psoriasis in HCV patients (Tables 8.A and B) [139, 172].

As for traditional 'nonbiologic' therapy, to the best of my knowledge, literature remains substantially silent with regard to acute flares of hepatitis deriving from treatment of psoriasis or other skin inflammatory conditions. I was able to find just one case of HCV reactivation occurring in a psoriatic patient after reduction of daily ciclosporin dosage [127]. By contrast, many cases of HCV reactivation have been reported during tapering of ciclosporin regimens in noncutaneous disease settings, such as bone marrow transplanted subjects [173]. In my opinion, reasons for possible underreporting in the dermatological literature of any drug-related liver undesired effects in the HCV setting are very likely to be the same as those discussed in paragraph 4.1.1.

As shown in Table 6, the management of moderate-to-severe psoriasis lies in a wide panel of agents which may often be a double-edged weapon owing to their broad immunosuppressive action. This concern is prompting continuous efforts to develop pharmacological agents (such as the new anti-interleukin-17 antibodies) [174-176] which are able to interfere with the TNFα cascade as downstream as possible, and are thus more likely to significantly lower the risk for side-effects related to impaired immune surveillance. Nevertheless, in more or less recent years (i.e., well after the breakthrough of 'TNFα inhibitor era') some faint interest has been renewed for traditional psoriasis treatment modalities, eg so-called *Goeckerman treatment* [177] or oral ciclosporin [178, 179]. In my view, the debate 'biologics *versus* nonbiologics' for management of skin inflammatory conditions is on the whole still highly controversial, and the decision-making process in daily clinical practice seems to be more conveniently left to the physician's wisdom.

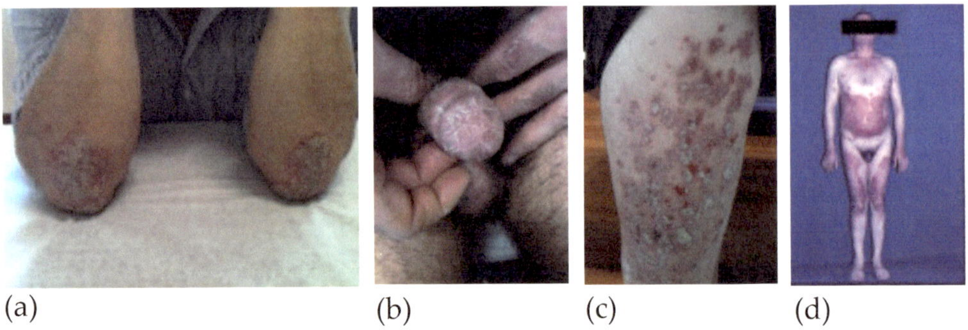

Figure 25. Psoriasis

-Methotrexate	-Alefacept
-Thioguanine	-Efalizumab
-Ciclosporin	-Ustekinumab
-Retinoids	-Ixekizumab
-Fumaric acid esters	-brodalumab
-Adalimumab	-secukinumab
-Etanercept	-tofacitinib
-Infliximab	

Table 6. Systemic therapy for psoriasis

Rank	Therapeutic option
1	UV-B narrowband
2	UV-B broadband
3	Topical corticosteroids
4	UV plus topical anthralin, or crude coal tar (*)
5	Topical steroids and calcipotriene
6	UV-A plus psoralen (P-UV-A)
7	UV plus acitretin
8	Efalizumab
9	Acitretin

UV = ultraviolet phototherapy; (*) Goeckerman treatment [177]

Table 7. Ranking of therapeutic options for treatment of moderate-to-severe psoriasis in chronic carriers of HBV. From: Strober et al [139], modified

Rank	Therapeutic option
1	Etanercept
2	UVB narrowband
3	TNF-inhibitor (without concern for any individual drug)
4	Adalimumab
5	UVB broadband
6	Infliximab
7	Topical corticosteroid in combination with calcipotriene
8	Topical corticosteroids
9	Efalizumab
10	Alefacept

A: From: Strober et al [139], *modified*

Rank	Therapeutic option
First line	UVB narrowband
	UVB broadband
	Topical therapies
Second line	Acitretin
	Etanercept
	Infliximab
	Adalimumab
	PUVA
Third line	Alefacept
	Cyclosporine
	Efalizumab
	Azathioprine

B: From: Frankel et al [180], *modified*

Table 8. Ranking of therapeutic options for treatment of moderate-to-severe psoriasis in chronic carriers of HCV

Author details

Mastrolonardo M.

Address all correspondence to: m.mastrolonardo@unifg.it

Department of Dermatology, University of Foggia, Foggia, Italy

References

[1] Hazin, R. Abu-Rajab Tamimi TI, Abuzetun JY, Zein NN. Recognizing and treating cutaneous signs of liver disease. Cleve Clin J Med (2009). Oct;, 76(10), 599-606.

[2] Nishioka, S, & Gyorkos, T. W. Tattoos as risk factors for transfusion-transmitted diseases. Int J Infect Dis (2001). , 5(1), 27-34.

[3] Jafari, S, Buxton, J. A, Afshar, K, Copes, R, & Baharlou, S. Tattooing and risk of hepatitis B: a systematic review and meta-analysis. Can J Public Health (2012). May;, 103(3), 207-212.

[4] Miyazaki, Y, Akizuki, S, Sakaoka, H, Yamamoto, S, & Terao, H. Disseminated infection of herpes simplex virus with fulminant hepatitis in a healthy adult. A case report. APMIS (1991). Nov;, 99(11), 1001-1007.

[5] Angarone, M, & Ison, M. G. Prevention and early treatment of opportunistic viral infections in patients with leukemia and allogeneic stem cell transplantation recipients. J Natl Compr Canc Netw (2008). Feb;, 6(2), 191-201.

[6] Sharma, S, & Mosunjac, M. Herpes simplex hepatitis in adults: a search for muco-cutaneous clues. J Clin Gastroenterol (2004). Sep;, 38(8), 697-704.

[7] Arkin, L. M, Castelo-Soccio, L, & Kovarik, C. Disseminated herpes simplex virus (HSV) hepatitis diagnosed by dermatology evaluation. Int J Dermatol (2009). Sep;, 48(9), 1020-1021.

[8] El-Serag, H. B, Hampel, H, Yeh, C, & Rabeneck, L. Extrahepatic manifestations of hepatitis C among United States male veterans. Hepatology (2002). Dec;, 36(6), 1439-1445.

[9] Rebora, A. Skin diseases associated with hepatitis C virus: facts and controversies. Clin Dermatol (2010). Sep;, 28(5), 489-496.

[10] Cacoub, P, Renou, C, Rosenthal, E, Cohen, P, Loury, I, Loustaud-ratti, V, et al. Extrahepatic manifestations associated with hepatitis C virus infection. A prospective multicenter study of 321 patients. The GERMIVIC. Groupe d'Etude et de Recherche en Medecine Interne et Maladies Infectieuses sur le Virus de l'Hepatite C. Medicine (Baltimore) (2000). Jan;, 79(1), 47-56.

[11] Sterling JC. Virus infections. In: Burns T, Breathmach S, Cox N, Griffiths C (ed.) Rook's Textbook of Dermatology. Oxford: Wiley-Blackwell; 2010. p33.1-81.

[12] Cecchi, R, Giomi, A, Tuci, F, Bartoli, L, & Seghieri, G. Pityriasis rubra pilaris, lichen planus, alopecia universalis and vitiligo in a patient with chronic viral hepatitis C. Dermatology (1994). , 188(3), 239-240.

[13] Ramos-casals, M, Mana, J, Nardi, N, Brito-zeron, P, Xaubet, A, Sanchez-tapias, J. M, et al. Sarcoidosis in patients with chronic hepatitis C virus infection: analysis of 68 cases. Medicine (Baltimore) (2005). Mar;, 84(2), 69-80.

[14] Lewiecki, E. M, & Rahman, F. Pruritus. A manifestation of iron deficiency. JAMA (1976). Nov 15;, 236(20), 2319-2320.

[15] Cribier, B, Samain, F, Vetter, D, Heid, E, & Grosshans, E. Systematic cutaneous examination in hepatitis C virus infected patients. Acta Derm Venereol (1998). Sep;, 78(5), 355-357.

[16] Soylu, S, Gul, U, & Kilic, A. Cutaneous manifestations in patients positive for anti-hepatitis C virus antibodies. Acta Derm Venereol (2007). , 87(1), 49-53.

[17] Soufir, N, Descamps, V, Crickx, B, Thibault, V, Cosnes, A, Becherel, P. A, et al. Hepatitis C virus infection in cutaneous polyarteritis nodosa: a retrospective study of 16 cases. Arch Dermatol (1999). Aug;, 135(8), 1001-1002.

[18] Keane, F. M. MacFarlane CS, Munn SE, Higgins EM. Pyoderma gangrenosum and hepatitis C virus infection. Br J Dermatol (1998). Nov;, 139(5), 924-925.

[19] Bockle, B. C, Baltaci, M, Ratzinger, G, Graziadei, I, Vogel, W, Sepp, N. T, & Hepatitis, C. and autoimmunity: a therapeutic challenge. J Intern Med (2012). Jan;, 271(1), 104-106.

[20] Abe, M, Kawakami, Y, Oyama, N, Nakamura-wakatsuki, T, & Yamamoto, T. A rare co-occurrence of primary localized cutaneous amyloidosis and chronic C type hepatitis. Int J Dermatol (2010). Aug;, 49(8), 960-962.

[21] Dessoukey, M. W, Abdel-dayem, H, Omar, M. F, & Al-suweidi, N. E. Pigmented purpuric dermatosis and hepatitis profile: a report on 10 patients. Int J Dermatol (2005). Jun;, 44(6), 486-488.

[22] Kono, T, Kobayashi, H, Ishii, M, Nishiguchi, S, & Taniguchi, S. Synchronous development of disseminated superficial porokeratosis and hepatitis C virus-related hepatocellular carcinoma. J Am Acad Dermatol (2000). Nov;43(5 Pt 2):966-968.

[23] Zechini, B, Teggi, A, Antonelli, M, Persechino, S, Pranteda, G, Versace, I, et al. A case report of pityriasis lichenoides in a patient with chronic hepatitis C. J Infect (2005). Aug;51(2):EE25., 23.

[24] Granel, B, Serratrice, J, Rey, J, Bouvier, C, Weiller-merli, C, Disdier, P, et al. Chronic hepatitis C virus infection associated with a generalized granuloma annulare. J Am Acad Dermatol (2000). Nov;43(5 Pt 2):918-919.

[25] Baglieri, F, & Scuderi, G. Disseminated Kaposi's sarcoma and HCV infection: only a casual relationship? A case report. G Ital Dermatol Venereol (2009). Jun;, 144(3), 317-320.

[26] Kapoor, R, & Johnson, R. A. Necrolytic acral erythema. N Engl J Med (2011). Apr 14;, 364(15), 1479-1480.

[27] Ramos-casals, M, Stone, J. H, Cid, M. C, & Bosch, X. The cryoglobulinaemias. Lancet (2012). Jan 28;, 379(9813), 348-360.

[28] Frank, J, & Poblete-gutierrez, P. Porphyria cutanea tarda--when skin meets liver. Best Pract Res Clin Gastroenterol (2010). Oct;, 24(5), 735-745.

[29] Chuang, T. Y, Brashear, R, & Lewis, C. Porphyria cutanea tarda and hepatitis C virus: a case-control study and meta-analysis of the literature. J Am Acad Dermatol (1999). Jul;, 41(1), 31-36.

[30] Gisbert, J. P, Garcia-buey, L, Pajares, J. M, & Moreno-otero, R. Prevalence of hepatitis C virus infection in B-cell non-Hodgkin's lymphoma: systematic review and meta-analysis. Gastroenterology (2003). Dec;, 125(6), 1723-1732.

[31] Ryan, C. F, Sendi, H, Bonkovsky, H. L, & Hepatitis, C. porphyria cutanea tarda and liver iron: an update. Liver Int (2012). Jul;, 32(6), 880-893.

[32] Breathmach S. Lichen planus and lichenoid disorders. In: Burns T, Breathmach S, Cox N, Griffiths C (ed.) Rook's Textbook of Dermatology. Oxford: Wiley-Blackwell; 2010. p41.1-28.

[33] Carrozzo, M. How common is oral lichen planus? Evid Based Dent (2008). , 9(4), 112-113.

[34] Carrozzo, M, Dametto, E, Fasano, M. E, Arduino, P, Bertolusso, G, et al. Cytokine gene polymorphisms in hepatitis C virus-related oral lichen planus. Exp Dermatol (2007). Sep;, 16(9), 730-736.

[35] Sontheimer, R. D. Lichenoid tissue reaction/interface dermatitis: clinical and histological perspectives. J Invest Dermatol (2009). May;, 129(5), 1088-1099.

[36] Farhi, D, & Dupin, N. Pathophysiology, etiologic factors, and clinical management of oral lichen planus, part I: facts and controversies. Clin Dermatol (2010). Jan;, 28(1), 100-108.

[37] Baccaglini L, Thongprasom K, Carrozzo M, Bigby M. Urban legends series: lichen planus. Oral Dis 2012; 19(2) 128-143.

[38] Lodi, G, Pellicano, R, & Carrozzo, M. Hepatitis C virus infection and lichen planus: a systematic review with meta-analysis. Oral Dis (2010). Oct;, 16(7), 601-612.

[39] Shengyuan, L, Songpo, Y, Wen, W, Wenjing, T, Haitao, Z, & Binyou, W. Hepatitis C virus and lichen planus: a reciprocal association determined by a meta-analysis. Arch Dermatol (2009). Sep;, 145(9), 1040-1047.

[40] Lapane, K. L, Jakiche, A. F, Sugano, D, Weng, C. S, & Carey, W. D. Hepatitis C infection risk analysis: who should be screened? Comparison of multiple screening strat-

egies based on the National Hepatitis Surveillance Program. Am J Gastroenterol (1998). Apr;, 93(4), 591-596.

[41] Van Dh, V, Antoine, J. L, & Lachapelle, J. M. Histopathological discriminant criteria between lichenoid drug eruption and idiopathic lichen planus: retrospective study on selected samples. Dermatologica (1989). , 179(1), 10-13.

[42] Breathmach SM. Drug reactions. In: Burns T, Breathmach S, Cox N, Griffiths C (ed.) Rook's Textbook of Dermatology. Oxford: Wiley-Blackwell; 2010. p75.1-177.

[43] Giuliani, M, Lajolo, C, Sartorio, A, Scivetti, M, Capodiferro, S, & Tumbarello, M. Oral lichenoid lesions in HIV-HCV-coinfected subjects during antiviral therapy: 2 cases and review of the literature. Am J Dermatopathol (2008). Oct;, 30(5), 466-471.

[44] Han, S. H. Extrahepatic manifestations of chronic hepatitis B. Clin Liver Dis (2004). May;, 8(2), 403-418.

[45] Terrier B, Cacoub P. Virus de l'hépatite B, manifestations extrahépatiques immunologiques et risque de réactivation virale [Hepatitis B virus, extrahepatic immunologic manifestations and risk of viral reactivation]. Rev Med Interne 2011; 32(10) 622-627.

[46] Cacoub, P, Saadoun, D, Bourliere, M, Khiri, H, Martineau, A, Benhamou, Y, et al. Hepatitis B virus genotypes and extrahepatic manifestations. J Hepatol (2005). Nov;, 43(5), 764-770.

[47] Shusterman, N, London, W. T, & Hepatitis, B. and immune-complex disease. N Engl J Med (1984). Jan 5;, 310(1), 43-46.

[48] Shusterman, N, London, W. T, & Hepatitis, B. and immune-complex disease. N Engl J Med (1984). Jan 5;, 310(1), 43-46.

[49] Han, S. H. Extrahepatic manifestations of chronic hepatitis B. Clin Liver Dis (2004). May;, 8(2), 403-418.

[50] Caroli, J. Serum-sickness-like prodromata in viral hepatitis: Caroli's triad. Lancet (1972). Apr 29;, 1(7757), 964-965.

[51] Tabata, N, Kato, T, Noguchi, K, Ueno, Y, & Tagami, H. Erythema multiforme following the exacerbation of hepatitis B virus infection. Int J Dermatol (1999). Jan;, 38(1), 52-53.

[52] van ARde Pagter AP, van Genderen PJ. Urticaria and periorbital edema as prodromal presenting signs of acute hepatitis B infection. J Travel Med (2011). May;, 18(3), 224-225.

[53] Wu, Y. L, Tsai, M. H, & Liu, L. L. Erythema nodosum and hepatitis B: a case report and literature review. J Microbiol Immunol Infect (2008). Oct;, 41(5), 437-439.

[54] Brandt, O, Abeck, D, Gianotti, R, & Burgdorf, W. Gianotti-Crosti syndrome. J Am Acad Dermatol (2006). Jan;, 54(1), 136-145.

[55] Haug, S, Schnopp, C, Ring, J, Folster-holst, R, & Abeck, D. Gianotti-Crosti syndrome following immunization]. Hautarzt (2002). Oct;, 53(10), 683-685.

[56] Karakas, M, Durdu, M, Tuncer, I, & Cevlik, F. Gianotti-Crosti syndrome in a child following hepatitis B virus vaccination. J Dermatol (2007). Feb;, 34(2), 117-120.

[57] Sagi, E. F, Linder, N, & Shouval, D. Papular acrodermatitis of childhood associated with hepatitis A virus infection. Pediatr Dermatol (1985). Nov;, 3(1), 31-33.

[58] Guibal, F, Buffet, P, Mouly, F, Morel, P, & Rybojad, M. Papular-purpuric gloves and socks syndrome with hepatitis B infection. Lancet (1996). Feb 17;347(8999):473.

[59] Turki, S, Guillevin, L, Dallot, A, Jarrousse, B, Vernier, I, Laroche, L, et al. Nodular and granulomatous form of periarteritis nodosa caused by the hepatitis B virus]. Ann Dermatol Venereol (1994). , 121(4), 325-327.

[60] Cox NH, Jorizzo JL, Bourke JF et al. Vasculitis, neutrophilic dermatoses and related disorders. In: Burns T, Breathmach S, Cox N, Griffiths C (ed.) Rook's Textbook of Dermatology. Oxford: Wiley-Blackwell; 2010. p50.1-138.

[61] Chrysomali, E, Piperi, E, & Sklavounou-andrikopoulou, A. Oral acanthosis nigricans in chronic hepatitis B with a 21-year follow up. J Dermatol (2011). Dec;, 38(12), 1172-1176.

[62] Askin, U, Durdu, M, & Senel, E. Generalized granuloma annulare in a patient with myelocytic leukemia and chronic hepatitis B virus infection. Indian J Dermatol Venereol Leprol (2009). May;, 75(3), 287-289.

[63] Birkenfeld, S, Dreiher, J, Weitzman, D, & Cohen, A. D. A study on the association with hepatitis B and hepatitis C in 1557 patients with lichen planus. J Eur Acad Dermatol Venereol (2011). Apr;, 25(4), 436-440.

[64] Bokor-bratic, M. Lack of evidence of hepatic disease in patients with oral lichen planus in Serbia. Oral Dis (2004). Sep;, 10(5), 283-286.

[65] Goolsby, P. L. Erythema nodosum after Recombivax HB hepatitis B vaccine. N Engl J Med (1989). Oct 26;, 321(17), 1198-1199.

[66] Wolf, F, Grezard, P, Berard, F, Clavel, G, & Perrot, H. Generalized granuloma annulare and hepatitis B vaccination. Eur J Dermatol (1998). Sep;, 8(6), 435-436.

[67] Tay, Y. K. Gianotti-Crosti syndrome following immunization. Pediatr Dermatol (2001). May;18(3):262.

[68] De KFNaeyaert JM, Hindryckx P, Elewaut D, Verplancke P, Peene I, et al. Immune-mediated pathology following hepatitis B vaccination. Two cases of polyarteritis nodosa and one case of pityriasis rosea-like drug eruption. Clin Exp Rheumatol (2000). Jan;, 18(1), 81-85.

[69] Calista, D, & Morri, M. Lichen planus induced by hepatitis B vaccination: a new case and review of the literature. Int J Dermatol (2004). Aug;, 43(8), 562-564.

[70] Stavrianeas, N. G, Katoulis, A. C, Kanelleas, A, Hatziolou, E, & Georgala, S. Papulonodular lichenoid and pseudolymphomatous reaction at the injection site of hepatitis B virus vaccination. Dermatology (2002). , 205(2), 166-168.

[71] Pham-ledard, A, Vergier, B, Doutre, M. S, & Beylot-barry, M. Disseminated cutaneous lymphoid hyperplasia of 12 years' duration triggered by vaccination. Dermatology (2010). , 220(2), 176-179.

[72] Cox NH, Coulson IH. Systemic disease and the skin. In: Burns T, Breathmach S, Cox N, Griffiths C (ed.) Rook's Textbook of Dermatology. Oxford: Wiley-Blackwell; 2010. p62.1-121.

[73] Jariwala, S, Vernon, N, & Shliozberg, J. Henoch-Schonlein purpura after hepatitis A vaccination. Ann Allergy Asthma Immunol (2011). Aug;, 107(2), 180-181.

[74] Mchutchison, J. G, Lawitz, E. J, Shiffman, M. L, Muir, A. J, Galler, G. W, Mccone, J, et al. Peginterferon alfa-2b or alfa-2a with ribavirin for treatment of hepatitis C infection. N Engl J Med (2009). Aug 6;, 361(6), 580-593.

[75] Ogawa, E, Furusyo, N, Kajiwara, E, Takahashi, K, Nomura, H, Tanabe, Y, et al. Evaluation of the adverse effect of premature discontinuation of pegylated interferon alpha-2b and ribavirin treatment for chronic hepatitis C virus infection: results from Kyushu University Liver Disease Study. J Gastroenterol Hepatol (2012). Jul;, 27(7), 1233-1240.

[76] Sookoian, S, Neglia, V, Castano, G, Frider, B, Kien, M. C, & Chohuela, E. High prevalence of cutaneous reactions to interferon alfa plus ribavirin combination therapy in patients with chronic hepatitis C virus. Arch Dermatol (1999). Aug;, 135(8), 1000-1001.

[77] Mistry, N, Shapero, J, & Crawford, R. I. A review of adverse cutaneous drug reactions resulting from the use of interferon and ribavirin. Can J Gastroenterol (2009). Oct;, 23(10), 677-683.

[78] Cacoub, P, Bourliere, M, Lubbe, J, Dupin, N, Buggisch, P, Dusheiko, G, et al. Dermatological side effects of hepatitis C and its treatment: patient management in the era of direct-acting antivirals. J Hepatol (2012). Feb;, 56(2), 455-463.

[79] Brok, J, Gluud, L. L, & Gluud, C. Ribavirin plus interferon versus interferon for chronic hepatitis C. Cochrane Database Syst Rev (2010). CD005445.

[80] Vazquez-lopez, F, Manjon-haces, J. A, Perez-alvarez, R, & Perez-oliva, N. Eczema-like lesions and disruption of therapy in patients treated with interferon-alfa and ribavirin for chronic hepatitis C: the value of an interdisciplinary assessment. Br J Dermatol (2004). May;, 150(5), 1046-1047.

[81] Lubbe, J, Kerl, K, Negro, F, & Saurat, J. H. Clinical and immunological features of hepatitis C treatment-associated dermatitis in 36 prospective cases. Br J Dermatol (2005). Nov;, 153(5), 1088-1090.

[82] Berth-Jones J. Eczema, lichenification, prurigo and erythroderma. In: Burns T, Breathmach S, Cox N, Griffiths C (ed.) Rook's Textbook of Dermatology. Oxford: Wiley-Blackwell; 2010. p23.1-51.

[83] Streiler JW. Skin-associated lymphoid tissues (SALT): origins and functions. J Invest Dermatol 1983; 80 (suppl) 12s-16s.

[84] Kim, B. S, Miyagawa, F, Cho, Y. H, Bennett, C. L, Clausen, B. E, & Katz, S. I. Keratinocytes function as accessory cells for presentation of endogenous antigen expressed in the epidermis. J Invest Dermatol (2009). Dec;, 129(12), 2805-2817.

[85] Von Andrian, U. H. Mackay CR. T-cell function and migration. Two sides of the same coin. N Engl J Med (2000). Oct 5;, 343(14), 1020-1034.

[86] Lodi, G, Scully, C, Carrozzo, M, Griffiths, M, Sugerman, P. B, & Thongprasom, K. Current controversies in oral lichen planus: report of an international consensus meeting. Part 1. Viral infections and etiopathogenesis. Oral Surg Oral Med Oral Pathol Oral Radiol Endod (2005). Jul;, 100(1), 40-51.

[87] Shiohara, T, & Mizukawa, Y. The immunological basis of lichenoid tissue reaction. Autoimmun Rev (2005). Apr;, 4(4), 236-241.

[88] Langhans, B, Nischalke, H. D, Arndt, S, Braunschweiger, I, Nattermann, J, Sauerbruch, T, et al. Ribavirin exerts differential effects on functions of Cd4+ Th1, Th2, and regulatory T cell clones in hepatitis C. PLoS One (2012). e42094.

[89] Jadali, Z. Dermatologic manifestations of hepatitis C infection and the effect of interferon therapy: a literature review. Arch Iran Med (2012). Jan;, 15(1), 43-48.

[90] Barritt, A. S, & Fried, M. W. Maximizing opportunities and avoiding mistakes in triple therapy for hepatitis C virus. Gastroenterology (2012). May;, 142(6), 1314-1323.

[91] Hayashi, N, Okanoue, T, Tsubouchi, H, Toyota, J, Chayama, K, & Kumada, H. Efficacy and safety of telaprevir, a new protease inhibitor, for difficult-to-treat patients with genotype 1 chronic hepatitis C. J Viral Hepat (2012). Feb;19(2):ee142., 134.

[92] Cunningham, M, & Foster, G. R. Efficacy and safety of telaprevir in patients with genotype 1 hepatitis C infection. Therap Adv Gastroenterol (2012). Mar;, 5(2), 139-151.

[93] Kumada, H, Toyota, J, Okanoue, T, Chayama, K, Tsubouchi, H, & Hayashi, N. Telaprevir with peginterferon and ribavirin for treatment-naive patients chronically infected with HCV of genotype 1 in Japan. J Hepatol (2012). Jan;, 56(1), 78-84.

[94] Jacobson, I. M, Mchutchison, J. G, & Dusheiko, G. Di Bisceglie AM, Reddy KR, Bzowej NH, et al. Telaprevir for previously untreated chronic hepatitis C virus infection. N Engl J Med (2011). Jun 23;, 364(25), 2405-2416.

[95] Zeuzem, S, Andreone, P, Pol, S, Lawitz, E, Diago, M, Roberts, S, et al. Telaprevir for retreatment of HCV infection. N Engl J Med (2011). Jun 23;, 364(25), 2417-2428.

[96] FDA Antiviral Drugs Advisory CommitteeTelaprevir Briefing Document April 28. (2011).

[97] Dupin, N, Mallet, V, Carlotti, A, Vallet-pichard, A, & Pol, S. Severe skin rash in case of readministration of telaprevir in a patient who previously experienced a non severe rash. Hepatology (2012). Jun;, 55(6), 2042-2043.

[98] Awwad, A, Renard, P, Pouzoulet, J, Sigal, M. L, & Mahe, E. Perianal ulcerations with telaprevir]. Ann Dermatol Venereol (2012). May;, 139(5), 391-392.

[99] Poordad, F, & Mccone, J. Jr., Bacon BR, Bruno S, Manns MP, Sulkowski MS, et al. Boceprevir for untreated chronic HCV genotype 1 infection. N Engl J Med (2011). Mar 31;, 364(13), 1195-1206.

[100] Bacon, B. R, Gordon, S. C, Lawitz, E, Marcellin, P, Vierling, J. M, Zeuzem, S, et al. Boceprevir for previously treated chronic HCV genotype 1 infection. N Engl J Med (2011). Mar 31;, 364(13), 1207-1217.

[101] Manns, M. P, Bourliere, M, Benhamou, Y, Pol, S, Bonacini, M, Trepo, C, et al. Potency, safety, and pharmacokinetics of the NS3/4A protease inhibitor BI201335 in patients with chronic HCV genotype-1 infection. J Hepatol (2011). Jun;, 54(6), 1114-1122.

[102] Sulkowski M, Bourliere M, Bronowicki J-P et al. SILEN-C2: early antiviral activity and safety or BI 201335 combined with peginterferon alfa-2a and ribavirin (PegIFN/RBV) in chronic HCV genotype-1 patients with non-response to PegIFN/RBV. J Hepatol 2010; 52 (suppl) s462-s643

[103] Zeuzem, S, Asselah, T, Angus, P, Zarski, J. P, Larrey, D, Mullhaupt, B, et al. Efficacy of the protease inhibitor BI 201335, polymerase inhibitor BI 207127, and ribavirin in patients with chronic HCV infection. Gastroenterology (2011). Dec;, 141(6), 2047-2055.

[104] Carosi, G, Rizzetto, M, Alberti, A, Cariti, G, Colombo, M, Craxi, A, et al. Treatment of chronic hepatitis B: update of the recommendations from the 2007 Italian Workshop. Dig Liver Dis (2011). Apr;, 43(4), 259-265.

[105] European Association for the Study of the Liver. EASL clinical practice guidelines: management of chronic hepatitis B. J Hepatol 2009; 50(1) 227-242

[106] De VSDe R, V, Sansonno D, Sorrentino D, Corte RL, Pivetta B, et al. Gastric mucosa as an additional extrahepatic localization of hepatitis C virus: viral detection in gas-

tric low-grade lymphoma associated with autoimmune disease and in chronic gastritis. Hepatology (2000). Jan;, 31(1), 182-189.

[107] Fletcher, N. F, & Mckeating, J. A. Hepatitis C virus and the brain. J Viral Hepat (2012). May;, 19(5), 301-306.

[108] Sansonno, D, Cornacchiulo, V, Iacobelli, A. R, Di, S. R, Lospalluti, M, & Dammacco, F. Localization of hepatitis C virus antigens in liver and skin tissues of chronic hepatitis C virus-infected patients with mixed cryoglobulinemia. Hepatology (1995). Feb;, 21(2), 305-312.

[109] Crowson, A. N, Nuovo, G, Ferri, C, & Magro, C. M. The dermatopathologic manifestations of hepatitis C infection: a clinical, histological, and molecular assessment of 35 cases. Hum Pathol (2003). Jun;, 34(6), 573-579.

[110] Kontochristopoulos, G, Stavrinos, C, Aroni, K, & Tassopoulos, N. C. Cutaneous necrosis by subcutaneous injection of a-interferon in a patient with chronic type B hepatitis. J Hepatol (1996). Aug;25(2):271.

[111] Kilic, M, Dogan, Y, Taskin, E, Sen, Y, & Kalpaklioglu, A. F. Desensitization protocol administered successfully with interferon-alpha 2a in a child with chronic hepatitis B infection. J Investig Allergol Clin Immunol (2010). , 20(5), 447-448.

[112] Milkiewicz, P, Yim, C, Pache, I, & Heathcote, J. Diffuse skin reaction in patient with hepatitis B, treated with two different formulations of pegylated interferon. Can J Gastroenterol (2005). Nov;, 19(11), 677-678.

[113] Barut, S, Yuksek, J, Sezer, E, Gunal, O, & Koseoglu, D. Morbilliform drug eruption due to pegylated alpha-interferon can show complete regression after switching to non-pegylated interferon. J Dermatol (2011). May;, 38(5), 479-481.

[114] Ketikoglou, I, Karatapanis, S, Elefsiniotis, I, Kafiri, G, & Moulakakis, A. Extensive psoriasis induced by pegylated interferon alpha-2b treatment for chronic hepatitis B. Eur J Dermatol (2005). Mar;, 15(2), 107-109.

[115] Seckin, D, Durusoy, C, & Sahin, S. Concomitant vitiligo and psoriasis in a patient treated with interferon alfa-2a for chronic hepatitis B infection. Pediatr Dermatol (2004). Sep;, 21(5), 577-579.

[116] Dalekos, G. N, Christodoulou, D, Kistis, K. G, Zervou, E. K, Hatzis, J, & Tsianos, E. V. A prospective evaluation of dermatological side-effects during alpha-interferon therapy for chronic viral hepatitis. Eur J Gastroenterol Hepatol (1998). Nov;, 10(11), 933-939.

[117] Ozdogan, M, Gur, G, Kadayifcilar, S, Boyacioglu, S, Ozgur, O, & Teletar, H. An unusual adverse effect of interferon: hypertrichosis of the eyelashes. J Interferon Cytokine Res (2000). Jul;, 20(7), 633-634.

[118] Kaptanoglu, A. F, & Kutluay, L. Ichthyosiform eruption associated with lamivudine in a patient with chronic hepatitis-B infection. Int J Clin Pract (2005). Oct;, 59(10), 1237-1238.

[119] Kim, S. B, & Seo, P. J. Baik dS, Yun SY, Kim BH, Shin JE, et al. [A case of severe skin eruption caused by lamivudine in a patient with chronic hepatitis B]. Korean J Gastroenterol (2006). Oct;, 48(4), 281-285.

[120] Atzori, L, Pinna, A. L, Pilloni, L, Ferreli, C, Pau, M, & Aste, N. Bullous skin eruption in an HIV patient during antiretroviral drugs therapy. Dermatol Ther (2008). Oct;21 Suppl 2:SS34., 30.

[121] Yamada, S, Sawada, Y, & Nakamura, M. Maculopapular-type drug eruption caused by entecavir. Eur J Dermatol (2011). Jul;, 21(4), 635-636.

[122] Sugiura, K, Sugiura, M, Takashi, T, Naoki, H, & Itoh, A. Immediate allergy, drug-induced eruption, by entecavir. J Eur Acad Dermatol Venereol (2009). Apr;, 23(4), 487-489.

[123] Lockhart, S. M, Rathbun, R. C, Stephens, J. R, Baker, D. L, Drevets, D. A, Greenfield, R. A, et al. Cutaneous reactions with tenofovir disoproxil fumarate: a report of nine cases. AIDS (2007). Jun 19;, 21(10), 1370-1373.

[124] Chattopadhyay, P, & Sarma, N. Adefovir-induced Stevens-Johnson syndrome and toxic epidermal necrolysis overlap syndrome. Singapore Med J (2011). Feb; 52(2):ee34., 31.

[125] Yang, C. H, Wu, T. S, & Chiu, C. T. Chronic hepatitis B reactivation: a word of caution regarding the use of systemic glucocorticosteroid therapy. Br J Dermatol (2007). Sep;, 157(3), 587-590.

[126] Kouba M, Rudolph SE, Hrdlicka P, Zuber MA. Hepatitis-B-Reaktivierung unter TNF-α-Blocker-Therapie mit Adalimumab bei Psoriasis-Arthritis [Hepatitis-B reactivation during treatment with tumor necrosis factor-alpha blocker adalimumab in a patient with psoriasis arthritis]. Dtsch Med Wochenschr 2012; 137(1-2) 23-26.

[127] Miura, H, Itoh, Y, Matsumoto, Y, Tani, M, Tanabe, N, Isonokami, M, et al. Long-term administration of cyclosporin A to HCV-antibody-positive patients with dermatologic diseases. Int J Dermatol (1999). Apr;, 38(4), 310-314.

[128] Nestle, F. O, Kaplan, D. H, & Barker, J. Psoriasis. N Engl J Med (2009). Jul 30;, 361(5), 496-509.

[129] Lecluse LL, Naldi L, Stern RS, Spuls PI. National registries of systemic treatment for psoriasis and the European 'Psonet' initiative. Dermatology 2009; 218(4) 347-356.

[130] Huerta, C, Rivero, E, & Rodriguez, L. A. Incidence and risk factors for psoriasis in the general population. Arch Dermatol (2007). Dec;, 143(12), 1559-1565.

[131] Rapp, S. R, Feldman, S. R, Exum, M. L, & Fleischer, A. B. Jr., Reboussin DM. Psoriasis causes as much disability as other major medical diseases. J Am Acad Dermatol (1999). Sep;41(3 Pt 1):401-407.

[132] Stern, R. S, Nijsten, T, Feldman, S. R, Margolis, D. J, & Rolstad, T. Psoriasis is common, carries a substantial burden even when not extensive, and is associated with widespread treatment dissatisfaction. J Investig Dermatol Symp Proc (2004). Mar;, 9(2), 136-139.

[133] Richards, H. L, Fortune, D. G, Sullivan, O, Main, T. M, & Griffiths, C. J. CE. Patients with psoriasis and their compliance with medication. J Am Acad Dermatol (1999). Oct;, 41(4), 581-583.

[134] Pathirana, D, Ormerod, A. D, Saiag, P, Smith, C, Spuls, P. I, Nast, A, et al. European S3-guidelines on the systemic treatment of psoriasis vulgaris. J Eur Acad Dermatol Venereol (2009). Oct;23 Suppl , 2, 1-70.

[135] Del, V. G-S, Gomez-camacho, F, Poyato-gonzalez, A, Iglesias-flores, E. M, De Dios-vega, J. F, & Sancho-zapatero, R. Infliximab therapy in a patient with Crohn's disease and chronic hepatitis B virus infection. Inflamm Bowel Dis (2004). Sep;, 10(5), 701-702.

[136] Cassano, N, Mastrandrea, V, Principi, M, & Loconsole, F. De TN, Di LA, et al. Anti-tumor necrosis factor treatment in occult hepatitis B virus infection: a retrospective analysis of 62 patients with psoriatic disease. J Biol Regul Homeost Agents (2011). Apr;, 25(2), 285-289.

[137] Vigano, M, Degasperi, E, Aghemo, A, Lampertico, P, & Colombo, M. Anti-TNF drugs in patients with hepatitis B or C virus infection: safety and clinical management. Expert Opin Biol Ther (2012). Feb;, 12(2), 193-207.

[138] Bongartz, T, Sutton, A. J, Sweeting, M. J, Buchan, I, Matteson, E. L, & Montori, V. Anti-TNF antibody therapy in rheumatoid arthritis and the risk of serious infections and malignancies: systematic review and meta-analysis of rare harmful effects in randomized controlled trials. JAMA (2006). May 17;, 295(19), 2275-2285.

[139] Strober, B, Berger, E, Cather, J, Cohen, D, Crowley, J. J, Gordon, K. B, et al. A series of critically challenging case scenarios in moderate to severe psoriasis: a Delphi consensus approach. J Am Acad Dermatol (2009). Jul;61(1 Suppl 1):SS46., 1.

[140] Garcia-doval, I, Carretero, G, Vanaclocha, F, Ferrandiz, C, Dauden, E, Sanchez-carazo, J. L, et al. Risk of serious adverse events associated with biologic and nonbiologic psoriasis systemic therapy: patients ineligible vs eligible for randomized controlled trials. Arch Dermatol (2012). Apr;, 148(4), 463-470.

[141] Brunasso, A. M, Puntoni, M, Gulia, A, & Massone, C. Safety of anti-tumour necrosis factor agents in patients with chronic hepatitis C infection: a systematic review. Rheumatology (Oxford) (2011). Sep;, 50(9), 1700-1711.

[142] Ostuni, P, Botsios, C, Punzi, L, Sfriso, P, & Todesco, S. Hepatitis B reactivation in a chronic hepatitis B surface antigen carrier with rheumatoid arthritis treated with infliximab and low dose methotrexate. Ann Rheum Dis (2003). Jul;, 62(7), 686-687.

[143] Wendling, D, Auge, B, Bettinger, D, Lohse, A, Le, H. G, Bresson-hadni, S, et al. Reactivation of a latent precore mutant hepatitis B virus related chronic hepatitis during infliximab treatment for severe spondyloarthropathy. Ann Rheum Dis (2005). May;, 64(5), 788-789.

[144] Madonia, S, Orlando, A, Scimeca, D, Olivo, M, Rossi, F, & Cottone, M. Occult hepatitis B and infliximab-induced HBV reactivation. Inflamm Bowel Dis (2007). Apr;, 13(4), 508-509.

[145] Stine, J. G, Bass, M, Ibrahim, D, Khokhar, O. S, & Lewis, J. H. Dermatologists' awareness of and screening practices for hepatitis B virus infection before initiating tumor necrosis factor-alpha inhibitor therapy. South Med J (2011). Dec;, 104(12), 781-788.

[146] Hartnell, N. R, & Wilson, J. P. Replication of the Weber effect using postmarketing adverse event reports voluntarily submitted to the United States Food and Drug Administration. Pharmacotherapy (2004). Jun;, 24(6), 743-749.

[147] http://www.psonet.eu.

[148] Roux, C. H, Brocq, O, Breuil, V, Albert, C, & Euller-ziegler, L. Safety of anti-TNF-alpha therapy in rheumatoid arthritis and spondylarthropathies with concurrent B or C chronic hepatitis. Rheumatology (Oxford) (2006). Oct;, 45(10), 1294-1297.

[149] Sakellariou, G. T, & Chatzigiannis, I. Long-term anti-TNFalpha therapy for ankylosing spondylitis in two patients with chronic HBV infection. Clin Rheumatol (2007). Jun;, 26(6), 950-952.

[150] Conde-taboada, A, Munoz, J. P, Munoz, L. C, & Lopez-bran, E. Infliximab treatment for severe psoriasis in a patient with active hepatitis B virus infection. J Am Acad Dermatol (2009). Jun;, 60(6), 1077-1080.

[151] Prignano, F, Zanieri, F, Milani, S, & Lotti, T. Switch from etanercept to efalizumab in a psoriatic patient with HCV infection: a case report. Dermatol Ther (2009). Jul;, 22(4), 386-390.

[152] Pritchard, C. Etanercept and hepatitis C. J Clin Rheumatol (1999). Jun;5(3):179.

[153] Cansu, D. U, Kalifoglu, T, & Korkmaz, C. Short-term course of chronic hepatitis B and C under treatment with etanercept associated with different disease modifying antirheumatic drugs without antiviral prophylaxis. J Rheumatol (2008). Mar;, 35(3), 421-424.

[154] Ferri, C, Ferraccioli, G, Ferrari, D, Galeazzi, M, Lapadula, G, Montecucco, C, et al. Safety of anti-tumor necrosis factor-alpha therapy in patients with rheumatoid arthritis and chronic hepatitis C virus infection. J Rheumatol (2008). Oct;, 35(10), 1944-1949.

[155] Kaur, P. P, Chan, V. C, & Berney, S. N. Histological evaluation of liver in two rheumatoid arthritis patients with chronic hepatitis B and C treated with TNF-alpha blockade: case reports. Clin Rheumatol (2008). Aug;, 27(8), 1069-1071.

[156] Li, S, Kaur, P. P, Chan, V, & Berney, S. Use of tumor necrosis factor-alpha (TNF-alpha) antagonists infliximab, etanercept, and adalimumab in patients with concurrent rheumatoid arthritis and hepatitis B or hepatitis C: a retrospective record review of 11 patients. Clin Rheumatol (2009). Jul;, 28(7), 787-791.

[157] Cecchi, R, & Bartoli, L. Psoriasis and hepatitis C treated with anti-TNF alpha therapy (etanercept). Dermatol Online J (2006).

[158] Linardaki, G, Katsarou, O, Ioannidou, P, Karafoulidou, A, & Boki, K. Effective etanercept treatment for psoriatic arthritis complicating concomitant human immunodeficiency virus and hepatitis C virus infection. J Rheumatol (2007). Jun;, 34(6), 1353-1355.

[159] De SCParadisi A, Capizzi R, Carbone A, Siciliano M, Amerio PL. Etanercept therapy in two patients with psoriasis and concomitant hepatitis C. J Am Acad Dermatol (2006). Jun;, 54(6), 1102-1104.

[160] Piccolo, D, Di, C. A, Fargnoli, M. C, Paoloni, M, Vecchiotti, S, & Peris, K. Effective control of psoriasis by etanercept in a patient with HCV-related diseases. Eur J Dermatol (2008). Jul;, 18(4), 459-460.

[161] Alcaide, A. J, Barrera, M. V, Habicheyn, S, Lopez, N, Mendiola, M. V, & Herrera, E. Safety of etanercept therapy in a patient with psoriasis, Down's syndrome and concomitant hepatitis C virus infection. J Eur Acad Dermatol Venereol (2008). Dec;, 22(12), 1514-1516.

[162] Behnam, S. E, Hindiyeh, R, Fife, D. J, & Jeffes, E. W. III, Wu JJ. Etanercept as prophylactic psoriatic therapy before interferon-alpha and ribavirin treatment for active hepatitis C infection. Clin Exp Dermatol (2010). Jun;, 35(4), 397-398.

[163] Ventura, F, Gomes, J, Duarte, M. L, Fernandes, J. C, & Brito, C. Efficacy and safety of etanercept in patients with psoriasis and hepatitis C. Eur J Dermatol (2010). Nov;, 20(6), 808-809.

[164] Rokhsar, C, Rabhan, N, & Cohen, S. R. Etanercept monotherapy for a patient with psoriasis, psoriatic arthritis, and concomitant hepatitis C infection. J Am Acad Dermatol (2006). Feb;, 54(2), 361-362.

[165] Paradisi, A, Caldarola, G, Capizzi, R, Siciliano, M, Annichiarico, E, Vecchio, F. M, et al. Safety of etanercept in patients with psoriasis and hepatitis C virus assessed by liver histopathology: preliminary data. J Am Acad Dermatol (2010). Jun;, 62(6), 1067-1069.

[166] Allen E, Hurley Y, Leonardi C. Etanercept therapy in psoriasis patients with underlying hepatitis C. J Am Acad Dermatol 2005; 52 (3) s1.

[167] Esposito M, Bianchi L, Mazzotta A et al. Influence of etanercept on serum-related liver related tests and viral load values in patients with psoriasis and hepatitis C infection. J Am Acad Dermatol 2007; 56 (Suppl 2) P2700.

[168] Magliocco, M. A, & Gottlieb, A. B. Etanercept therapy for patients with psoriatic arthritis and concurrent hepatitis C virus infection: report of 3 cases. J Am Acad Dermatol (2004). Oct;, 51(4), 580-584.

[169] Gisondi, P, Prignano, F, Grossi, P, Lotti, T, & Girolomoni, G. Treatment of psoriasis with efalizumab in patients with hepatitis C viral infection: report of five cases. Dermatology (2009). , 219(2), 158-161.

[170] Thaci, D, Patzold, S, Kaufmann, R, & Boehncke, W. H. Treatment of psoriasis with alefacept in patients with hepatitis C infection: a report of two cases. Br J Dermatol (2005). May;, 152(5), 1048-1050.

[171] Zein, N. N. Etanercept as an adjuvant to interferon and ribavirin in treatment-naive patients with chronic hepatitis C virus infection: a phase 2 randomized, double-blind, placebo-controlled study. J Hepatol (2005). Mar;, 42(3), 315-322.

[172] Frankel, A. J, Van Voorhees, A. S, Hsu, S, Korman, N. J, Lebwohl, M. G, Bebo, B. F, et al. Treatment of psoriasis in patients with hepatitis C: from the Medical Board of the National Psoriasis Foundation. J Am Acad Dermatol (2009). Dec;, 61(6), 1044-1055.

[173] Akiyama, H, Yoshinaga, H, Tanaka, T, Hiruma, K, Tanikawa, S, Sakamaki, H, et al. Effects of cyclosporin A on hepatitis C virus infection in bone marrow transplant patients. Bone Marrow Transplantation Team. Bone Marrow Transplant (1997). Dec;, 20(11), 993-995.

[174] Leonardi, C, Matheson, R, Zachariae, C, Cameron, G, Li, L, Edson-heredia, E, et al. Anti-interleukin-17 monoclonal antibody ixekizumab in chronic plaque psoriasis. N Engl J Med (2012). Mar 29;, 366(13), 1190-1199.

[175] Papp, K. A, Leonardi, C, Menter, A, Ortonne, J. P, Krueger, J. G, Kricorian, G, et al. Brodalumab, an anti-interleukin-17-receptor antibody for psoriasis. N Engl J Med (2012). Mar 29;, 366(13), 1181-1189.

[176] Hueber, W, Patel, D. D, Dryja, T, Wright, A. M, Koroleva, I, Bruin, G, et al. Effects of AIN457, a fully human antibody to interleukin-17A, on psoriasis, rheumatoid arthritis, and uveitis. Sci Transl Med (2010). Oct 6;2(52):52ra72.

[177] Serrao, R, & Davis, M. D. Goeckerman treatment for remission of psoriasis refractory to biologic therapy. J Am Acad Dermatol (2009). Feb;, 60(2), 348-349.

[178] Brunasso AMGCyclosporine as monotherapy for psoriasis in the setting of chronic HCV infection. In: Michetti P FLea, ed. 12 ed. (2012). , 52-349.

[179] Di, L, & Albertini, V. G. Treatment of psoriasis with cyclosporine in patients with hepatitis C infection: risk or opportunity? J Am Acad Dermatol (2010). Aug;, 63(2), 342-343.

[180] Frankel, A. J, Van Voorhees, A. S, Hsu, S, Korman, N. J, Lebwohl, M. G, Bebo, B. F, et al. Treatment of psoriasis in patients with hepatitis C: from the Medical Board of the National Psoriasis Foundation. J Am Acad Dermatol (2009). Dec;, 61(6), 1044-1055.

Chapter 11

Chronic C Hepatitis, Interferon and Psychiatric Disorders

Giuseppe Valerio Torres, Emanuela Apicella,
Elisa D'Alterio, Angela Chiara Cecere and
Antonello Bellomo

Additional information is available at the end of the chapter

http://dx.doi.org/10.5772/54748

1. Introduction

The following chapter deals with the clinical management of mental and behavioural disorders that may occur in patients with chronic viral hepatitis C during alpha-interferon therapy.

Actually, in clinical experience, psychopharmacological and psychological interventions are frequently found in patients with HCV-related chronic hepatitis. These interventions are often requested by clinicians with hepatologic and infectious diseases competence, who deliver the ambulatory care for the treatment of interferon in general hospitals.

These interventions are always complex due to several reasons:

a. they are multidisciplinary interventions that require a great collaboration between all specialists involved and high patients management skills.

The clinician has to deal with complex and multi-problematic situations for both the underlying disease and its complications and both the onset of psychiatric disorders, especially anxiety and depressive symptoms. Psychotic symptoms are occasional, instead.

b. there are no specific treatment guidelines for mental disorders related to chronic viral hepatitis. Therefore, the management of these patients can be different according to the internal organization of a psychiatric service and to the one of the general hospital that rarely provide a specific ambulatory care for the treatment and management of psychiatric side effects during alpha-interferon treatment.

c. The clinical picture is often blurred reported and is characterized by heterogeneous symptoms of anxiety and depression that vary from mild to severe degree and may also have a pejorative evolution.

d. The most common criteria for psychiatric diagnosis used in the international clinical practice and scientific research are those of the DSM IV TR [1]. This means provides diagnostic categories whose inclusion criteria are very restrictive. Mental disorders due to a general medical condition and substance-induced mental disorders are included in these diagnostic categories. This last diagnostic category even includes mental disorders induced by drugs. Nevertheless, there is no explicit reference to either HCV or interferon therapy in both diagnostic categories.

Moreover, the underlying causes of mental disorders in patients with chronic HCV hepatitis seem to be very complex.

In Psychiatry it is widely recognized as valid the bio-psycho-social paradigm according to which the causes of mental illness must be found not only in genetic and constitutional reasons but also in psychological and environmental factors. This paradigm is even more appropriate when the mental illness and the organic illness are present at the same time.

The psychological impact of diagnosis of HCV-related chronic hepatitis, interferon treatment and hcv neurotoxicity are definitely important in the genesis of symptoms.

2. HCV infection as life event

The role of stressful psychosocial events or "life events" in the unleashing of psychic pathology is generally accepted by most clinicians. As a matter of fact, it is difficult to document a causal link between life events and mental illness and it is hard to think of a real direct causality between these two factors. Some authors have proposed a model based on a circular relationship between the event and the psychopathological manifestation, rather than a model based on a linear cause-effect relationship [2]. Available researches, moreover, show that only some individuals will develop a specific psychiatric disorder at the presence of the same life events [3].

Different regulation scales are used to define the events that can be considered as stressful and to value their psychological burden. A personal illness, especially if chronic, is certainly an event characterized by great emotional and psychological impact [4]. Moreover, symptoms such as mood changes and anxiety, which are commonly observed in patients affected by HCV, can be related to the awareness of suffering from a chronic progressive disease and to the past or current substance abuse [5].

As we have said, the aetiology of psychiatric disorders is multifactorial and several factors can lead to the development of the manifestations: genetic factors, evolutionary factors, environmental factors and life events. The onset of an organic diseases can lead to the outbreak of a psychiatric disorder, not only for the psychological impact that the disease has but even due to the changes in the immune system that can establish in certain medical conditions.

Depressive symptoms are often found in pathologies such as AIDS [6], diabetes mellitus [7], multiple sclerosis [8] and cardiovascular disorders [9].

3. Proinflammatory cytokines and neurotransmitter systems

It is well known that the assumption of interferon α (IFN α) is associated with the onset of depressive symptoms, similar to those observed in major depression [10], in fact, from 30% to 50% of patients receiving IFN develop depression during treatment [11].Many data in literature show the very important role of pro-inflammatory cytokines in the onset of the Depression [12,13-14,15].Since the 90s, several studies have highlighted that in certain cases the alterations of the immune system can contribute to the development of depressive symptoms, favouring the acquisition of new knowledge about the so-called Psychoneuroimmunology [16].

The Neuro- Endocrine System (SNE) and the Immune System (SI) are part of a totally integrated biological circuit, in fact, the same biochemical signals are used both for the exchange of information between the components of the same system both for communications between the two systems. Numerous researches, in fact, have shown that the SI is able to modify its responses, either through automatic mechanisms of regulation either by signals coming from the Central Nervous System (CNS) and endocrine system (SE). In turn, the cells of the SI, sending signals to the central nervous system and to the SE, trigger specific neuroendocrine and behavioural responses. Pro-inflammatory cytokines are ones of the main messengers employed by SI to communicate directly with the SNE, in particular, they stimulate the activity of the locus coeruleus (LC) and the hypothalamic secretion of Corticotrophin-Releasing Factor (CRF) [17].

The immune cells communicate with the SNE also by means of several neuropeptides and neuro-hormones, such as the CRF, adrenocorticotropic hormone (ACTH), the Growth Hormone (GH), the Thyrotropin-Releasing Hormone (TRH), prolactin, the β-endorphin, etc.; immune cells, in fact, possess specific membrane receptors, both for these mediators both for neurotransmitters such as adrenaline, serotonin, histamine, GABA [18].

The existence of a bi-directional network of communication between SNE and SI is extremely important since it allows to SNE to receive and respond to a wide range of non-cognitive stimuli, which include stresses-induced stimuli and infectious, autoimmune or neoplastic nature-stimuli, that it could not perceive otherwise. The relationship between the nervous system, endocrine system and immune system has been highlighted by several studies. The baseline concentration of soluble receptors for TNF and IL-6 were linked with the development of depression during therapy with IFN α [19]. Moreover it was found that patients suffering from cancer and depression showed higher levels of interleukin 6 (IL6) compared to patients affected by cancer but without depression [20]. In patients suffering from HCV, concentrations of receptors for IL-2, IL-6 and IL-10 are significantly higher in patients who develop a depressive symptomatology during therapy with IFN, compared to patients who did not develop it. Therefore, a greater activation of the immune system may be predictive of the development of depression during IFN therapy [21,22].

Let's look now at the way through pro-inflammatory cytokines, in particular IFN α, act in the genesis of psychiatric interest symptoms. It's well known that serotonergic and dopaminergic neurotransmitter systems are involved in depressive disorders and anxiety disorders. In clinical practice, drugs that act on the neurotransmitter systems are commonly used. The role of IFNα in the development of depression and anxiety may be partly due to the action on serotonin metabolism. The administration of selective serotonin reuptake inhibitors (SSRIs), in fact, inhibits the development of depression in patients treated with IFN α [22]. The administration of paroxetine (SSRI) reduces to approximately 4 times the risk of onset of depression during therapy with IFN α [23]. The IFNα and cytokines in general, would contribute to the alteration of serotonin metabolism through the activation of an enzyme called indoleamine 2-3 deoxigenase (IDO), which converts tryptophan, an amino acid precursor of serotonin, in kynurenine [24], leading to a reduction in the synthesis of serotonin. In fact, it has been demonstrated that, patients treated with IFN α, who develop depression, have lower blood concentrations of tryptophan [25,26]. Patients who develop major depression during IFN-α therapy, compared with patients who did not develop, show in the peripheral blood significantly reduced level of tryptophan and increased levels of kynurenine [27]. These data would support the hypothesis according to which the reduction of levels of tryptophan and, consequently the reduction of the synthesis of serotonin, are consequent to activation of the IDO.

Another mechanism involved in the reduction of levels of serotonin induced by cytokines is the activation of a protein kinase, called MAPK, by themselves.

The IFNα is a potent inducer of p38 MAPK; the activation of this protein kinase increases the expression and synthesis of serotonin transporters [28,29], thus resulting in the increase of serotonin reuptake, with consequent reduction of the neurotransmitter in the synaptic cleft. Recent studies have linked the increased function of serotonin transporters with seasonal affective disorder [30].In addition to the reduction of serotonin, alterations in metabolism of dopamine (DA), would also contribute to the onset of symptoms such as psychomotor retardation and fatigue. In fact, the IFN and, more generally, pro-inflammatory cytokines, act on the metabolism of DA, especially at the level of the basal ganglia, causing a symptomatology characterized by neuro-vegetative symptoms, anhedonia, psychomotor retardation, fatigue [31,32-33].

Dopamine is involved in different circuits in mood, reward and motivation, motor activity, sleep-wake rhythm, cognitive processes [34,35].

It has been shown that IFN α induces motor slowing and this slowing down is correlated, significantly, to the development of depression and fatigue [31].

The mechanisms by which the IFN would act resulting in a reduction of DA in the synaptic cleft are manifold; primarily cytokines, and therefore the IFN α as well, induce an increase of nitric oxide (NO), which causes a reduction of tetrahydrobiopterin (BH4) that is a co-enzyme for tyrosine hydroxylase, which converts tyrosine to L-DOPA, this causes a reduction in the synthesis of DA [27].

It has also been shown that the action of IFN on BH4 is mediated by nitric oxide, in fact, treatments that inhibit the synthesis of NO, block the inhibitory effect mediated by IFN on the concentration, at the level of the central nervous system, of tetrahydrobiopterin (BH4) and DA [36]. It was also demonstrated that the IL6 (whose blood concentrations increase after administration of IFN α), reduces the tetrahydrobiopterin at the neuronal level [37].

Another mechanism by which the IFN α works reducing the levels of DA in the synaptic cleft involves the Kynurenic acid (KA). As we have already said, with regard to the effect of cytokines on the metabolism of serotonin, the IFN determines an activation of the enzyme indoleamine 2,3 dioxygenase (IDO), which cleaves the tryptophan in kynurenic acid (KA). KA reduces the release of glutamate. The glutamate, as well known, stimulates the release of dopamine [37,38-39]. The final effect is, in this case as well, a reduction of the levels of DA in the synaptic cleft. Finally, the IFN α, as we mentioned above, can activate some protein kinase, the MAPK pathway, which results in the increase in the expression of those genes coding for transporters of DA, this causes an increased DA reuptake with consequent reduction of the available levels of DA in the synaptic cleft [40].

It is worth pointing out that, in addition to depressive and autonomic manifestations, symptoms of anxiety and irritability may also occur during therapy with IFN α.

Several studies have shown that a significant number of patients develop anxiety symptoms 1 or 2 hours after taking the interferon therapy [41]. Some neuroimaging studies have shown that one of the mechanisms by which cytokines may cause anxiety and hyper arousal, is related to the increased activation of neural circuits in dorsal anterior cingulate cortex [42,43].

4. Neurotoxicity of HCV

With regard to the aetio- pathogenesis the third aspect to consider is the one of specific neurotoxicity of HCV.

In the last years it has been supposed that psychiatric disorders that occur in patients affected by HCV are due to a direct effect of the virus.

In particular, it has been suggested that there is no link between the onset of depressive disorders in patients with HCV infection and the IFN α- therapy [44].

An interesting study using magnetic resonance spectroscopy (MRS), a non-invasive technique that allows to get localized biochemical information from tissues and organs, has pointed out several alterations of cerebral metabolites in patients with HCV infection [45]. These alterations are very similar to those caused by HIV virus which can be found in the central nervous system during the overt disease. [46,47]. These studies support the hypothesis according to which, even the HCV would be able to infect cells of the central nervous system, causing changes in the brain [48]. According to this hypothesis, the virus after infecting monocytes in circulation, is introduced into the CNS thanks to a mechanism known as "Trojan Horse," resulting in neuronal dysfunction. This hypothesis is supported by recent studies that have demonstrated the presence of HCV gene sequences in post-mortem examined brain tissue [49]. Another important aspect that rises from data in literature is that different viral genotypes correlate with a different response to the antiviral therapy with IFN-α. Up to now, according to differences in nucleotide sequence, 7 different genotypes of HCV (in turn subdivided into several subtypes) have been identified, with a different geographical prevalence. The most common genotypes in Europe are 1a, 1b, 2a, 2b and 3 while in the USA is genotype 1a. Many people believe that the genetic heterogeneity of the virus strains is the basis of the differences in the development of disease and in the responsiveness to treatment. It is well known, in fact, that the genotypes 1, 5 and 6 have a lower response to antiviral treatment. In particular, the virus 1b leads to a more rapid progression to cirrhosis. In contrast, viral genotypes 2 and 3 have a better response to antiviral treatment [50].

5. Psychological aspects of the diagnosis of hepatitis C and consultation – Liaison psychiatry

What has been argued so far gives an account of how much weight may have, in a bio-psycho-social dimension, the diagnosis of HCV. The patient has, in fact, to live a chronic medical condition, often without any physical and psychological resource to manage it, whose treatment is not always effective and has serious side effects; in addition, an uncontrollable factor, the constitutive genetic component indeed, may be decisive to a successful treatment.

The meeting with an illness, whatever it is, brings about such a big change of life to threaten the own sense of identity so that the disease can be lived with deep anguish, hate, anxiety and depression.

Organic disease, whatever is the form in which it may manifest, acute or chronic, mild or severe, always represents a more or less significant break of the individual cycle of life and therefore, it involves the psychological sphere.

Several times we have emphasized the complexity of the Psychiatrist role in patients with HCV-related chronic hepatitis. Actually, these patients live a condition of severe insecurity, both physical and psychological. They are forced to change their lifestyle, putting in practice new behaviours and careful conduct rules in personal, social and relational context.

They live together with the fear of serious complications and death. The many disorders related to hepatitis, depressive symptoms and interferon treatment, make them lose their physical and mental energy to manage their disease condition. Typically, in fact, depressive symptoms reported by this type of patients, are purely somatic; fatigue, muscle ache, tiredness are the most common symptoms that cause great discomfort to patients and most influence their quality of life. They are "carriers" of a deep sufferance but they have no more own energy to deal with it. It is clear that these people are able to encourage the clinician to work harder in order to match medical experience with psychological and relational competence. They are also able to lead the clinician to overcome the so-called "mind-body dichotomy" and get a new clinic view focused on the suffering person and not just on the disease. This aspect is really important because it makes actual an ethical problem that all health care professionals have to face in everyday clinical life:

a sterile biological reductionism to the detriment of the centrality of the person [51]. The Consultation and Liaison Psychiatry deals with the application of psychiatric theories and practices for the care of patients with organic disease treated in hospitals and health care services (e.g., primary care). The request for assistance from colleagues belonging to other specializations is so high that since the mid 70's specific consultation-liaison units have been provided within the departments of psychiatry even more frequently.

Specific areas of Consultation Psychiatry include the study, the diagnosis, the treatment and the prevention of psychiatric morbidity in patients affected by organic disease or somatic symptoms.

The continuous attention to the phenomena of the organic and psychological interaction between body and mind is the operative height of the psychiatrist who operates outside the psychiatric setting [52]. The Consultation and Liaison Psychiatry has been defined as a branch of psychiatry that focuses on diagnosis, treatment, study and prevention of the psychiatric morbidity in patients with organic diseases and in those who have somatic symptoms. It also provides to organize psychiatric consultations, liaison activities and training for non-psychiatric operators who belong to all types of clinical setting, especially in the general hospital [53].

It must be said that the setting of the psychiatrist's intervention is very different from the usual one, and actually, it consists of a general hospital, inside of which should always be present a consultation-liaison unit and, inside of it, it must be present an ambulatory for the management of patients with chronic C hepatitis and IFN treatment or at least, specialized and trained personnel to the management of this kind of patients.

In everyday clinical practice, psychiatric work consists of two types of intervention: the psychiatric consultation and liaison. The consultation focuses primarily on diagnosis and therapy. The diagnosis relies on means such as the clinical interview and psycho-diagnostic tests.

The treatment involves both pharmacologic and psychotherapy interventions.

The specificity of the consultant psychiatrist is therefore, based on his training that allows him to value the interactions between biological, psychological, social and psychodynamic variables in clinical practice, in diagnostics, in the treatment plan and prognosis of a mental disorder [49]. The consultant psychiatrist may also, if he deems it necessary, take charge of the patient in a continuous way, going beyond the single psychiatric consultation [54]. This possibility is not uncommon within the psychiatric ambulatories for the management of patients with HCV in IFN treatment. Many of these patients already have a basic psychiatric disorder, usually it is a medium degree disorder, never gone to the observation of psychiatrists. This psychiatric disorder will reoccur or worsen after the diagnosis of HCV or during IFN treatment, making continuous psychiatric cares necessary. In this regard, it should be said that patients are hopeful when it is given a chance of cure to them, on the other hand, they are frightened by the possibility of a therapeutic failure, the length of treatment and the possibility of serious side effects, including psychiatric symptoms. Actually, patients are really frightened of these latter symptoms because they have to face the spectrum of madness that, in their fantasies, drives them to the anguish of losing the ownership of their actions and thoughts.

Fairly often when they come to the psychiatric interview they feel concerned, sometimes distrustful. They often hide their fears and try to be light-hearted and cheerful. The classic joke is: "Doctor, am I mad?

Whatever is the way they face the interview, the spectrum of madness, the anguish of losing the integrity of their mind, after having already lost their physical integrity, shine through their words. Sending patients to the psychiatry ambulatory is just a crucial moment. The hepatologist should always motivate the consultation request, properly informing the patient about the therapy that he is going to take. What is more, he should inform the patient of the possible psychiatric side effects, reassuring him at the same time. Reassuring a patient does not mean to say "do not worry, it's nothing" but it means to be empathetic and show understanding and affectivity to themselves. An empathetic attitude together with clarity of information and precision to show the therapeutic path, are interventions that reassure themselves the patient. It is important, therefore, to pursue an empathetic attitude, that is trying to get as close as possible to emotional experience and the experiences of the other person, trying to perceive feelings and personal meanings experienced by the patient and communicate him understanding. Empathic listening is, therefore, a psychological structure of hospitality that is used to establish trust and strong therapeutic alliance [55].

Clinical experience shows that all patients and, in particular the multi- diagnosed ones, get the most comfort from knowing that they are at the centre of an integrated and multidisciplinary system of interventions. Confirming them the importance of their centrality, building around the patient a set of integrated and coordinated interventions, certainly has positive effects on collaboration, motivation and, finally, on the outcomes of the interventions.

The Liaison is a more complex and continuous type of intervention, which arises from the request made by the doctors of department to the psychiatrist or to the clinical psychologist. It consists of a great collaboration with the treating team that requested the consultation in order to share the management of the patient's problems. The psychiatrist will discuss with colleagues from other specialties about therapeutic strategies, he will involve all health professionals in the care and in the project, he will deal with the relationship problems that may occur into the staff or between the team and the patient, he will work to promote bio-psycho-social cultural models within the department. [56] Therefore, interventions addressed to one or more operators are the true liaison and they can focus on a specific case or on the overall method of intervention adopted by the consultants. Interventions vary from simple advice on the attitude to get in the therapeutic relationship to the interpretations of dynamics that may develop between the patient and the treating team, up to the training programs [57].

Motivations that drive the hepatologist to ask a psychiatric consultation are:

1. a consultation focused on the patient who has already started a therapy with interferon α.

2. a consultation focused on the patient who is "candidate" for a therapy with interferon α.

In the first case, the aim is the one of defining the clinical manifestations and, if possible, the formulation of the diagnosis and the treatment plan.

In the second case, they are problematic patients since they have a personal story of psychiatric disorders, a story of past or current psychopharmacological treatments, a story of abuse or substance dependence. The consultation, therefore, has the purpose to set the patient from a diagnostic and personological point of view, in order to support the requesting colleague in his choice or orientating him towards different treatment choices. The psychiatrist could, for example, suggest to postpone, if possible, the starting of interferon therapy after an appropriate period of psychopharmacological treatment or even suggest to avoid interferon therapy. Any decision must be shared by the patient and, if possible, one member of his family at least. This kind of patients often needs to be taken in charge by the psychiatric service, for both pharmacological and psychotherapeutic aspects.

It is clear that each component of the medical team will manage the situation with important ethical implications. The ease of relationship, in terms of respect and recognition of roles, responsibilities and tasks within the team, is the secret for all health care professionals to take any decision with greater confidence.

Psychiatric consultation, therefore, can also be directed to the consultant: the patient will not be visited since the focus is a diagnostic, therapeutic and relational problem.

6. Diagnosis and treatment of mental disorders in patients with HCV infection during interferon treatment

In the following section we analyse the psychiatric symptoms most frequently found in these patients.

According to literature, many studies concerning the onset of psychiatric disorders in patients suffering from HCV, show that depressive symptoms are commonly found despite of the assumption of antiviral therapy based on Interferon alpha (IFNα) and Ribavirin [58]. It has been demonstrated that 35% of 293 patients suffering from HCV reported an increase of the scores of depression even before starting antiviral therapy [59]. Also, it is well known the interferon α therapy may induce depressive symptoms.

The most important symptoms include: depressive symptoms, anxiety symptoms, cognitive symptoms, autonomic and somatic symptoms [11].

The autonomic and somatic symptoms tend to occur early during treatment with IFN-α and persist over time; the symptoms relating to mood, anxiety and cognitive symptoms tend to occur later during treatment [60,61].

The onset of neuro-vegetative symptoms (e.g. psychomotor retardation) and depressive symptoms prior to antiviral treatment would increase the likelihood of developing depressive symptoms [62,63-64,65].

The management of patients with HCV, candidate for therapy with interferon-α, is a vexed question, considering the prevalence of hepatitis C, the likely presence of problems related to substance abuse, the psychological question that the impact of the diagnosis of a disease with poor prognosis determines and multi-systemic side effects that the therapy itself may cause.

Many studies have shown, in fact, that the impairment of quality of life in these patients is both linked to the severity of the disease [45] and to the previous substance abuse and side effects of treatment [66.67]. On the other hand, it is also true that interferon therapy, slowing down and, in some cases, arresting the progression of the disease, could improve the quality of life of patients suffering from hepatitis C virus [68].

Psychiatric disorders more frequently found in HCV patients treated with interferon α include: sleep disorders, fatigue, irritability, anxiety disorders, cognitive disorders with impairment of concentration and memory, depressive episodes (mild, moderate or severe), confusion, delirium, psychotic disorder, mania, craving (alcohol, drugs). It is worth stressing that Depression does not just mean deflection of mood; this clinical picture, in fact, is characterized by a collection of disorders, involving emotional, cognitive and neuro-vegetative changes, which may occur in several combinations but usually tend to occur all together, resulting in the so-called depressive spectrum. Some studies have highlighted that depression related to interferon therapy is significantly different from Major Depression itself. The differences would involve the ideational sphere mainly. Patients on interferon therapy, in fact, do not present depressive ideations of guilt and ruin, ideas of inadequacy and worthlessness [69], typically experienced by patients with major depression. The hypothesis might be that depression occurring during interferon therapy should be included in the diagnostic category of "Mood Disorder due to a general medical condition" or "substance-induced disorder", according to the classification in the DSM IV TR [70]. According to the DSM IV TR, in fact, a Mood Disorder due to a general medical condition, is "a significant and persistent alteration in mood that is believed to be due to direct physiological effects of a general medical condition", including degenerative neurological diseases, metabolic conditions, viral infections or other infections as well. With regards to "Substances-Induced Mood Disorder", this is a condition that can be induced not only by drugs of abuse but also by medication, toxins. These conditions are not only characterized by a purely depressive symptomatology but also include symptoms such as high, expansive or irritable mood. It is shown that manic symptoms [71] and psychotic disorders [72] may also occur in patients receiving interferon.

It is also interesting to note that cognitive deficits often occur in patients suffering from chronic hepatitis C [73, 74].

It should also be noted that drug addicts with hepatitis C are affected by psychopathological alterations to a far greater extent than those who did not abuse substances [75].

In the guidelines of the EASL (European Association for the Study of Liver) [76] it states that depression is the leading cause of discontinuation of antiviral treatment with interferon α. According to these guidelines, patients with a documented story of depression should be evaluated by a psychiatrist before the start of antiviral therapy, so that it could be assessed the presence of possible psychiatric contraindications. These patients should be followed throughout the treatment to find out the onset of depression immediately and then, must be treated with antidepressants-based pharmacotherapy, when depressive symptoms are recognized.

Some studies have evaluated the possible use of antidepressants, in particular SSRIs, for "preventative" purposes, showing actually a reduction in the incidence of depression during treatment with interferon-α [77].

Regarding the abuse of alcohol, the EASL guidelines recommend not to exclude alcoholic patients from any antiviral therapy, these patients should receive counselling interventions to reduce and then stop the consumption of alcohol, as well as psychological support in order to encourage the compliance with therapies. With regard to addicted patients, guidelines say that these patients should have stopped the assumption of drugs or should be taking replacement therapy from 6-12 months. In both cases, it is recommended a close follow up by a multidisciplinary team composed of the hepatologist, the psychiatrist and the psychologist.

The psychiatrist's figure in a multidisciplinary team for the care of patients with HCV is therefore essential to evaluate before beginning the treatment: the presence of current anxiety or depressive episode, history of anxiety or depression or other past psychiatric disorders, previous psychiatric hospitalisations, history of abuse or dependence on alcohol, drugs and medication, family history of anxiety disorders, depression or suicide attempts, the presence or absence of a social support network. Patient must be informed on the risks of psychiatric symptoms linked to the assumption of IFN-α, showing him all treatment options that are available in case of psychiatric disorders. If psychiatric disorders were found under way, they should be treated before starting any antiviral therapy.

Self-administered tests can be used as diagnostic tools for psychiatric assessment, for example, the Zung Self Rating Depression Scale (ZSDS), the Zung Self Rating Anxiety Scale (ZSAS), other tests that can be administered are the Hamilton Depression Rating Scale (HAM D) and the Hamilton Anxiety Rating Scale (HAM A). These tests may be helpful to monitor patient during therapy.

Regarding any interventions to take in case of psychopathological disorders, such as anxiety disorders or depressive disorders, it should be said that they must be implemented as early as possible. The best first choice in treating anxiety disorders is the one of anxiolytics (BDZ). Among the benzodiazepine, those with little or no hepatic metabolism (oxazepam, lorazepam) should be chosen. A brief psychotherapeutic intervention may be decisive in case of reactive anxiety symptoms. SSRIs are the first choice for depressive disorders, especially paroxetine, sertraline, citalopram, that is, those with the best tolerability profile, the fewer interactions, the best demonstrated efficiency. If the severity of depressive condition is mild or moderate, antiviral treatment can be continued. Even in this case psychotherapeutic support interventions are suggested. If depressive symptoms persist and therapy does not work (by 2-4 weeks), it should be considered the use of another antidepressant with a different mechanism of action, or the reduction or discontinuation of IFN treatment; this decision could be made jointly by the infectious disease specialist, the consultant psychiatrist, the patient and a familiar at least. If psychotic symptoms occurred, IFN therapy should be discontinued and, if necessary, started again, only after the patient has been properly treated with antipsychotic drugs.

Depression induced by IFN α responds well to treatment with SSRIs, as it would be mainly due to alterations involving the serotonergic circuits, while the so-called Neuro-vegetative

Syndrome induced by IFN, characterized by fatigue, anorexia, pain and psychomotor retardation, which is often found in association with depressive symptoms, would benefit from drugs such as SNRIs (venlafaxine) and Bupropion [78].

Confusional episodes characterized by disorientation, somnolence, psychomotor retardation, psychotic symptoms have also been documented in patients treated with IFN α [79, 80]. In these cases it is necessary to discontinue therapy and administer neuroleptics or atypical antipsychotics, including especially olanzapine[81].

It should also be considered the degree of hepatic impairment in these patients in order to determine the optimal dosage of the drugs. In general, drugs should be used at the lowest effective dose. It should be pointed out that paroxetine, fluoxetine and fluvoxamine may reduce the metabolism of other drugs, increasing their blood levels.

It is also useful to consider that some side effects of antidepressants may be exploited for the patient's benefit; such as weight gain and drowsiness that occurred during treatment with mirtazapine may be useful in those patients affected by HCV, in which therapy with IFN α and ribavirin caused hyporexia / anorexia and insomnia.

Another psychiatric symptom that may be found during therapy with IFN α, as already said, is mania [82,83]. It is important to note that irritability which very often occurs in these patients is a classic symptom of mania [84]. It seems that manic or hypomanic symptoms develop in approx. 20% of HCV-positive patients treated with IFN-α and ribavirin [85]. It is very important to recognize dysphoric mania carefully. It is a clinical situation in which both elements related to manic activation and depressive elements may occur together. The use of antidepressants in dysphoric mania would induce the worsening of the manic picture. Indeed, it is common that dysphoria may be sometimes confused with a depressive symptom and that is why the opinion of the psychiatrist should be asked whenever a picture of psychopathological alterations is suspected.

Finally, we must not forget that interferon therapy may increase the risk of suicide although studies in this field are still few and results don't appear unique [86, 87]. It is clear that the prognosis of viral disease itself, which, as well known, can result in cirrhosis and hepatocellular carcinoma, may cause psychological reactions of despair that can lead to depression and suicidal ideation. It is worth noting that, according to the DSM IV TR "Mood Disorder due to a general medical condition increases the risk of suicide attempts and suicide" [1]. Even in case of suicide then, we must consider several risk factors, ranging from psychological consequences of diagnosis and prognosis to depression caused by the therapy.

7. Conclusions

In view of these considerations, it is understandable that the management of patients with HCV treated or not with IFN α, requires several specialized figures that can deal with the many aspects that this condition brings with it. The guidelines and literature recommend the presence of a multidisciplinary team, in which the psychiatrist plays a key role for the great incidence of psychiatric disorders in these patients.

In a Consensus Conference held by European specialists in 2005 it was established that, in case of psychiatric disorders, it is not necessary to delay or forego treatment if this is complemented by a global care, where several specialists are involved, such as: Gastroenterologist, Infectious disease specialist, Psychiatrist, Addiction Service Operators, Psychologist – Counsellor [88]. Then, in case of psychiatric disorders, treatment with IFN is strongly recommended, keeping in mind that the psychological state must be stabilized before starting antiviral therapy.

Some studies have shown that psychiatric disorders may also occur several months after discontinuation of therapy with IFN α and ribavirin [89], or may still persist even after discontinuation of therapy [90]. It would be good practice then, that the control of the mental state of patient continued even after discontinuation of antiviral treatment.

In view of these considerations, it is certain that interferon therapy acts causing mental status changes that include mainly changes in mood and anxiety. The widespread of C virus is a ubiquitous problem and therefore, it requires a strong attention that helps to do more and more to deal with any organic and psychic problems "orbiting" around this condition. It would be desirable that these patients may have assistance which allows them to continue antiviral therapy, coping with possible side effects that would probably be a contraindication to continue therapy, "condemning" the patient to a forced coexistence with the virus.

Author details

Giuseppe Valerio Torres[1], Emanuela Apicella[2], Elisa D'Alterio[3], Angela Chiara Cecere[2] and Antonello Bellomo[4]

1 Department of Mental Health ASL FG, University of Foggia, Italy

2 University of Foggia, Italy

3 University of Naples, Italy

4 Department of Medical Occupational Sciences, University of Foggia, Italy

References

[1] Diagnostic, A. A. V. V. and statistical manual of mental disorder: DSM IV TR. American Psychiatric Pub. 4ª ed;(2000).

[2] Lteif, G. N, & Mavissakalion, M. R. Life events and panic disorders/agoraphobia. Compreh. Psychiatry (1995).

[3] Kessler, R. C. Sociology and Psychiatry. In: Kaplan H.I., Sadock B.J. Comprehensive Textbook of Psychiatry. Williams & Wilkins; (1989).

[4] Paykel, E. S. The interview for recent life events. Psycol. Med (1997). , 27(2), 301-310.

[5] Carta, M. G. Hardoy MC at al. Association of chronic hepatitis C with major depressive disorders: irrespective of interferon-alpha therapy. Clinical Practice and Epidemiology in Mental Health (2007).

[6] Voss, J. G. Dodd, Portillo C, Holzemer W. Theories of fatigue: application in HIV/AIDS. J. Assoc. Nurses AIDS Care (2006). , 17-37.

[7] Astle, F. Diabetes and depression: a review of the literature. Nurs Clin North Am. (2007). , 42-67.

[8] Gold, S. M, & Irwin, M. R. Depression and immunity: inflammation and depressive symptoms in multiple sclerosis. Neurol. Clin.(2006). , 24-507.

[9] Ranjit, N, Diez-roux, A. V, Shea, S, Cushman, M, Seeman, T, Jackson, S. A, & Ni, H. Psychosocial factors and inflammation in the multi-ethnic study of atherosclerosis. Arch. Intern. Med. (2007). , 167-174.

[10] Dieperink, E, Willenbring, M, & Ho, S. B. Neuropsychiatric symptoms associated with hepatitis C and interferon alpha: a review. Am J Psychiatry (2000). , 157-867.

[11] Lotrich, F. E, Rabinovitz, M, et al. Depression following pegylated interferon-alpha: Characteristics and vulnerability. Journal of Psychosomatic Research (2007). , 63-131.

[12] Licinio, J, & Wong, M. L. The role of inflammatory mediators in the biology of major depression: central nervous system cytokines modulate the biological substrate of depressive symptoms, regulate stress-responsive systems, and contribute to neurotoxicity and neuroprotection. Mol. Psychiatry (1993). , 4-317.

[13] Loftis, J. M, & Hauser, P. The phenomenology and treatment of interferoninduced depression. J. Affect Disord. (2004). , 82-175.

[14] Raison, C. L, Capuron, L, & Miller, A. H. Cytokines sing the blues: inflammation and the pathogenesis of depression. Trends Immunol. (2006). , 27-24.

[15] Schiepers, O. J, Wichers, M. C, & Maes, M. Cytokines and major depression. Prog. Neuropsychopharmacol. Biol. Psychiatry (2005). , 29-201.

[16] Andreoli, A. V, Keller, S. E, Rabaeus, M, Marin, P, Bartlett, J. A, & Taban, C. Depression and immunity: age, severity, and clinical course. Brain. Behav. Immun. (1993). , 7-279.

[17] Leonard, B. E, & Myint, A. The psychoneuroimmunology of depression. Hum Psychopharmacol (2009). Apr;, 24(3), 165-175.

[18] Turnbull, A. V, & Rivier, C. L. Regulation of the hypothalamic-pituitary-adrenal axis by cytokines: actions and mechanisms of action. Physiol Rev (1999). Jan;, 79(1), 1-71.

[19] Friebe, A, Schwarz, M. J, Schmid-wendtner, M, Volkenandt, M, Schmidt, F, Horn, M, Janssen, G, & Schaefer, M. Pre-treatment levels of sTNF-R1 and sIL-6R are associated with a higher vulnerability for IFN-alpha-induced depressive symptoms in patients with malignant melanoma. J. Immunother (1997). , 30-333.

[20] Musselman, D. L, Miller, A. H, Porter, M. R, Manatunga, A. K, Gao, F, Penna, S, Pearce, B. D, Landry, J, Glover, S, Mcdaniel, J. S, & Nemeroff, C. B. Higher than normal plasma interleukin-6 concentrations in cancer patients with depression: preliminary findings. Am. J. Psychiatry (2001). , 158-1252.

[21] Wichers, M. C, Kenis, G, Leue, C, Koek, G, Robaeys, G, & Maes, M. Baseline immune activation as a risk factor for the onset of depression during interferon-alpha treatment. Biol. Psychiatry (2006). , 60-77.

[22] Morasco, B. J, & Rifai, M. A. A randomized trial of paroxetine to prevent interferon-α-induced depression in patients with hepatitis C. Journal of Affective Disorders (2007). , 103-83.

[23] Musselman, D. L, Lawson, D. H, Gumnick, J. F, Manatunga, A. K, Penna, S, Goodkin, R. S, Greiner, K, Nemeroff, C. B, & Miller, A. H. Paroxetine for the prevention of depression induced by high-dose interferon alpha. N. Engl. J. Med. (2001). , 344, 961-966.

[24] Dantzer, R, Connor, O, Freund, J. C, Johnson, G. G, & Kelley, R. W. K.W. From inflammation to sickness and depression: when the immune system subjugates the brain. Nat. Rev. Neurosci. (2008). , 9-46.

[25] Capuron, L, Ravaud, A, Neveu, P. J, Miller, A. H, Maes, M, & Dantzer, R. Association between decreased serum tryptophan concentrations and depressive symptoms in cancer patients undergoing cytokine therapy. Mol. Psychiatry (2002b). , 7-468.

[26] Maes, M, Bonaccorso, S, Marino, V, Puzella, A, Pasquini, M, Biondi, M, Artini, M, Almerighi, C, & Meltzer, H. Treatment with interferon-alpha (IFN alpha) of hepatitis C patients induces lower serum dipeptidyl peptidase IV activity, which is related to IFN alpha-induced depressive and anxiety symptoms and immune activation. Mol. Psychiatry (2001). , 6-475.

[27] Miller, A. H. Mechanisms of cytokine-induced behavioral changes: Psychoneuroimmunology at the translational interface. Brain, Behavior, and Immunity (2009). , 23-149.

[28] Zhu, C. B, Carneiro, A. M, Dostmann, W. R, Hewlett, W. A, & Blakely, R. D. p. MAPK activation elevates serotonin transport activity via a traffickingindependent, protein phosphatase 2A-dependent process. J. Biol. Chem. (2005). , 280-15649.

[29] Zhu, C. B, Blakely, R. D, & Hewlett, W. A. The proinflammatory cytokines interleukin-1beta and tumor necrosis factor-alpha activate serotonin transporters. Neuropsychopharmacology (2006). , 31-2121.

[30] Willeit, M, Sitte, H. H, Thierry, N, Michalek, K, Praschak-rieder, N, Zill, P, Winkler, D, Brannath, W, Fischer, M. B, Bondy, B, Kasper, S, & Singer, E. A. Enhanced serotonin

transporter function during depression in seasonal affective disorder. Neuropsychopharmacology (2008). , 33, 1503-1513.

[31] Majer, M, Welberg, L. A, Capuron, L, Pagnoni, G, Raison, C. L, & Miller, A. H. IFNalpha-induced motor slowing is associated with increased depression and fatigue in patients with chronic hepatitis C. Brain Behav. Immun. (2008). , 22-870.

[32] Horikawa, N, Yamazaki, T, Sagawa, M, & Nagata, T. A case of akathisia during interferon-alpha therapy for chronic hepatitis type C. Gen. Hosp. Psychiatry (1999). , 21-134.

[33] Kamata, M, Higuchi, H, Yoshimoto, M, Yoshida, K, & Shimizu, T. Effect of single intracerebroventricular injection of alpha-interferon on monoamine concentrations in the rat brain. Eur. Neuropsychopharmacol. (2000). , 10-129.

[34] Salamone, J. D, Correa, M, Mingote, S. M, & Weber, S. M. Beyond the reward hypothesis: alternative functions of nucleus accumbens dopamine. Curr. Opin. Pharmacol. (2005). , 5-34.

[35] Schultz, W. Multiple dopamine functions at different time courses. Annu. Rev. Neurosci. (2007). , 30-259.

[36] Kitagami, T, Yamada, K, Miura, H, Hashimoto, R, Nabeshima, T, & Ohta, T. Mechanism of systemically injected interferon-alpha impeding monoamine biosynthesis in rats: role of nitric oxide as a signal crossing the blood-brain barrier. Brain Res. (2003). , 978-104.

[37] Capuron, L, Neurauter, G, Musselman, D. L, Lawson, D. H, Nemeroff, C. B, Fuchs, D, & Miller, A. H. Interferon-alpha-induced changes in tryptophan metabolism. Relationship to depression and paroxetine treatment. Biol. Psychiatry (2003a). , 54-906.

[38] Wu, H. Q, Rassoulpour, A, & Schwarcz, R. Kynurenic acid leads, dopamine follows: a new case of volume transmission in the brain? J. Neural. Transm. (2007). , 114, 33-41.

[39] Moron, J. A, Zakharova, I, Ferrer, J. V, Merrill, G. A, Hope, B, Lafer, E. M, Lin, Z. C, Wang, J. B, Javitch, J. A, Galli, A, & Shippenberg, T. S. Mitogen-activated protein kinase regulates dopamine transporter surface expression and dopamine transport capacity. J. Neurosci. (2003). , 23, 8480-8488.

[40] Capuron, L, Pagnoni, G, Demetrashvili, M, Woolwine, B. J, Nemeroff, C. B, Berns, G. S, & Miller, A. H. Anterior cingulate activation and error processing during interferon-alpha treatment. Biol. Psychiatry (2005). , 58, 190-196.

[41] Reichenberg, A, Yirmiya, R, Schuld, A, Kraus, T, Haack, M, Morag, A, & Pollmacher, T. Cytokine-associated emotional and cognitive disturbances in humans. Arch. Gen. Psychiatry (2001). , 58, 445-452.

[42] Ursu, S, Stenger, V. A, Shear, M. K, Jones, M. R, & Carter, C. S. Overactive action monitoring in obsessive-compulsive disorder: evidence from functional magnetic resonance imaging. Psychol. Sci. (2003)., 14, 347-353.

[43] Grassi, L, Satriano, J, Serra, A, Biancosino, B, Zotos, S, Sighinolfi, L, & Ghinelli, F. Emotional stress, psychosocial variables and coping associated with haepatitis C virus and human immunodeficiency virus infections in intravenous drug users. Psychother Psychosom (2002)., 71-342.

[44] Carta, M. G. Hardoy MC at al. Association of chronic hepatitis C with major depressive disorders: irrespective of interferon-alpha therapy. Clinical Practice and Epidemiology in Mental Health (2007).

[45] Forton, D. M, Allsop, J. M, Main, J, Foster, G. R, Thomas, H. C, & Taylor-robinson, S. D. Evidence for a cerebral effect of the hepatitis C virus. Lancet (2001)., 358-38.

[46] Chang, L, Ernst, T, Witt, M. D, Ames, N, Gaiefsky, M, & Miller, E. Relationships among brain metabolites, cognitive function, and viral loads in antiretroviral-naive HIV patients. Neuroimage (2002)., 17-1638.

[47] Chang, L, Lee, P. L, Yiannoutsos, C. T, Ernst, T, Marra, C. M, Richards, T, Kolson, D, Schifitto, G, Jarvik, J. G, Miller, E. N, Lenkinski, R, Gonzalez, G, & Navia, B. A. HIV MRS Consortium: A multicenter in vivo proton- MRS study of HIV-associated dementia and its relationship to age. Neuroimage (2004)., 23-1336.

[48] Thomas, H. C, Torok, M. E, Forton, D. M, & Taylor-robinson, S. D. Possible mechanisms of action and reasons for failure of antiviral therapy in chronic hepatitis C. J Hepatol (1999)., 31(1), 152-159.

[49] Radkowski, M, Wilkinson, J, Nowicki, M, Adair, D, Vargas, H, Ingui, C, Rakela, J, & Laskus, T. Search for hepatitis C virus negative-strand RNA sequences and analysis of viral sequences in the central nervous system: evidence of replication. J Virol (2002)., 76-600.

[50] Shepherd, J, Brodin, H, Cave, C, Waugh, N, Price, A, & Gabbay, J. Pegylated interferon-2a and-2b in combination with ribavirin in the treatment of chronic hepatitis C: a systematic review and economic evaluation. Health Technology Assessment (2004).

[51] Invernizzi, G, Gala, C, & Bressi, C. La Psichiatria di Consultazione nell'Ospedale Generale. CIC Ed. Internazionali, Roma;(1997).

[52] De Bertolini, C, Rigatelli, M, & Rizzardo, R. Psichiatria di consultazione e collegamento. In:Pavan L. Trattato italiano di psichiatria. Masson;(1999).

[53] Lipowski, Z. J. Consultation-Liaison Psychiatry at century's end. Psychosomatics (1992).

[54] Kaplan, H. I, Sadoch, B. J, & Grebb, J. A. Psichiatria.Manuale di scienze del comportamento e psichiatria clinica. Centro Scientifico Internazionale (2001)., 818-819.

[55] Orsi, E. Comunicazione efficace: l'approccio empatico nelle relazioni d'aiuto. In: Bellomo A. Psicologia Medica e abilità relazionali. Edizioni Minerva Medica (2004). , 79-80.

[56] Mayou, R. A. Consultation-liaison psychiatry: panoramica internazionale. Upiohn International inc (1988).

[57] Fulcheri, M, Bellino, S, & Zizza, M. Di Lorenzo R, Bogetto F. La Psichiatria di consultazione e collegamento::modelli e dati della letteratura. Rivista di Psichiatria (2001).

[58] Angelino, A. F, & Treisman, G. J. Evidence-informed assessment and treatment of depression in HCV and interferon-treated patients. Int. Rev. Psychiatry (2005). , 17-471.

[59] Fireman, M, Indest, D. W, Blackwell, A, Whitehead, A, & Hauser, P. Addressing tri-morbidity (hepatitis C, psychiatric disorders, and substance use): the importance of routine mental health screening as a component of a comanagement model of care. Clin. Infect. Dis. (2005). , 40(5), 286-291.

[60] Capuron, L, Gumnick, J. F, Musselman, D. L, Lawson, D. H, Reemsnyder, A, Nemeroff, C. B, & Miller, A. H. Neurobehavioral effects of interferon-alpha in cancer patients: phenomenology and paroxetine responsiveness of symptom dimensions. Neuropsychopharmacology (2002). , 26-643.

[61] Capuron, L, & Miller, A. H. Cytokines and psychopatology :lessons from interferon-alpha.Biol.Psichiatry (2004). , 56-819.

[62] Capuron, L, & Miller, A. H. Cytokines and psychopathology: lessons from interferon-alpha. Biol. Psychiatry (2004). Capuron L, Ravaud A, Dantzer R. Timing and specificity of the cognitive changes induced by interleukin-2 and interferon-alpha treatments in cancer patients. Psychosom. Med. 2001;63 376-386., 56-819.

[63] Capuron, L, & Ravaud, A. Prediction of the depressive effects of interferon alpha therapy by the patient's initial affective state. N. Engl. J. Med. (1999).

[64] Majer, M, Welberg, L. A, Capuron, L, Pagnoni, G, Raison, C. L, & Miller, A. H. IFNalpha-induced motor slowing is associated with increased depression and fatigue in patients with chronic hepatitis C. Brain Behav. Immun. (2008). , 22-870.

[65] Raison, C. L, Borisov, A. S, Broadwell, S. D, Capuron, L, Woolwine, B. J, Jacobson, I. M, Nemeroff, C. B, & Miller, A. H. Depression during pegylated interferonalpha plus ribavirin therapy: prevalence and prediction. J. Clin. Psychiatry (2005). , 66-41.

[66] Hussain, K, Fontana, R, Moyer, C, Su, G. L, Sneed-pee, N, & Lok, A. S. F. Comorbid illness is an important determinant of health-related quality of life in patients with chronic hepatitis C. Am J Gastroenterol. (2001). , 96-2737.

[67] Spiegel, B, Younossi, Z, Hays, R, Hays, R. D, Revicki, D, Robins, S, et al. Impact of hepatitis C on health related quality of life: a systematic review and quantitative assessment. Hepatology. (2005). , 41-790.

[68] Kamal, S. M, Ahmed, A, et al. Enhanced efficacy of pegylated interferon alpha-2a over pegylated interferon and ribavirin in chronic hepatitis C genotype 4A randomized trial and quality of life analysis. Liver Int. (2011). Mar;, 31(3), 401-11.

[69] Pasquini, M, Speca, A, et al. Differences in depressive thougths between major depressive disorder, IFN-α-induced depression, and depressive disorders among cancer patients. Journal of Psychosomatic Research (2008). , 65-153.

[70] Gregory, M, et al. Interferon-Induced Depression in CHC. J Clin Gastroenterol. (2006).

[71] Giunta, B, Somboonwit, C, et al. Psychiatric implications of hepatitis-C infection. Crit Rev Neurobiol. (2007).

[72] Silverman, B. C, Kim, A. Y, & Freudenreich, O. Interferon-induced psychosis as a "psychiatric contraindication" to hepatitis C treatment: a review and case-based discussion. Psychosomatics. (2010). Jan-Feb;, 51(1), 1-7.

[73] Forton, D. M, Thomas, H. C, et al. Hepatitis C and cognitive impairment in a cohort of patients with mild liver disease. Hepatology (2002). , 3-433.

[74] Forton, D. M, Taylor-robinson, S. D, & Thomas, H. C. Cerebral dysfumction in chronic hepatitis C infection. J Viral Hepatitis (2003). , 10-81.

[75] Johnson, M. E, Fisher, D. G, et al. Hepatitis C virus and depression in drug users. Am J Gastroenterol. (1998). , 93-785.

[76] European Association for the Study of the LiverEASL Clinical Practice Guidelines: Management of hepatitis C virus infection. Journal of Hepatology (2011).

[77] Bezemer, G, Van Gool, A. R, Drenth, J. P, & Hansen, B. E. Fortuyn HAD, Weegink CJ, et al. A double blind, placebo-controlled trial with escitalopram to prevent psychiatric adverse events during treatment with pegylated interferonalpha and ribavirin for chronic hepatitis c: the ''prevention of psychiatric side effects (Pops)-study''. Hepatology (2008). A.

[78] Charles, L. Raison Marina Demetrashvili, Lucile Capuron and Andrew H. Miller. Neuropsychiatric Adverse Effects of Interferon-α Recognition and Management. CNS Drugs. (2005). , 19(2), 105-123.

[79] Rohatiner, A. Z, Prior, P. F, Burton, A. C, et al. Central nervous system toxicity of interferon. Br J Cancer. (1983). , 47(3), 419-22.

[80] Poutiainen, E, Hokkanen, L, Niemi, M. L, et al. Reversible cognitive decline during high-dose α-interferon treatment. Pharmacol Biochem Behav. (1994). , 47(4), 901-5.

[81] Hoffman, R. G, Cohen, M. A, Alfonso, C. A, et al. Treatment of interferon-induced psychosis in patients with comorbid hepatitis C and HIV. Psychosomatics. (2003). , 44(5), 417-20.

[82] Carpiniello, B, Orru, M. G, Baita, A, et al. Mania induced by withdrawal of treatment with interferon alfa. Arch Gen Psychiatry. (1998). , 55(1), 88-9.

[83] Kanno, A, Yamada, M, Abe, M, et al. A case of interferon α-induced manic psychosis in chronic hepatitis C. Tohoku J Exp Med. (1999). , 187(1), 79-82.

[84] Raison, C. L, & Miller, A. H. The neuroimmunology of stress and depression. Semin Clin Neuropsychiatry (2001). , 6(4), 277-94.

[85] Gould, R. A, Ball, S, Kaspi, S. P, et al. Prevalence and correlates of anger attacks: a two site study. J Affect Disord. (1996). , 39(1), 31-8.

[86] Sockalingam, S, Links, P. S, & Abbey, S. E. Suicide risk in hepatitis C and during interferon-alpha therapy: a review and clinical update. J Viral Hepat. (2011). Mar;, 18(3), 153-60.

[87] Debien, C. De Chouly De Lenclave MB, Foutrein P, Bailly D. [Alpha-interferon and mental disorders]. Encephale. (2001). Jul-Aug;, 27(4), 308-17.

[88] Alberti, A, Clumeck, N, Collins, S, Gerlich, W, Lundgren, J, Palù, G, Reiss, P, Thiebaut, R, Weiland, O, & Yazdanpanah, Y. Zeuzem S (The ECC Jury). Short statement of the first European consensus conference on the treatment of chronic hepatitis B and C in HIV co-infected patients. Journal of Hepatology (2005). , 42-615.

[89] Nickel, T, et al. Depression during therapy with interferon alpha-how long should an antidepressant treatment last? Pharmacopsychiatry (2005). , 38-102.

[90] Meyers, C. A, et al. Persistent neurotoxicity of systemically administered interferon-alpha. Neurology (1991). , 41-672.

Section 3

Complications and Patient Education

Chapter 12

HCV, Mixed Cryoglobulinemia and Malignant Lymphoproliferation

Gianfranco Lauletta

Additional information is available at the end of the chapter

http://dx.doi.org/10.5772/55474

1. Introduction

Hepatitis C virus (HCV) is a member of the family *Flaviviridae*, genus *Hepacivirus*, and about 200 million people worldwide are thought to be infected [1]. Some 80% of HCV-infected individuals will develop chronic hepatitis, with 10–20% eventually developing cirrhosis and 1–5% progressing to hepatocarcinoma [2]. The HCV genome is about 9,600 kb in length and encodes a single protein from an open reading frame of over 9024 nucleotides. This single polyprotein is subsequently cleaved into several structural and non-structural proteins. The structural proteins consist of the *core* and two envelope proteins (E1 and E2), starting from the 5′ end [1]. The ion-channel protein p7 derives from E2 cleavage [3] and is followed by the six non-structural proteins, namely, NS2, NS3, NS4A, NS4B, NS5A, and NS5B. During the replicative stage, HCV genomic RNA is transcribed into a complementary RNA strand. This "negative" strand constitutes a template for new genomic synthesis and its identification in an infected host provides convincing evidence of active viral replication [4]. Viral proteins are the result of the co- and post-translational cleavage of a single polyprotein, while host peptidases catalyze the cleavage of structural proteins. The HCV particles form a membrane-associated replication complex; after genome amplification and protein expression, progeny virions are assembled and released [5, 6].

Although HCV is primarily hepatotropic, clinically it is characterized by the emergence of several extrahepatic manifestations. In fact, after the identification of HCV as the etiologic agent of non-A, non-B chronic hepatitis and the availability in the early 1990s of a serologic test for the demonstration of IgG anti-HCV, several authors described an intriguing association between HCV infection and "essential" mixed cryoglobulinemia (MC), an immune complex-mediated vasculitis involving small vessels, with some geographic differences [7-9]. This association was subsequently confirmed by the detection of viral genome in the sera of cryoglobulinemic patients, with a selective concentration of viral RNA in cryoprecipitates [10, 11]. The incidence of HCV infection in MC ranges from 40 to 90% [12] whereas HCV-negative MC accounts for about 5–10% of the total cases [13].

Since B-cell clonal expansion is a hallmark of MC [14], the malignant evolution of these cells may reflect the occurrence of additional genetic accidents [15].

Here, we discuss the currently accepted pathogenetic mechanisms underlying cryoglobulinemic vasculitis and its specific clinical manifestations, the molecular events proposed to explain the potentially malignant evolution of MC, the many clinical features of the disease, and the currently available therapeutic options for the treatment of MC and B-cell NHLs.

2. Mixed cryoglobulinemia: Clinical features

Cryoglobulins are immunoglobulins (Igs) that are insoluble at low temperature (below 37°C) but redissolve after warming. In 1933, Wintrobe and Buell first described the phenomenon of cryoprecipitation in the serum of a patient with multiple myeloma [16], although the term "cryoglobulin" was introduced in 1947 by Lerner and Watson [17]. Meltzer *et al.*, in a study of 29 patients, associated cryoglobulin production with a clinical picture characterized by a typical symptomatologic triad of purpura, weakness, and arthralgias. These patients were also observed to have increased serum levels of rheumatoid factor (RF) and/or organ dysfunction [18].

According to Brouet's immunochemically based classification, cryoglobulins are either single (type I) or mixed (type II and III) in their composition [19]. Thus, type I cryoglobulinemia consists of a monoclonal Ig, usually of IgM or IgG isotype. IgM cryoglobulins occur in ~6% of malignant IgM paraproteinemias and IgG cryoglobulins in ~2% of all myelomas. Type I IgA cryoglobulins are rare [20]. In type II MC, which accounts for 50–60% of all cryoglobulins, there is an IgM monoclonal component, frequently consisting of light k chains, and polyclonal IgG. IgM molecules have RF activity and are thus capable of reacting with intact IgG and/or its F(ab)2' fragment [21]. In type III MC, which accounts for 30-40% of cryoglobulins, a monoclonal component is lacking. According to some authors, this type represents a transitional form that evolves into type II MC [22].

Mixed cryoglobulins are potentially present in connective tissue and autoimmune diseases and in chronic infections [23, 24]. The term "essential" defines cryoglobulinemic syndromes without an underlying identifiable etiology. It is now accepted that MC most often occurs in patients chronically infected with HCV [25], as the result of specific interactions between the virus and the host immune system [11]. Thus, while initially considered as "essential", MC is now recognized as the most common HCV-related extrahepatic disease. It has been estimated that 40–60% of chronically HCV-infected patients produce cryoglobulins, but only15–20% will develop the full-blown clinical features of MC [26].

The prevalence of MC shows great heterogeneity in terms of geographic distribution. The disease seems to be more common in Southern Europe and in the Mediterranean basin than in Northern Europe and North America [27]. Although MC is considered to be a rare disorder, with an estimated prevalence of approximately of 1:100,000 (with a F:M ratio of 3:1), its true prevalence is unknown because of a failure by the treating physician to recognize the clinical symptoms such that patients are referred to several specialists and are often incorrectly diagnosed.

Cryoglobulinemic syndrome can be considered an immune-mediated systemic vasculitis preferentially affecting the small and medium-sized vessels. Although Meltzer's symptomatologic triad of purpura, weakness, and arthralgias is considered diagnostic, the clinical spectrum of cryoglobulinemic vasculitis varies depending on the exact organ involvement.

2.1. Skin tissue

Cutaneous manifestations are the most typical clinical sign of cryoglobulinemic vasculitis; they range from palpable purpura of the lower limbs to chronic torpid cutaneous ulcers typically located in the supramalleolar regions. Usually, the clinical course of the purpura consists of recurrent flares in which the lesions spontaneously heal but leave a characteristic brown pigmentation due to residual hemosiderin deposits. Less frequently, purpura can extend from the abdomen, upper limbs, and thorax. Although small petechial lesions are typically seen on the skin, other manifestations have been described, including Raynaud's phenomenon, *livedo reticularis,* urticaria, and edema. The cutaneous involvement is often complicated by the occurrence of chronic leg ulcers with little or no tendency to heal and which spontaneously cause pain and severe discomfort to the patient (Figure 1) [28].

The histopathologic features of palpable purpura include a non-specific inflammatory infiltrate involving the small vessels (leukocytoclastic vasculitis), sometimes with a mononuclear cells infiltration of the vessel walls. Endoluminal thrombi and fibrinoid necrosis of the arteriolar walls have also been described [29].

As previously reported, skin lesions are almost invariable associated with arthralgias, which often symmetrically involve the hands and knees. Weakness is nearly always present.

2.2. Kidney

Kidney involvement is a common feature of an immune-complex-mediated systemic vasculitis. Renal injury complicates MC in almost 30% of the cases and is present at the time of diagnosis in 20% [12, 30, 31]. In about 50% of the cases, renal failure follows an indolent course, whereas nephritic or nephrotic syndrome occurs in 14% and 21% of MC patients, respectively [32]. The most common clinical features are hypertension, proteinuria, microhematuria, and red blood cell casts. A definitive cryoglobulinemic glomerulonephritis evolves into chronic renal failure in 14% of patients after a mean follow-up of 6 years [33].

Although kidney involvement is a common feature of systemic vasculitis, cryoglobulinemic nephropathy is considered a distinct clinical and pathological entity and the etiological role of HCV in the disease has been extensively investigated [34]. Type I membranoproliferative glomerulonephritis is predominantly associated with HCV infection [35, 36]. Light microscopy

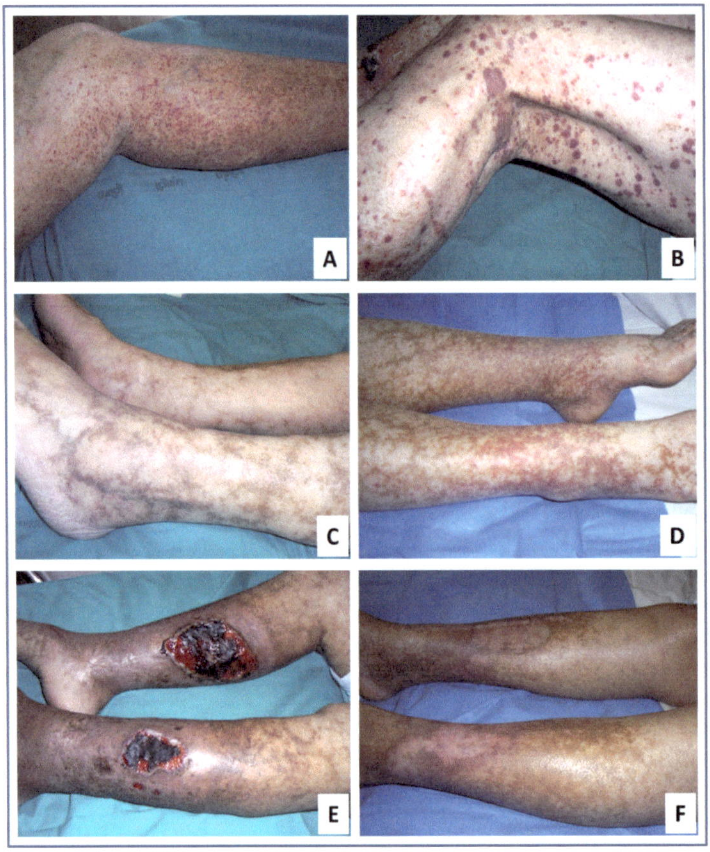

Figure 1. Clinical manifestation of cryoglobulinemic vasculitis. (A) Typical purpuric lesions, seen here on the legs, may become confluent (B). (C) and (D): livedo reticularis. (E) Chronic leg ulcers. (F) Ulcers healing after therapy

of biopsy samples shows a pronounced glomerular lobulation with a diffuse thickening of the glomerular capillary walls and a monocytic infiltration. PAS-positive hyaline thrombi may be observed inside capillary lumina [35, 37]. The mechanism of HCV-induced renal damage is unclear. However, HCV core protein has been detected in a homogeneous distribution along the glomerular capillary wall and tubulo-interstitial blood vessels [38] in association with an anti-core activity, suggesting a major role for these immune complexes in the pathogenesis of renal damage [39].

2.3. Nervous system

The involvement of the nervous system in the course of HCV-related MC ranges from 17% to 60% [40]. In some cases, however, peripheral neuropathy is the first clinical sign of cryoglobulinemia [41]. Peripheral nervous system involvement may complicate MC by causing a sensory-motor neuropathy, especially of the lower limbs, with paresthesias as well as loss of strength, pain, and burning sensations [42]. Central nervous system involvement, characterized by transient dysarthria, hemiplegia, and confusional state, is less frequently seen [43].

2.4. Liver

As HCV infection represents the underlying condition characterizing MC, the liver is involved in almost 70% of cases. In the majority, the clinical picture consists of a chronic hepatitis with the histopathologic features of chronic active hepatitis, potentially leading to cirrhosis and hepatocellular carcinoma [7, 44].

2.5. Gastroenteric and pulmonary systems

Gastrointestinal and pulmonary involvement are less common, occurring in 2–6% and 5% of cases, respectively. Intestinal ischemia may arise, with acute abdominal pain. Intestinal perforation and symptoms that mimic cholecystitis and/or pancreatitis have also been described [45].

Lung involvement in MC is characterized by interstitial pneumopathy; these patients typically present with dyspnea and dry cough. An acute alveolar hemorrhage with hemoptysis, respiratory failure, and a radiologic demonstration of multiple infiltrates occurs only rarely [46, 47].

2.6. Classification of cryoglobulinemic vasculitis

Currently, there are no commonly accepted classification criteria for cryoglobulinemic vasculitis, even if accurate diagnosis and staging are crucial in order to establish a more precise clinical and therapeutic approach to this multifaceted disease. Recently, the Italian Study Group on Cryoglobulinemia (GISC) proposed preliminary classification criteria for cryoglobulinemic vasculitis [48]. Drawing on other classification systems designed to assess autoimmune diseases such as Sjögren's syndrome, the preliminary criteria for the classification of cryoglobulinemic vasculitis include a questionnaire as well as clinical and laboratory parameters. This approach yields good sensitivity and sensibility but it remains to be formally validated.

3. Pathogenesis of HCV-induced MC

For many years, an infectious agent was thought to be the etiologic factor underlying MC. This hypothesis gained significant support from the study of Meltzer and Franklin [18], in which the pathogenetic role of a hepatotropic virus was suggested. Levo et al. [49] proposed hepatitis B virus as the causative agent but this was ruled out because HBV viremia was rarely observed in MC patients and anti-HBV antibody expression varies widely among different MC populations. Currently, HBV is considered as a causative agent of MC only in about 5% of cases [50].

In the early 1990s, after the identification of HCV as the major etiologic agent of non-A, non-B hepatitis, several authors reported the high prevalence of anti-HCV antibodies in MC patients [9, 51]. This correlation was subsequently confirmed by the detection of HCV genomic sequences, especially in the cryoprecipitates versus the corresponding supernatants [10]. In addition, HCV-related proteins were demonstrated in the liver, skin, and kidneys of MC patients [29, 38] as well as in their lymph nodes and circulating CD34+ hematopoietic progenitor cells [52, 53].

The intrinsic mechanism by which HCV promotes cryoglobulin production remains unclear. Viral persistence may provide a continuous stimulus for the host immune system, which is unable to synthesize neutralizing antibodies [54, 55]. According to this scheme, cryoglobulins may be considered the result of these interactions and the presence of IgM molecules with RF activity a crucial event in the cryoprecipitating process [12]. These IgM molecules are almost always associated with light chain 17.109 and heavy chain G6 [56] cross-idiotypes, considered to be the product of a restricted expression of germline genes [24]. In the course of chronic HCV infection, the IgM-17.109 RF immune complexes bind anti-HCV IgG [57]. Among viral antigens, core protein plays a crucial role in cryoglobulin formation as it is the relevant ligand for IgG (Figure 2) [39].

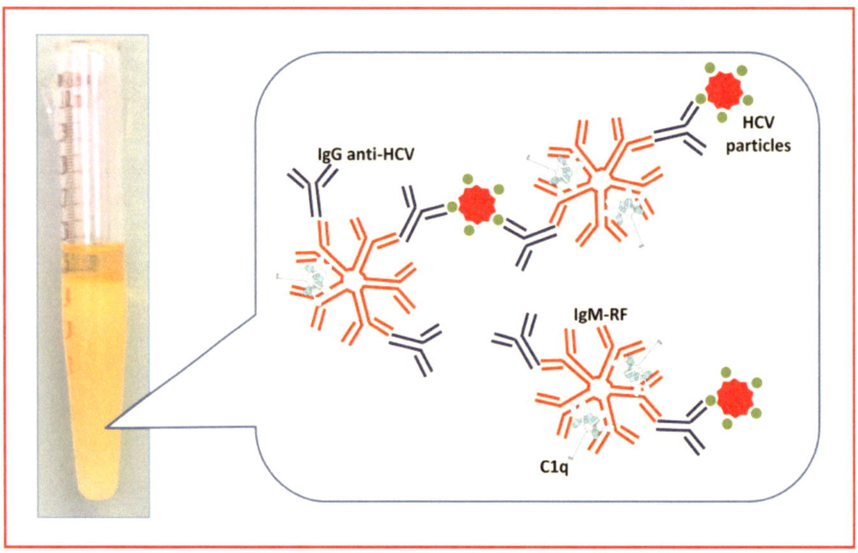

Figure 2. Serum cryoprecipitation at low temperature (+4°C) in a Wintrobe's tube. Cryoprecipitating immune complexes are typified by IgM-RF, which binds IgG with anti-HCV specificity. Of crucial importance is the role of complement fractions such as C1q.

The interaction between HCV and lymphocytes results in the modulation of cell functions. In particular, the *in vivo* activation and expansion of CD5-positive B cells is considered the major source of IgM RF molecules in type III MC [58, 59]. It has been postulated that the initial activation of these cells is followed by the emergence of a dominant clone that synthesizes a monoclonal RF, resulting in the development of type II MC after a transition phase in which an IgM clonal heterogeneity reflects a type II–type III variant [22]. In the peripheral blood of a subset of HCV-positive patients with MC, a clonal expansion of $IgM^{+}CD27^{+}$ B cells expressing hyper-mutated RF-like Ig has been demonstrated in association with V_H 1-69/J_H4 and V_H 3-20 gene segment restriction [60]. These findings have been interpreted as a B-cell proliferation induced by specific antigen stimulation, thus sustaining the notion that persistent B-cell stimulation is a first step in the malignant evolution of MC [61].

An important role in the nature of cryoprecipitating immune complexes is played by the complement system. Generally, complement binding reduces the size of immune complexes, thus maintaining them in solution [62]. In the sera of MC patients, two different compartments can be identified in which C3 and C4 fractions are present in larger amounts in the soluble phase but are barely detectable in cryoprecipitates [12]. By contrast, C1q protein and C1q binding activity are significantly enriched in cryoprecipitates [39]. These data support the hypothesis that an efficient engagement of C1q protein by cryoglobulins is a crucial factor in the pathogenesis of MC (Figure 2).

The receptor for the globular domain of C1q (gC1q-R) directly interacts with HCV core protein, thereby altering host T- and B-cell immunity. Specifically, the gC1q-R/HCV core protein interaction has been shown to modulate T-cell immune responses whereas circulating HCV core protein engagement with gC1q-R expressed on the surface of B-lymphocytes allows the virus to directly affect host immunity [63-65]. The widespread expression of gC1q-R on the surface of circulating blood immunocytes and endothelial cells may determine specific binding to HCV core protein containing immune complexes. Moreover, it was recently demonstrated that higher levels of soluble gC1q-R reflect a higher specific mRNA expression by the blood mononuclear cells of MC patients [66]. Soluble gC1q-R was shown to circulate as a complexed form containing both C1q and HCV core protein binding to two different sites of the molecule.

Serum C4d protein levels were found to be lower in MC patients than in either chronic HCV carriers or healthy subjects [66]. C4d is a low molecular weight fragment derived from the cleavage of C4 complement fraction as part of the classical pathway of complement activation. Deposits of the protein are present in almost all skin biopsy samples of patients with cryoglobulinemic vasculitis, suggesting that low circulating C4d levels are derived from sequestered fragments in the vascular bed.

HCV core protein, in the presence of high levels of circulating gC1q-R, can exacerbate the inflammatory state by activating the complement cascade, thus determining endothelial cell activation and initiating an *in situ* inflammatory response. From a biological point of view, the clinical response to antiviral therapy consists of a significant reduction in soluble gC1q-R in association with increased levels of C4d and a lower viral load [66].

4. Clinical outcome

Cryoglobulinemic syndrome (CS) is a systemic vasculitis that changes the clinical outcome of HCV-infected patients but its long-term impact on the course of HCV infection has not been assessed. In 2004, Ferri et al. reported a significantly lower cumulative 10-year survival from the time of diagnosis in their series of 231 cryoglobulinemic patients age and sex-matched with individuals from the general population [41]. Other factors recognized as associated with a poor prognosis are renal involvement, widespread vasculitis, and infectious processes [67, 68].

Recently, we completed a prospective study of a cohort of 950 chronically HCV-infected patients who were referred to our department over a period of about 15 years starting from 1990. MC was determined in 246 patients (28%), 184 (74.8%) of whom also had cryoglobulinemic vasculitis. The rate of progression of liver fibrosis was lower in patients with CS than in those without but the probability of developing cirrhosis and hepatocellular carcinoma was higher in the latter group (24.9% vs. 14.2%, $p<0.005$ and 20.3% vs. 7.5%, $p=0.003$, respectively). Extrahepatic complications such as renal failure, neurological impairment, and the evolution to a B-cell malignancy were more frequent in patients with CS than in those without (32.6% vs. 3%, $p < 0.0001$; 31.2% vs. 4.8%, $p < 0.0001$ and 15% vs. 7.1%, $p = 0.003$, respectively; unpublished data, manuscript submitted). However, the 15-year survival rate was similar in HCV-infected patients with or without CS, despite differences in morbidity and causes of death (70.2% vs. 71.7%).

5. Therapy

In the pre-HCV era, the management of MC was conventionally based on the use of corticosteroids and immunosuppressive drugs such as cyclophosphamide, with the aim of preventing irreversible organ failure, reducing pain, and improving patients' quality of life. In 1987, recombinant IFN-α was empirically tested in seven patients with "essential" MC [69]. With the subsequent demonstration of the pathogenetic role of HCV [11], IFN-α became a rational therapeutic strategy. The introduction of pegylated IFN-α and subsequently of ribavirin changed the therapeutic scenario for chronic hepatitis C, by increasing the virological response [70-72]. This combination was shown to also be remarkably effective in HCV-related MC, resulting in a complete clinical response and a sustained virological response (SVR) in 78% of the patients [73]. In addition, serum levels of C3 and C4 complement fractions normalized in 80% of the treated patients and cryoglobulins disappeared in 56%. However, even if antiviral treatment results in a resolution of the vasculitis, for patients with neuropathy or glomerulonephritis there is no or only partial improvement, suggesting that the clinical outcome is conditioned by factors other than the virus [12].

Extra-hepatic manifestations of chronic HCV infection such as MC are characterized by B-cell clonal expansions (including RF-synthesizing B-cells) [12, 74-76], which have been demonstrated in at least three different compartments, namely, liver, bone marrow, and the circulation. Consequently, the deletion of B-cell clonalities may provide a further approach to the treatment of MC. It is well known that CD20 antigen, a transmembrane protein, is selectively expressed on pre-B and mature lymphocytes and that CD20-positive cells are greatly expanded and activated in patients with MC [77, 78].

On the basis of the demonstrated effectiveness of Rituximab (RTX), a chimeric monoclonal antibody specifically directed at CD20 antigen, in autoimmune and lymphoproliferative disorders [79-81], its use seemed logical in the treatment of HCV-related MC in patients refractory to, or relapsing after, conventional antiviral therapy. Indeed, RTX was shown to be effective, safe, and well tolerated in MC patients, both in those resistant to previous treatments and in those with recurrent disease [82, 83]. Thus, several papers subsequently addressed the issue of using RTX in this setting, either alone or in combination with steroids [84, 85].

Since an increased viremia has been frequently reported in responsive patients, we proposed a triple therapeutic approach (pIFN-α plus RBV plus RTX), designated with the acronym PIRR [86]. This drug combination was administered to 22 HCV-positive MC patients whereas 15 additional patients with the same pathology received pIFN-α plus RBV with the exclusion of RTX. All patients were followed for 36 months from the end of treatment. A complete response was determined in 54.5% of the patients treated with PIRR, but in only 33.3% of those on pIFN-α plus RBV without RTX ($p<0.05$). Even more interesting were the observations that: a) in the large majority (83.3%) of the responders in the PIRR-treated group, B-cell populations in the liver, bone marrow, and peripheral blood compartments underwent a conversion from oligoclonal to polyclonal; b) CR was maintained in all patients in the PIRR group throughout the follow-up period whereas this was the case in only 40% of those in the control group. However, whether RTX should be administered to patients with cryoglobulinemic vasculitis as first- or second-line therapy remains to be established [87].

Of particular interest are MC patients who do not achieve a SVR and those in whom there is continuous cryoglobulin production despite viral eradication. In the former, the use of the new direct-acting antivirals (DAAs) such as Telaprevir or Boceprevir (recently approved by the FDA for the treatment of HCV genotype 1 chronic infection) may offer a further therapeutic option [88]. The persistence of MC vasculitis in patients achieving a SVR represents an emerging picture following antiviral and B-cell-depleting combined therapies [89, 90]. In these patients differences in the immunochemical structure of circulating immune-complexes may be postulated and the use of corticosteroids, cyclophosphamide, RTX, or novel anti-CD20 monoclonal antibodies such as Ofatumomab may be considered as alternative therapeutic options [91]. Therapeutic apheresis is a palliative procedure that can be extremely useful for the treatment of severe, life-threatening vasculitis [87] as well as for chronic leg ulcers in patients resistant to other therapies [92].

Additional therapeutic approaches to MC, including the tyrosine kinase inhibitor imatinib and anti-angiogenic drugs such as thalidomide, bortezomib (a proteasome inhibitor), and IL-2 have been proposed but their therapeutic effectiveness in patients with MC remains to be determined in controlled studies [93, 94].

6. HCV infection and malignant lymphoproliferation

About 15% of all human tumors are of viral origin. The percentage of virus-related cancer is three-fold higher in developing than in developed countries, reflecting the higher prevalence of infection with oncogenic viruses rather than exposure to tumor-enhancing co-factors [95]. The pathogenetic role of some viruses in human tumors has been clearly described. This is the case for Epstein-Barr virus (EBV), which is etiologically linked to Burkitt's lymphoma and probably other tumors [96]. Other such viruses include human papillomavirus (HPV), associated with cervical, ano-genital, skin and head and neck cancers [97]; human T-cell leukemia virus type 1 (HTLV-1), which causes adult T-cell leukemia [98]; and human herpes virus type 8 (HHV-8), which may be involved in Kaposi's sarcoma, primary effusion lymphoma, and multicentric Castelman's disease [99].

Among hepatotropic viruses, the role of both hepatitis B (HBV) and hepatitis C (HCV) viruses in the etiopathogenesis of hepatocellular carcinoma (HCC) is well defined, although HBV and HCV-induced cancerogenesis proceeds by quite different mechanisms. For HCV, initial observations regarding the causative association between infection with the virus and NHL [100] were subsequently confirmed in a large number of studies [101, 102]. In a meta-analysis evaluating 15 studies [103], the relative risk (RR) of all NHL among HCV-positive patients was 2.5, with a 95% confidence interval (CI) considering case control studies, and a RR of 2.0 (95% CI) in cohort studies. Early studies reported the prevalence of extranodal NHLs and histotypes such as lymphoplasmacytic lymphomas in HCV-positive patients. These findings can be ascribed to the occurrence of malignant lymphomas in HCV-positive patients with other low-grade lymphoproliferative disorders such as MC (Figure 3) [104].

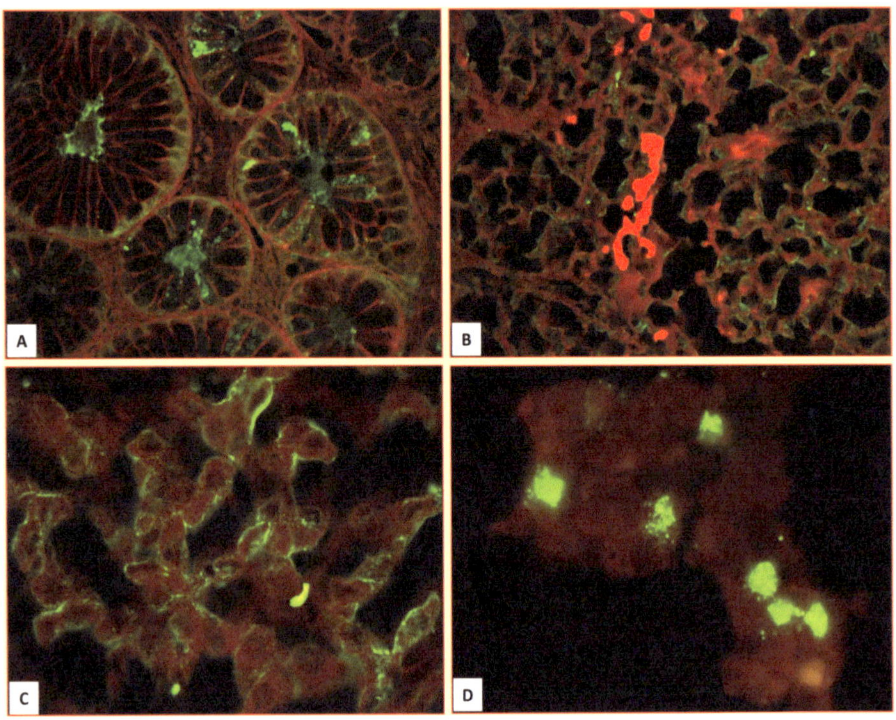

Figure 3. Demonstration of HCV E2 protein by immunofluorescence in the neoplastic B-cells of mucosa-associated lymphoid tissue (MALT)-like gastric lymphoma (A), a neoplastic lymph node (B), splenic lymphoma (C) and bone marrow infiltrates (D).

Currently, there are no clear differences concerning the association between HCV and major histologic B-cell NHL subtypes such as diffuse large B-cell (DLBC), follicular, marginal zone, and chronic lymphocytic leukemia/small lymphocytic lymphomas [105]. However, lymphoma subtypes that do not originate from germinal center or post-germinal center B-cells, such as mantle cell (MC)-NHL, Burkitt's lymphoma, T-cell lymphoma, and Hodgkin's lymphoma, have not been consistently linked to HCV infection [106]. This finding is in line with the notion that the proliferation of specific B-cell clones following chronic antigenic stimulation is the mechanism that drives the determination of NHL subtypes.

7. Clinical and histopathological features of HCV-associated NHLs

As previously stated, both clinical and biological observations strongly suggest a role for HCV in a variety of extrahepatic disorders, including dermatologic, hematologic, endocrinologic, and autoimmune diseases. Of interest here is the striking association between HCV infection and MC, which has been convincingly demonstrated. However, MC can also develop as an indolent B-cell lymphoproliferative disorder, with a potentially malignant evolution [12]. In a long-term analysis, progression to NHL was demonstrated in 5–10% of HCV-infected patients. Symptoms indicative of progression are usually mild and comprise an expanding spectrum of autoimmune phenomena, including hemolytic anemia, thrombocytopenia, and granulocytopenia [107-109].

It has been calculated that about 13% of patients with B-NHLs are HCV-positive [110] and that about 10% of patients with HCV-associated MC will develop a B-NHL within the following ten years [111]. Two different subsets of HCV-associated B-cell NHLs can be distinguished, presenting as distinct clinical and pathological entities. The first is a low-grade NHL evolving from MC, with possible bone marrow involvement and further evolution into an aggressive phenotype. The second is an aggressive NHL without an underlying MC and with bone marrow involvement [100, 107].

A peculiar feature of HCV-associated lymphomas is the extranodal involvement, with the liver, salivary glands, bone marrow, and spleen most often affected [112]. The most common histotypes are marginal zone lymphomas, lymphoplasmacytic lymphomas, and DLBC lymphomas [113]. Splenic marginal zone lymphoma in particular seems to have a high prevalence in HCV-infected patients with MC [114]. In addition, follicular and MC lymphomas may also be associated with HCV infection [113], as can MALT lymphoma, in which HCV is detected in about 35% of the non-gastric forms of these tumors [115].

8. Pathogenesis of HCV-associated NHLs

The chronic persistence of HCV provides a continuous stimulus for the host immune system sustaining B-cell clonal expansions [15]. Thus, the monoclonal IgM RF synthesis that characterizes MC can be ascribed to the expression of one such single dominant clone [22, 59]. Accordingly, the capacity of HCV to directly modulate B- and T-cell function [116] can be considered as one of the necessary criteria needed to define HCV as an etiologic factor in lymphomagenesis.

Among the different cell-surface receptors that have been described as possible binding sites for HCV [117, 118], the most well-studied is CD81, a tetraspanin present on the surface of B-lymphocytes (Figure 4) [119].

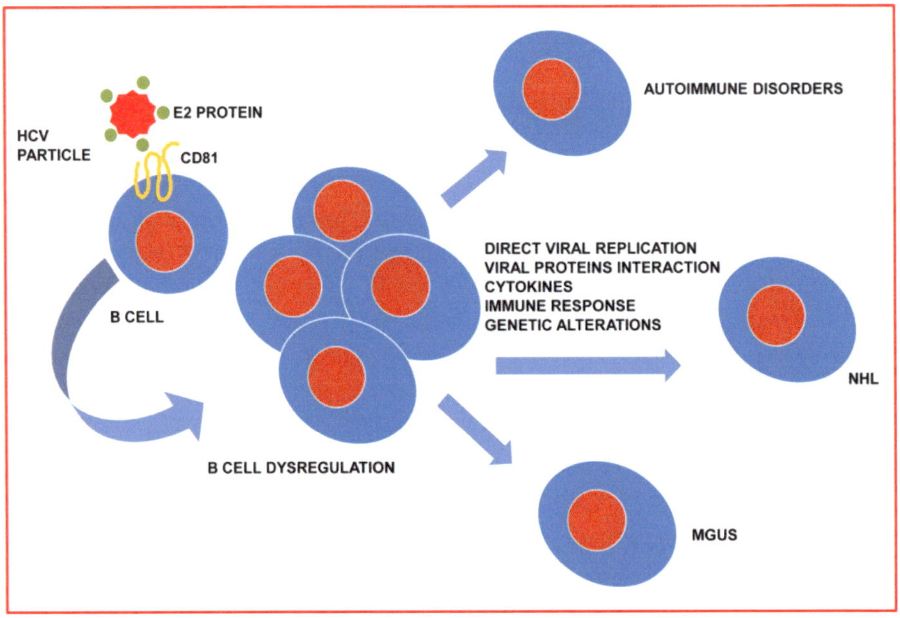

Figure 4. Schematic representation of the interactions between HCV and B cells. CD81, which binds E2 protein, is the best-studied cellular receptor. Active HCV replication in B-lymphocytes, in addition to continuous stimulation of the host immune system, may lead to a "B-cell deregulation," which eventually gives rise to oligo/monoclonal expansions. Clinical evolution into autoimmune disease or monoclonal gammopathy of undetermined significance (MGUS) as well as frank lymphoma may be conditioned by other factors, either alone or in combination, e.g., active viral replication, viral protein interactions, cytokines, the host immune response, and genetic factors.

Interestingly, a higher cell-associated viral load due to the enrichment of HCV RNA in circulating lymphocytes has been demonstrated in cryoglobulinemic patients [77] and appears to reflect either a higher receptor density on the cell surface or the polymorphism of receptor genes [120-122].

In addition, a direct stimulus for lymphocyte proliferation can be provided by direct infection with HCV and active replication of the virus inside B-cells [123], further evidence that HCV is an oncogenic virus. Since HCV is a single-stranded RNA virus with an RNA-dependent RNA polymerase, detection of the viral RNA minus strand is the only molecular marker of an active viral replication whereas detection of the plus strand RNA may be the result of passive cellular contamination by circulating virions. A direct correlation between active HCV infection of B cells and MC was established using a highly specific and sensitive method for HCV RNA minus strand detection [124]. These results demonstrated the lymphotropism of HCV, in which peripheral blood lymphocytes are another productive compartment of HCV infection in addition to serving as a circulating reservoir of the virus (Figure 4) [125].

A distinguishing feature seen in cryoglobulinemic patients is the presence of clonally expanded, RF-synthesizing B-cells [126]. By means of PCR amplification techniques, immunoglobulin variable region (IgV) genomic sequences, as a molecular marker of B cell progeny, were analyzed, providing evidence of an antigen-driven B cell clonal expansion. Heavy- and light-chain IgV gene analysis indicated a high mutation rate as usually occurs from a germinal or post-germinal center origin [127]. Little is known about the viral antigens capable of inducing this clonal expansion and no viral protein identified thus far seems to be a specific ligand for the B-cell receptor [128]. All expanded B-cell clones characterized by the somatic hypermutation of IgV genes seem capable of recognizing a single epitope, suggesting that they arise from a pool of cells selected for non-self antigens, probably in the course of a germinal center reaction [127]. Interestingly, many expanded B-cell clones display a complementarity determining region-3 (CDR-3) resembling CDR-3 of rheumatoid factor (RF CDR-3), suggesting that they derive from autoimmune-oriented precursors with anti-IgG specificity.

B-cell proliferation is characterized by a continuous rearrangement of IgV genes that gives rise to different mutants. PCR amplification of the VDJ region identifies the unique combinations of N regions with DH and JH regions that can be considered as a clonal marker of cellular progeny. This method was used to show that B-cell clonal expansions are present in the liver tissue, rather than in the blood and bone marrow compartments, of almost 90% of HCV-positive MC patients [126]. The detection of inflammatory infiltrates of the portal tracts resembling follicle-like structures with a functionally active germinal center is a diagnostic feature of liver biopsies from patients chronically infected with HCV [129, 130]. In addition, the VDJ patterns determined in these patients show oligoclonality or monoclonality, thus demonstrating that intrahepatic B cell expansions derive from a few cells or a single cell; morevoer, each focus may derive from a different B-cell, resulting in the development of unrelated clones [129, 130].

Intrahepatic B-cell clonal expansions are almost invariably associated with extrahepatic manifestations such as MC, high serum levels of RF activity, monoclonal gammopathy of undetermined significance, and B-cell malignancy. Sequence analyses of the IgH CDR-3 gene segments of intraportal B-cell clonalities revealed a wide range of variations, suggesting that they are also the result of an antigen-driven response [131]. Accordingly, it can be inferred that B-cell clones begin to expand in the liver as the result of an IgH-VDJ upregulated mutational activity, with subsequent migration of the cells to the peripheral blood and bone marrow [74].

Given that the liver is not only the primary target of HCV infection but also the main site of inflammation, B-cell recruitment and expansion, identification of the factor(s) contributing to the establishment and progression of this complex clinical spectrum is of crucial importance. In this context, research focused on the molecules capable of prolonging B-cell survival is particularly relevant. Among the compounds identified thus far, B-cell activating factor (BAFF), a chemokine belonging to the tumor necrosis factor (TNF) family, seems to play an important role in B-cell survival [30]. The most important effect of BAFF is probably the inhibition of B-cell apoptosis. BAFF expression was shown to be higher in the intraportal lymphoid aggregates and skin tissue of cryoglobulinemic patients. Synthesis is thought to start in inflammatory sites such as the liver and skin and then arise the circle [132].

One of the most important anti-apoptotic factors is Bcl-2 protein. Its upregulation due to t(14; 18) chromosomal translocation, is a specific feature of follicular B-NHLs and it also has been described in cryoglobulinemic patients [133]. However, in an our previous study, Bcl-2/IgH amplification was not detected in intraportal inflammatory infiltrates isolated from HCV-positive patients by means of laser microdissection of liver biopsy tissue [134], suggesting that heavy chain Ig gene rearrangement is not associated with Bcl-2/IgH chromosomal translocation in the liver compartment. This discrepancy could reflect ethnic and/or environmental factors in that Bcl-2/IgH rearrangement is less common in the Mediterranean region than in northern Europe [134]. Alternatively, in non-neoplastic conditions such as MC, Bcl-2/IgH rearrangement could be a transient effect due to the persistence of viral infection [134].

Activation-induced cytidine deaminase (AID) is an enzyme involved in the degradation of pyrimidine nucleotides. It is also essential for somatic hypermutation and class-switching recombination of immunoglobulin genes in B-cells [135]. Some studies have proposed a pathogenetic role of AID in B-cell lymphomagenesis, in particular during the initiation and progression of B-NHL because a deregulation in either of these two processes can determine a chromosomal translocation and/or an aberrant somatic hypermutation, two of the main causes of B-NHL-associated genetic accidents [136, 137]. It has been postulated that AID is triggered by HCV core protein in human hepatocytes *via* NFkB activation (Figure 5) [138].

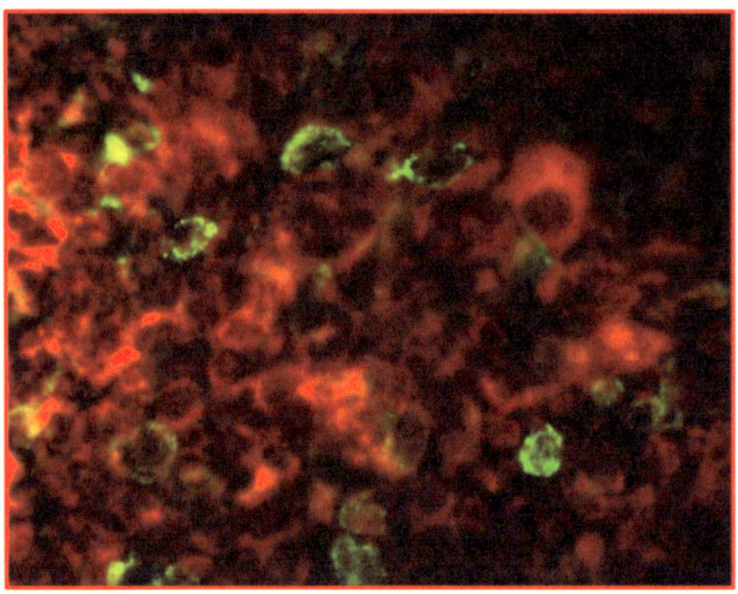

Figure 5. Detection of activation-induced cytidine deaminase (AID) protein in the lymph node of a patient with HCV-associated B-cell NHL.

Together, these data support epidemiological observations of an association between HCV chronic infection and B-NHL. Nonetheless, further studies will be necessary to better evaluate the pathogenetic mechanisms and optimize the therapeutic approaches.

9. HCV related NHLs: Therapeutic opportunities

As previously described, HCV chronic infection may well be a risk factor for the development of "indolent" lymphoproliferative disease such as MC as well as for frank B-cell NHL, albeit with a wide geographical variability.

The induction of a SVR following an effective antiviral therapy with pegylated interferon plus ribavirin should exert a preventive effect on lymphomagenesis in patients chronically infected with HCV [139]. In addition, based on the observation of gastric MALT lymphoma regression after the eradication of *H. pylori* infection, antiviral therapy should induce the regression of NHL.

The efficacy of antiviral therapy was described by Hermine *et al.* [140] in patients with villous lymphocytes splenic lymphoma, with complete remission achieved in eight of the nine HCV-positive patients. Further studies confirmed these data. In a systematic review by Gisbert et al. [141], about 75% of HCV-infected patients with a lymphoproliferative disorder achieved a complete remission following antiviral treatment.

Recently, Arcaini et al. assessed the role of antiviral therapy in HCV-associated indolent B-cell lymphomas [142]. According to the WHO classification, indolent lymphomas are poorly symptomatic diseases belonging to low-grade lymphoma [143]. They include follicular lymphoma, small lymphocytic lymphoma, marginal zone lymphomas, splenic marginal zone lymphoma, primary nodal marginal zone lymphoma, extranodal marginal zone lymphoma of mucosa-associated tissue (MALT), and lymphoplasmacytic lymphoma. In almost all such patients a hematologic response was obtained subsequent to the virological response, reinforcing the evidence for a causative link between HCV and lymphomas [142]. Further studies will be necessary to establish the efficacy of novel direct antiviral agents, such as boceprevir and telaprevir, which increase SVR rates in genotype 1 HCV infection while also increasing the hematologic response rate of patients with more resistant infection. On the basis of therapeutic regimens for HCV-associated MC that consist of a combination of RTX and antiviral therapy [86, 144] a similar approach may be successful also in HCV patients with indolent B-cell lymphomas.

The use of antiviral therapy in patients with HCV-positive aggressive B-cell lymphomas such as DLBC and mantle cell lymphomas appears to be less effective. This lack of a response may be related to the antigen-independent phase of lymphomagenesis, in which malignant evolution occurs irrespective of viral persistence. These lymphomas require an adequate chemotherapy with or without RTX, even if the development of hepatitis flares has been described [145]. However, there are also some papers showing a clinical remission of DLBCL [146] and mantle cell lymphoma [147] after antiviral therapy. While a combination of antiviral therapy and immunochemotherapy has been proposed to prevent or treat hepatitis flares [148], combination therapy consisting of interferon plus ribavirin usually results in an increased hematologic toxicity, as previously reported [149]. A more interesting strategy may be a sequential schedule consisting of immune-chemotherapy followed by pegylated interferon plus ribavirin. The aim is to induce a SVR in patients obtaining a complete remission of their lymphoma after chemotherapy, in order to prevent hepatitis reactivation and to achieve long-term control of their NHL [150], effectively and with good tolerance. However, this approach needs further validation in larger prospective studies.

10. Conclusions

HCV infection should not be considered as a major cause only of liver disease; instead, several different biological compartments are involved. In particular, B-lymphocytes are an important site in which HCV may actively replicate, thereby serving as a viral reservoir.

Viral persistence represents a continuous stimulus for the host immune system, leading to B-cell selection and clonal expansion as evidenced by the synthesis of IgM autoantibodies with RF activity (IgM-RF), which characterizes MC. This process seems to occur in a microenvironment such as that provided by intraportal lymphoid follicles due to distinct selection events probably supported by cytokine signaling, thereby sustaining B-cell activation and proliferation. The unique clinical features of MC are the result of the biological activities of the immune complexes constituted by IgM-RF, anti-HCV IgG, viral antigens, and complement fractions. Of particular interest is the role played by C1q and the globular domain of the C1q receptor (gC1q-R), which, in combination with viral proteins such as core protein, modulates immune complex deposition in the vascular bed, leading to cryoglobulinemic vasculitis. The involvement of viral proteins also has been suggested for B-cell proliferation.

Thus, MC may be considered a low-grade, indolent, benign lymphoproliferative disease reflecting an antigen-dependent B-cell clonal expansion with potential evolution into a malignant phenotype. HCV-related malignant NHLs may accordingly derive from a benign lymphoproliferation such as MC and usually occur as low grade/indolent lymphomas but, over time, their phenotypes may become more aggressive. Alternatively, they may arise directly, often involving extranodal sites, with an indolent phenotype similar to that of MALT lymphomas or as highly aggressive lymphomas.

The definition of HCV as an etiologic agent in both benign and malignant lymphoproliferations suggests the efficacy of antiviral therapy both in MC and in NHLs. The combination of antiviral therapy with B-cell depletion, with its ability to induce long-term clinical, immunologic, and virologic remission, may be considered the standard of care for cryoglobulinemic vasculitis. In addition, a clinical remission of low-grade NHLs after antiviral treatments has also been described. These results confirm the pathogenetic role of HCV in lymphoproliferative diseases and offer new therapeutic options even if further studies are mandatory. Antiviral therapy may also have a role in high grade NHLs in which the pathogenetic process can be considered antigen-independent. In these patients, who require immune-chemotherapy, antiviral treatment may be useful in preventing hepatitis flares as well as NHL relapse if a SVR is obtained.

In conclusion, HCV infection should be considered a multifaceted disease, with a potentially malignant evolution involving not only the liver compartment (i.e., hepatocellular carcinoma), but also other targets, such as lymphoid tissue. However, there are several further aspects that need to be clarified regarding the pathogenetic mechanisms of HCV-induced lymphomagenesis. In this regard, an evaluation of the impact of new direct antiviral agents as well as novel target-therapies inducing B-cell depletion will be of great interest in the prevention of HCV-related malignancies.

Acknowledgements

This article was made possible by the support and assistance of Dr. Vincenza Conteduca, Dr. Sabino Russi, Mr. Vito De Gennaro, Dr. Fabio Pavone, and Dr. Ida Sebastiani.

Funding was provided by the University of Bari and AIFA (Agenzia Italiana del Farmaco, funds for independent studies, 2007, contract no. FARM7SJX)

Author details

Gianfranco Lauletta

Address all correspondence to: gianfranco.lauletta@uniba.it

Department of Biomedical Sciences and Human Oncology, Section of Internal Medicine and Clinical Oncology,Liver Unit, University of Bari Medical School, Bari, Italy

References

[1] Choo QL, Richman KH, Han JH, Berger K, Lee C, Dong C, et al. Genetic organization and diversity of the hepatitis C virus. Proc Natl Acad Sci U S A 1991;88(6) 2451-2455.

[2] Hoofnagle JH. Course and outcome of hepatitis C. Hepatology 2002;36(5 Suppl 1) S21-29.

[3] Pavlovic D, Neville DC, Argaud O, Blumberg B, Dwek RA, Fischer WB, et al. The hepatitis C virus p7 protein forms an ion channel that is inhibited by long-alkyl-chain iminosugar derivatives. Proc Natl Acad Sci U S A 2003;100(10) 6104-6108.

[4] Rosenberg S. Recent advances in the molecular biology of hepatitis C virus. J Mol Biol 2001;313(3) 451-464.

[5] Lohmann V, Hoffmann S, Herian U, Penin F, Bartenschlager R. Viral and cellular determinants of hepatitis C virus RNA replication in cell culture. J Virol 2003;77(5) 3007-3019.

[6] Heller T, Saito S, Auerbach J, Williams T, Moreen TR, Jazwinski A, et al. An in vitro model of hepatitis C virion production. Proc Natl Acad Sci U S A 2005;102(7) 2579-2583.

[7] Dammacco F, Sansonno D. Antibodies to hepatitis C virus in essential mixed cryoglobulinaemia. Clin Exp Immunol 1992;87(3) 352-356.

[8] Ferri C, Greco F, Longombardo G, Palla P, Moretti A, Marzo E, et al. Antibodies to hepatitis C virus in patients with mixed cryoglobulinemia. Arthritis Rheum 1991;34(12) 1606-1610.

[9] Agnello V, Chung RT, Kaplan LM. A role for hepatitis C virus infection in type II cryoglobulinemia. N Engl J Med 1992;327(21) 1490-1495.

[10] Dammacco F, Sansonno D, Cornacchiulo V, Mennuni C, Carbone R, Lauletta G, et al. Hepatitis C virus infection and mixed cryoglobulinemia: a striking association. Int J Clin Lab Res 1993;23(1) 45-49.

[11] Dammacco F, Sansonno D, Piccoli C, Tucci FA, Racanelli V. The cryoglobulins: an overview. Eur J Clin Invest 2001;31(7) 628-638.

[12] Sansonno D, Dammacco F. Hepatitis C virus, cryoglobulinaemia, and vasculitis: immune complex relations. Lancet Infect Dis 2005;5(4) 227-236.

[13] Sansonno D, Carbone A, De Re V, Dammacco F. Hepatitis C virus infection, cryoglobulinaemia, and beyond. Rheumatology (Oxford) 2007;46(4) 572-578.

[14] Agnello V. The aetiology of mixed cryoglobulinaemia associated with hepatitis C virus infection. Scand J Immunol 1995;42(2) 179-184.

[15] Dammacco F, Sansonno D, Piccoli C, Racanelli V, D'Amore FP, Lauletta G. The lymphoid system in hepatitis C virus infection: autoimmunity, mixed cryoglobulinemia, and Overt B-cell malignancy. Semin Liver Dis 2000;20(2) 143-157.

[16] Wintrobe MM, Buell MV. Hyperproteinemia associated with multiple myeloma. Bull Johns Hopkins Hosp 1933;52(10.

[17] Lerner AB, Watson CJ. Studies of cryoglobulins; unusual purpura associated with the presence of a high concentration of cryoglobulin (cold precipitable serum globulin). Am J Med Sci 1947;214(4) 410-415.

[18] Meltzer M, Franklin EC. Cryoglobulinemia--a study of twenty-nine patients. I. IgG and IgM cryoglobulins and factors affecting cryoprecipitability. Am J Med 1966;40(6) 828-836.

[19] Brouet JC, Clauvel JP, Danon F, Klein M, Seligmann M. Biologic and clinical significance of cryoglobulins. A report of 86 cases. Am J Med 1974;57(5) 775-788.

[20] Denman AM. Cryoglobulins and the immunopathological manifestations of autoimmune disease. Clin Exp Immunol 1992;87(2) 169-171.

[21] Wang AC, Wells JV, Fudenberg HH. Chemical analyses of cryoglobulins. Immunochemistry 1974;11(7) 341-345.

[22] Tissot JD, Schifferli JA, Hochstrasser DF, Pasquali C, Spertini F, Clement F, et al. Two-dimensional polyacrylamide gel electrophoresis analysis of cryoglobulins and identification of an IgM-associated peptide. J Immunol Methods 1994;173(1) 63-75.

[23] Montagnino G. Reappraisal of the clinical expression of mixed cryoglobulinemia. Springer Semin Immunopathol 1988;10(1) 1-19.

[24] Gorevic PD, Frangione B. Mixed cryoglobulinemia cross-reactive idiotypes: implications for the relationship of MC to rheumatic and lymphoproliferative diseases. Semin Hematol 1991;28(2) 79-94.

[25] Trendelenburg M, Schifferli JA. Cryoglobulins are not essential. Ann Rheum Dis 1998;57(1) 3-5.

[26] Pawlotsky JM, Ben Yahia M, Andre C, Voisin MC, Intrator L, Roudot-Thoraval F, et al. Immunological disorders in C virus chronic active hepatitis: a prospective case-control study. Hepatology 1994;19(4) 841-848.

[27] Dammacco F, Sansonno D. Mixed cryoglobulinemia as a model of systemic vasculitis. Clin Rev Allergy Immunol 1997;15(1) 97-119.

[28] Ramos-Casals M, Stone JH, Cid MC, Bosch X. The cryoglobulinaemias. Lancet 2012;379(9813) 348-360.

[29] Sansonno D, Cornacchiulo V, Iacobelli AR, Di Stefano R, Lospalluti M, Dammacco F. Localization of hepatitis C virus antigens in liver and skin tissues of chronic hepatitis C virus-infected patients with mixed cryoglobulinemia. Hepatology 1995;21(2) 305-312.

[30] Matignon M, Cacoub P, Colombat M, Saadoun D, Brocheriou I, Mougenot B, et al. Clinical and morphologic spectrum of renal involvement in patients with mixed cryoglobulinemia without evidence of hepatitis C virus infection. Medicine (Baltimore) 2009;88(6) 341-348.

[31] Alpers CE, Smith KD. Cryoglobulinemia and renal disease. Curr Opin Nephrol Hypertens 2008;17(3) 243-249.

[32] Roccatello D, Fornasieri A, Giachino O, Rossi D, Beltrame A, Banfi G, et al. Multicenter study on hepatitis C virus-related cryoglobulinemic glomerulonephritis. Am J Kidney Dis 2007;49(1) 69-82.

[33] Tarantino A, Campise M, Banfi G, Confalonieri R, Bucci A, Montoli A, et al. Long-term predictors of survival in essential mixed cryoglobulinemic glomerulonephritis. Kidney Int 1995;47(2) 618-623.

[34] Beddhu S, Bastacky S, Johnson JP. The clinical and morphologic spectrum of renal cryoglobulinemia. Medicine (Baltimore) 2002;81(5) 398-409.

[35] D'Amico G. Renal involvement in hepatitis C infection: cryoglobulinemic glomerulonephritis. Kidney Int 1998;54(2) 650-671.

[36] Cordonnier DJ, Renversez JC, Vialtel P, Dechelette E. The kidney in mixed cryoglobulinemias. Springer Semin Immunopathol 1987;9(4) 395-415.

[37] Jennette JC, Olson JL, Schwartz MM, Silva FG, Heptinstall's Pathology of the Kidney. 6th ed. 2007, Philadelphia, Pa, USA.

[38] Sansonno D, Gesualdo L, Manno C, Schena FP, Dammacco F. Hepatitis C virus-related proteins in kidney tissue from hepatitis C virus-infected patients with cryoglobulinemic membranoproliferative glomerulonephritis. Hepatology 1997;25(5) 1237-1244.

[39] Sansonno D, Lauletta G, Nisi L, Gatti P, Pesola F, Pansini N, et al. Non-enveloped HCV core protein as constitutive antigen of cold-precipitable immune complexes in type II mixed cryoglobulinaemia. Clin Exp Immunol 2003;133(2) 275-282.

[40] Authier FJ, Pawlotsky JM, Viard JP, Guillevin L, Degos JD, Gherardi RK. High incidence of hepatitis C virus infection in patients with cryoglobulinemic neuropathy. Ann Neurol 1993;34(5) 749-750.

[41] Ferri C, Sebastiani M, Giuggioli D, Cazzato M, Longombardo G, Antonelli A, et al. Mixed cryoglobulinemia: demographic, clinical, and serologic features and survival in 231 patients. Semin Arthritis Rheum 2004;33(6) 355-374.

[42] Gemignani F, Melli G, Inglese C, Marbini A. Cryoglobulinemia is a frequent cause of peripheral neuropathy in undiagnosed referral patients. J Peripher Nerv Syst 2002;7(1) 59-64.

[43] Origgi L, Vanoli M, Carbone A, Grasso M, Scorza R. Central nervous system involvement in patients with HCV-related cryoglobulinemia. Am J Med Sci 1998;315(3) 208-210.

[44] Saadoun D, Asselah T, Resche-Rigon M, Charlotte F, Bedossa P, Valla D, et al. Cryoglobulinemia is associated with steatosis and fibrosis in chronic hepatitis C. Hepatology 2006;43(6) 1337-1345.

[45] Terrier B, Saadoun D, Sene D, Scerra S, Musset L, Cacoub P. Presentation and outcome of gastrointestinal involvement in hepatitis C virus-related systemic vasculitis: a case-control study from a single-centre cohort of 163 patients. Gut 2010;59(12) 1709-1715.

[46] Ramos-Casals M, Robles A, Brito-Zeron P, Nardi N, Nicolas JM, Forns X, et al. Life-threatening cryoglobulinemia: clinical and immunological characterization of 29 cases. Semin Arthritis Rheum 2006;36(3) 189-196.

[47] Retamozo S, Diaz-Lagares C, Bosch X, De Vita S, Ramos Casals M, Life-threatening cryoglobulinemia, in Autoimmune diseases: acute and complex situations., M.A.

Khamashta and M. Ramos Casals, Editors. 2011, Springer-Verlag: London. p. 133-162.

[48] De Vita S, Soldano F, Isola M, Monti G, Gabrielli A, Tzioufas A, et al. Preliminary classification criteria for the cryoglobulinaemic vasculitis. Ann Rheum Dis 2011;70(7) 1183-1190.

[49] Levo Y, Gorevic PD, Kassab HJ, Zucker-Franklin D, Franklin EC. Association between hepatitis B virus and essential mixed cryoglobulinemia. N Engl J Med 1977;296(26) 1501-1504.

[50] Mascia MT, Ferrari D, Campioli D, Sandri G, Mussini C, Ferri C. Non HCV-related mixed cryoglobulinemia. Dig Liver Dis 2007;39 Suppl 1(S61-64.

[51] Pascual M, Perrin L, Giostra E, Schifferli JA. Hepatitis C virus in patients with cryoglobulinemia type II. J Infect Dis 1990;162(2) 569-570.

[52] Sansonno D, De Vita S, Cornacchiulo V, Carbone A, Boiocchi M, Dammacco F. Detection and distribution of hepatitis C virus-related proteins in lymph nodes of patients with type II mixed cryoglobulinemia and neoplastic or non-neoplastic lymphoproliferation. Blood 1996;88(12) 4638-4645.

[53] Sansonno D, Lotesoriere C, Cornacchiulo V, Fanelli M, Gatti P, Iodice G, et al. Hepatitis C virus infection involves CD34(+) hematopoietic progenitor cells in hepatitis C virus chronic carriers. Blood 1998;92(9) 3328-3337.

[54] Rehermann B. Hepatitis C virus versus innate and adaptive immune responses: a tale of coevolution and coexistence. J Clin Invest 2009;119(7) 1745-1754.

[55] Dustin LB, Rice CM. Flying under the radar: the immunobiology of hepatitis C. Annu Rev Immunol 2007;25(71-99.

[56] Chen PP, Fong S, Goni F, Silverman GJ, Fox RI, Liu MF, et al. Cross-reacting idiotypes on cryoprecipitating rheumatoid factor. Springer Semin Immunopathol 1988;10(1) 35-55.

[57] Sansonno D, Iacobelli AR, Cornacchiulo V, Lauletta G, Distasi MA, Gatti P, et al. Immunochemical and biomolecular studies of circulating immune complexes isolated from patients with acute and chronic hepatitis C virus infection. Eur J Clin Invest 1996;26(6) 465-475.

[58] Curry MP, Golden-Mason L, Doherty DG, Deignan T, Norris S, Duffy M, et al. Expansion of innate CD5pos B cells expressing high levels of CD81 in hepatitis C virus infected liver. J Hepatol 2003;38(5) 642-650.

[59] Newkirk MM. Rheumatoid factors: host resistance or autoimmunity? Clin Immunol 2002;104(1) 1-13.

[60] Charles ED, Green RM, Marukian S, Talal AH, Lake-Bakaar GV, Jacobson IM, et al. Clonal expansion of immunoglobulin M+CD27+ B cells in HCV-associated mixed cryoglobulinemia. Blood 2008;111(3) 1344-1356.

[61] Lauletta G, Russi S, Conteduca V, Sansonno L. Hepatitis C virus infection and mixed cryoglobulinemia. Clin Dev Immunol 2012;2012(502156.

[62] Lindahl G, Sjobring U, Johnsson E. Human complement regulators: a major target for pathogenic microorganisms. Curr Opin Immunol 2000;12(1) 44-51.

[63] Kittlesen DJ, Chianese-Bullock KA, Yao ZQ, Braciale TJ, Hahn YS. Interaction between complement receptor gC1qR and hepatitis C virus core protein inhibits T-lymphocyte proliferation. J Clin Invest 2000;106(10) 1239-1249.

[64] Yao ZQ, Ray S, Eisen-Vandervelde A, Waggoner S, Hahn YS. Hepatitis C virus: immunosuppression by complement regulatory pathway. Viral Immunol 2001;14(4) 277-295.

[65] Yao ZQ, Prayther D, Trabue C, Dong ZP, Moorman J. Differential regulation of SOCS-1 signalling in B and T lymphocytes by hepatitis C virus core protein. Immunology 2008;125(2) 197-207.

[66] Sansonno D, Tucci FA, Ghebrehiwet B, Lauletta G, Peerschke EI, Conteduca V, et al. Role of the receptor for the globular domain of C1q protein in the pathogenesis of hepatitis C virus-related cryoglobulin vascular damage. J Immunol 2009;183(9) 6013-6020.

[67] Landau DA, Scerra S, Sene D, Resche-Rigon M, Saadoun D, Cacoub P. Causes and predictive factors of mortality in a cohort of patients with hepatitis C virus-related cryoglobulinemic vasculitis treated with antiviral therapy. J Rheumatol 2010;37(3) 615-621.

[68] Della Rossa A, Tavoni A, D'Ascanio A, Catarsi E, Marchi F, Bencivelli W, et al. Mortality rate and outcome factors in mixed cryoglobulinaemia: the impact of hepatitis C virus. Scand J Rheumatol 2010;39(2) 167-170.

[69] Bonomo L, Casato M, Afeltra A, Caccavo D. Treatment of idiopathic mixed cryoglobulinemia with alpha interferon. Am J Med 1987;83(4) 726-730.

[70] Reddy KR, Wright TL, Pockros PJ, Shiffman M, Everson G, Reindollar R, et al. Efficacy and safety of pegylated (40-kd) interferon alpha-2a compared with interferon alpha-2a in noncirrhotic patients with chronic hepatitis C. Hepatology 2001;33(2) 433-438.

[71] Glue P, Fang JW, Rouzier-Panis R, Raffanel C, Sabo R, Gupta SK, et al. Pegylated interferon-alpha2b: pharmacokinetics, pharmacodynamics, safety, and preliminary efficacy data. Hepatitis C Intervention Therapy Group. Clin Pharmacol Ther 2000;68(5) 556-567.

[72] Shepherd J, Brodin H, Cave C, Waugh N, Price A, Gabbay J. Pegylated interferon alpha-2a and -2b in combination with ribavirin in the treatment of chronic hepatitis C: a systematic review and economic evaluation. Health Technol Assess 2004;8(39) iii-iv, 1-125.

[73] Cacoub P, Saadoun D, Limal N, Sene D, Lidove O, Piette JC. PEGylated interferon alfa-2b and ribavirin treatment in patients with hepatitis C virus-related systemic vasculitis. Arthritis Rheum 2005;52(3) 911-915.

[74] Sansonno D, Lauletta G, De Re V, Tucci FA, Gatti P, Racanelli V, et al. Intrahepatic B cell clonal expansions and extrahepatic manifestations of chronic HCV infection. Eur J Immunol 2004;34(1) 126-136.

[75] Vallat L, Benhamou Y, Gutierrez M, Ghillani P, Hercher C, Thibault V, et al. Clonal B cell populations in the blood and liver of patients with chronic hepatitis C virus infection. Arthritis Rheum 2004;50(11) 3668-3678.

[76] Fan HB, Zhu YF, Chen AS, Zhou MX, Yan FM, Ma XJ, et al. B-cell clonality in the liver of hepatitis C virus-infected patients. World J Gastroenterol 2009;15(13) 1636-1640.

[77] Sansonno D, Lauletta G, Montrone M, Tucci FA, Nisi L, Dammacco F. Virological analysis and phenotypic characterization of peripheral blood lymphocytes of hepatitis C virus-infected patients with and without mixed cryoglobulinaemia. Clin Exp Immunol 2006;143(2) 288-296.

[78] Charles ED, Brunetti C, Marukian S, Ritola KD, Talal AH, Marks K, et al. Clonal B cells in patients with hepatitis C virus-associated mixed cryoglobulinemia contain an expanded anergic CD21low B-cell subset. Blood 2011;117(20) 5425-5437.

[79] Cheung MC, Haynes AE, Meyer RM, Stevens A, Imrie KR, Members of the Hematology DSGotCCOPiE-BC. Rituximab in lymphoma: a systematic review and consensus practice guideline from Cancer Care Ontario. Cancer Treat Rev 2007;33(2) 161-176.

[80] Sanz I, Anolik JH, Looney RJ. B cell depletion therapy in autoimmune diseases. Front Biosci 2007;12(2546-2567.

[81] Barcellini W, Zanella A. Rituximab therapy for autoimmune haematological diseases. Eur J Intern Med 2011;22(3) 220-229.

[82] Sansonno D, De Re V, Lauletta G, Tucci FA, Boiocchi M, Dammacco F. Monoclonal antibody treatment of mixed cryoglobulinemia resistant to interferon alpha with an anti-CD20. Blood 2003;101(10) 3818-3826.

[83] Zaja F, De Vita S, Mazzaro C, Sacco S, Damiani D, De Marchi G, et al. Efficacy and safety of rituximab in type II mixed cryoglobulinemia. Blood 2003;101(10) 3827-3834.

[84] Visentini M, Ludovisi S, Petrarca A, Pulvirenti F, Zaramella M, Monti M, et al. A phase II, single-arm multicenter study of low-dose rituximab for refractory mixed

cryoglobulinemia secondary to hepatitis C virus infection. Autoimmun Rev 2011;10(11) 714-719.

[85] Ferri C, Cacoub P, Mazzaro C, Roccatello D, Scaini P, Sebastiani M, et al. Treatment with rituximab in patients with mixed cryoglobulinemia syndrome: results of multi-center cohort study and review of the literature. Autoimmun Rev 2011;11(1) 48-55.

[86] Dammacco F, Tucci FA, Lauletta G, Gatti P, De Re V, Conteduca V, et al. Pegylated interferon-alpha, ribavirin, and rituximab combined therapy of hepatitis C virus-related mixed cryoglobulinemia: a long-term study. Blood 2010;116(3) 343-353.

[87] Pietrogrande M, De Vita S, Zignego AL, Pioltelli P, Sansonno D, Sollima S, et al. Recommendations for the management of mixed cryoglobulinemia syndrome in hepatitis C virus-infected patients. Autoimmun Rev 2011;10(8) 444-454.

[88] Lok AS, Gardiner DF, Lawitz E, Martorell C, Everson GT, Ghalib R, et al. Preliminary study of two antiviral agents for hepatitis C genotype 1. N Engl J Med 2012;366(3) 216-224.

[89] Levine JW, Gota C, Fessler BJ, Calabrese LH, Cooper SM. Persistent cryoglobulinemic vasculitis following successful treatment of hepatitis C virus. J Rheumatol 2005;32(6) 1164-1167.

[90] Landau DA, Saadoun D, Halfon P, Martinot-Peignoux M, Marcellin P, Fois E, et al. Relapse of hepatitis C virus-associated mixed cryoglobulinemia vasculitis in patients with sustained viral response. Arthritis Rheum 2008;58(2) 604-611.

[91] Cheson BD. Ofatumumab, a novel anti-CD20 monoclonal antibody for the treatment of B-cell malignancies. J Clin Oncol 2010;28(21) 3525-3530.

[92] Ramunni A, Lauletta G, Brescia P, Saliani MT, Montrone M, Chironna M, et al. Double-filtration plasmapheresis in the treatment of leg ulcers in cryoglobulinemia. J Clin Apher 2008;23(3) 118-122.

[93] Talamo G, Zangari M, Novel therapeutic approaches to cryoglobulinemia: imatinib, infliximab, bortezomib, and beyond, in HCV infection and mixed cryoglobulinemia, F. Dammacco, Editor. 2012, Springer: Milan. p. 349-355.

[94] Saadoun D, Rosenzwajg M, Joly F, Six A, Carrat F, Thibault V, et al. Regulatory T-cell responses to low-dose interleukin-2 in HCV-induced vasculitis. N Engl J Med 2011;365(22) 2067-2077.

[95] Butel JS. Viral carcinogenesis: revelation of molecular mechanisms and etiology of human disease. Carcinogenesis 2000;21(3) 405-426.

[96] Raab-Traub N, Epstein-Barr virus, lymphoproliferative disease and nasopharingeal carcinoma., in Microbes and Malignancy. Infection and cause of human cancers., J. Parsonnet, Editor. 1999, Oxford University Press: Oxford. p. 180-206.

[97] Martin D, Gutkind JS. Human tumor-associated viruses and new insights into the molecular mechanisms of cancer. Oncogene 2008;27 Suppl 2(S31-42.

[98] Boxus M, Willems L. Mechanisms of HTLV-1 persistence and transformation. Br J Cancer 2009;101(9) 1497-1501.

[99] Ganem D. KSHV and the pathogenesis of Kaposi sarcoma: listening to human biology and medicine. J Clin Invest 2010;120(4) 939-949.

[100] Dammacco F, Gatti P, Sansonno D. Hepatitis C virus infection, mixed cryoglobulinemia, and non-Hodgkin's lymphoma: an emerging picture. Leuk Lymphoma 1998;31(5-6) 463-476.

[101] Ferri C, Caracciolo F, Zignego AL, La Civita L, Monti M, Longombardo G, et al. Hepatitis C virus infection in patients with non-Hodgkin's lymphoma. Br J Haematol 1994;88(2) 392-394.

[102] Pozzato G, Mazzaro C, Crovatto M, Modolo ML, Ceselli S, Mazzi G, et al. Low-grade malignant lymphoma, hepatitis C virus infection, and mixed cryoglobulinemia. Blood 1994;84(9) 3047-3053.

[103] Dal Maso L, Franceschi S. Hepatitis C virus and risk of lymphoma and other lymphoid neoplasms: a meta-analysis of epidemiologic studies. Cancer Epidemiol Biomarkers Prev 2006;15(11) 2078-2085.

[104] Mussini C, Ghini M, Mascia MT, Giovanardi P, Zanni G, Lattuada I, et al. Monoclonal gammopathies and hepatitis C virus infection. Blood 1995;85(4) 1144-1145.

[105] Martyak LA, Yeganeh M, Saab S. Hepatitis C and lymphoproliferative disorders: from mixed cryoglobulinemia to non-Hodgkin's lymphoma. Clin Gastroenterol Hepatol 2009;7(8) 900-905.

[106] Matsuo K, Kusano A, Sugumar A, Nakamura S, Tajima K, Mueller NE. Effect of hepatitis C virus infection on the risk of non-Hodgkin's lymphoma: a meta-analysis of epidemiological studies. Cancer Sci 2004;95(9) 745-752.

[107] De Vita S, Sacco C, Sansonno D, Gloghini A, Dammacco F, Crovatto M, et al. Characterization of overt B-cell lymphomas in patients with hepatitis C virus infection. Blood 1997;90(2) 776-782.

[108] Ryan J, Wallace S, Jones P, Taggart G, Dudley F. Primary hepatic lymphoma in a patient with chronic hepatitis C. J Gastroenterol Hepatol 1994;9(3) 308-310.

[109] Vallisa D, Berte R, Rocca A, Civardi G, Giangregorio F, Ferrari B, et al. Association between hepatitis C virus and non-Hodgkin's lymphoma, and effects of viral infection on histologic subtype and clinical course. Am J Med 1999;106(5) 556-560.

[110] Giordano TP, Henderson L, Landgren O, Chiao EY, Kramer JR, El-Serag H, et al. Risk of non-Hodgkin lymphoma and lymphoproliferative precursor diseases in US veterans with hepatitis C virus. JAMA 2007;297(18) 2010-2017.

[111] Sene D, Ghillani-Dalbin P, Thibault V, Guis L, Musset L, Duhaut P, et al. Longterm course of mixed cryoglobulinemia in patients infected with hepatitis C virus. J Rheumatol 2004;31(11) 2199-2206.

[112] Viswanatha DS, Dogan A. Hepatitis C virus and lymphoma. J Clin Pathol 2007;60(12) 1378-1383.

[113] de Sanjose S, Benavente Y, Vajdic CM, Engels EA, Morton LM, Bracci PM, et al. Hepatitis C and non-Hodgkin lymphoma among 4784 cases and 6269 controls from the International Lymphoma Epidemiology Consortium. Clin Gastroenterol Hepatol 2008;6(4) 451-458.

[114] Saadoun D, Suarez F, Lefrere F, Valensi F, Mariette X, Aouba A, et al. Splenic lymphoma with villous lymphocytes, associated with type II cryoglobulinemia and HCV infection: a new entity? Blood 2005;105(1) 74-76.

[115] Arcaini L, Burcheri S, Rossi A, Paulli M, Bruno R, Passamonti F, et al. Prevalence of HCV infection in nongastric marginal zone B-cell lymphoma of MALT. Ann Oncol 2007;18(2) 346-350.

[116] Saadoun D, Bieche I, Maisonobe T, Asselah T, Laurendeau I, Piette JC, et al. Involvement of chemokines and type 1 cytokines in the pathogenesis of hepatitis C virus-associated mixed cryoglobulinemia vasculitis neuropathy. Arthritis Rheum 2005;52(9) 2917-2925.

[117] Scarselli E, Ansuini H, Cerino R, Roccasecca RM, Acali S, Filocamo G, et al. The human scavenger receptor class B type I is a novel candidate receptor for the hepatitis C virus. EMBO J 2002;21(19) 5017-5025.

[118] Agnello V, Abel G, Elfahal M, Knight GB, Zhang QX. Hepatitis C virus and other flaviviridae viruses enter cells via low density lipoprotein receptor. Proc Natl Acad Sci U S A 1999;96(22) 12766-12771.

[119] Petracca R, Falugi F, Galli G, Norais N, Rosa D, Campagnoli S, et al. Structure-function analysis of hepatitis C virus envelope-CD81 binding. J Virol 2000;74(10) 4824-4830.

[120] Zuckerman E, Kessel A, Slobodin G, Sabo E, Yeshurun D, Toubi E. Antiviral treatment down-regulates peripheral B-cell CD81 expression and CD5 expansion in chronic hepatitis C virus infection. J Virol 2003;77(19) 10432-10436.

[121] Laporte J, Bain C, Maurel P, Inchauspe G, Agut H, Cahour A. Differential distribution and internal translation efficiency of hepatitis C virus quasispecies present in dendritic and liver cells. Blood 2003;101(1) 52-57.

[122] Kronenberger B, Sarrazin C, Hofmann WP, von Wagner M, Herrmann E, Welsch C, et al. Mutations in the putative HCV-E2 CD81 binding regions and correlation with cell surface CD81 expression. J Viral Hepat 2004;11(4) 310-318.

[123] Pal S, Sullivan DG, Kim S, Lai KK, Kae J, Cotler SJ, et al. Productive replication of hepatitis C virus in perihepatic lymph nodes in vivo: implications of HCV lymphotropism. Gastroenterology 2006;130(4) 1107-1116.

[124] Sansonno D, Tucci FA, Lauletta G, De Re V, Montrone M, Troiani L, et al. Hepatitis C virus productive infection in mononuclear cells from patients with cryoglobulinaemia. Clin Exp Immunol 2007;147(2) 241-248.

[125] Dahari H, Feliu A, Garcia-Retortillo M, Forns X, Neumann AU. Second hepatitis C replication compartment indicated by viral dynamics during liver transplantation. J Hepatol 2005;42(4) 491-498.

[126] Sansonno D, De Vita S, Iacobelli AR, Cornacchiulo V, Boiocchi M, Dammacco F. Clonal analysis of intrahepatic B cells from HCV-infected patients with and without mixed cryoglobulinemia. J Immunol 1998;160(7) 3594-3601.

[127] Aarts WM, Bende RJ, Steenbergen EJ, Kluin PM, Ooms EC, Pals ST, et al. Variable heavy chain gene analysis of follicular lymphomas: correlation between heavy chain isotype expression and somatic mutation load. Blood 2000;95(9) 2922-2929.

[128] De Re V, De Vita S, Marzotto A, Rupolo M, Gloghini A, Pivetta B, et al. Sequence analysis of the immunoglobulin antigen receptor of hepatitis C virus-associated non-Hodgkin lymphomas suggests that the malignant cells are derived from the rheumatoid factor-producing cells that occur mainly in type II cryoglobulinemia. Blood 2000;96(10) 3578-3584.

[129] Ishak KG. Chronic hepatitis: morphology and nomenclature. Mod Pathol 1994;7(6) 690-713.

[130] Mosnier JF, Degott C, Marcellin P, Henin D, Erlinger S, Benhamou JP. The intraportal lymphoid nodule and its environment in chronic active hepatitis C: an immunohistochemical study. Hepatology 1993;17(3) 366-371.

[131] Racanelli V, Sansonno D, Piccoli C, D'Amore FP, Tucci FA, Dammacco F. Molecular characterization of B cell clonal expansions in the liver of chronically hepatitis C virus-infected patients. J Immunol 2001;167(1) 21-29.

[132] Cheema GS, Roschke V, Hilbert DM, Stohl W. Elevated serum B lymphocyte stimulator levels in patients with systemic immune-based rheumatic diseases. Arthritis Rheum 2001;44(6) 1313-1319.

[133] Zignego AL, Ferri C, Giannelli F, Giannini C, Caini P, Monti M, et al. Prevalence of bcl-2 rearrangement in patients with hepatitis C virus-related mixed cryoglobulinemia with or without B-cell lymphomas. Ann Intern Med 2002;137(7) 571-580.

[134] Sansonno D, Tucci FA, De Re V, Lauletta G, Montrone M, Libra M, et al. HCV-associated B cell clonalities in the liver do not carry the t(14;18) chromosomal translocation. Hepatology 2005;42(5) 1019-1027.

[135] Durandy A. Activation-induced cytidine deaminase: a dual role in class-switch recombination and somatic hypermutation. Eur J Immunol 2003;33(8) 2069-2073.

[136] Kuppers R, Dalla-Favera R. Mechanisms of chromosomal translocations in B cell lymphomas. Oncogene 2001;20(40) 5580-5594.

[137] Pasqualucci L, Neumeister P, Goossens T, Nanjangud G, Chaganti RS, Kuppers R, et al. Hypermutation of multiple proto-oncogenes in B-cell diffuse large-cell lymphomas. Nature 2001;412(6844) 341-346.

[138] Chiba T, Marusawa H. A novel mechanism for inflammation-associated carcinogenesis; an important role of activation-induced cytidine deaminase (AID) in mutation induction. J Mol Med (Berl) 2009;87(10) 1023-1027.

[139] Kawamura Y, Ikeda K, Arase Y, Yatsuji H, Sezaki H, Hosaka T, et al. Viral elimination reduces incidence of malignant lymphoma in patients with hepatitis C. Am J Med 2007;120(12) 1034-1041.

[140] Hermine O, Lefrere F, Bronowicki JP, Mariette X, Jondeau K, Eclache-Saudreau V, et al. Regression of splenic lymphoma with villous lymphocytes after treatment of hepatitis C virus infection. N Engl J Med 2002;347(2) 89-94.

[141] Gisbert JP, Garcia-Buey L, Pajares JM, Moreno-Otero R. Systematic review: regression of lymphoproliferative disorders after treatment for hepatitis C infection. Aliment Pharmacol Ther 2005;21(6) 653-662.

[142] Arcaini L, Merli M, Volpetti S, Rattotti S, Gotti M, Zaja F. Indolent B-cell lymphomas associated with HCV infection: clinical and virological features and role of antiviral therapy. Clin Dev Immunol 2012;2012(638185.

[143] Isaacson PG, Piris MA, Berger F, Swerdlow SH, Thieblemont C, Pittaluga S, et al., Splenic B-cell marginal zone lymphoma, in WHO classification of tumours of haematopoietic and lymphoid tissues., S.H. Swerdlow, et al., Editors. 2008, IARC Press: Lyon. p. 85-187.

[144] Saadoun D, Resche Rigon M, Sene D, Terrier B, Karras A, Perard L, et al. Rituximab plus Peg-interferon-alpha/ribavirin compared with Peg-interferon-alpha/ribavirin in hepatitis C-related mixed cryoglobulinemia. Blood 2010;116(3) 326-334; quiz 504-325.

[145] Pellicelli AM, Marignani M, Zoli V, Romano M, Morrone A, Nosotti L, et al. Hepatitis C virus-related B cell subtypes in non Hodgkin's lymphoma. World J Hepatol 2011;3(11) 278-284.

[146] Iannitto E, Ammatuna E, Tripodo C, Marino C, Calvaruso G, Florena AM, et al. Long-lasting remission of primary hepatic lymphoma and hepatitis C virus infection achieved by the alpha-interferon treatment. Hematol J 2004;5(6) 530-533.

[147] Levine AM, Shimodaira S, Lai MM. Treatment of HCV-related mantle-cell lymphoma with ribavirin and pegylated interferon Alfa. N Engl J Med 2003;349(21) 2078-2079.

[148] Ennishi D, Maeda Y, Niitsu N, Kojima M, Izutsu K, Takizawa J, et al. Hepatic toxicity and prognosis in hepatitis C virus-infected patients with diffuse large B-cell lymphoma treated with rituximab-containing chemotherapy regimens: a Japanese multicenter analysis. Blood 2010;116(24) 5119-5125.

[149] Musto P, Dell'Olio M, La Sala A, Mantuano S, Cascavilla N. Diffuse B-Large Cell Lymphomas (DBLCL) with Hepatitis-C Virus (HCV) Infection: Clinical Outcome and Preliminary Results of a Pilot Study Combining R-CHOP with Antiviral Therapy. Blood 2005;106(11) 2447.

[150] La Mura V, De Renzo A, Perna F, D'Agostino D, Masarone M, Romano M, et al. Antiviral therapy after complete response to chemotherapy could be efficacious in HCV-positive non-Hodgkin's lymphoma. J Hepatol 2008;49(4) 557-563.

Chapter 13

Surgical Management of HCC

R Lochan, HL Reeves and DM Manas

Additional information is available at the end of the chapter

http://dx.doi.org/10.5772/55743

1. Introduction

Hepatocellular cancer (HCC) accounts for approximately 80% of all primary liver cancers. It is the fifth most common cancer worldwide and is the third leading cause of cancer related deaths across the world, with a case fatality rate of 0.93 making it one of the most lethal malignancies [1]. In the majority of cases, HCC develops in the setting of cirrhosis and treatment with curative intent is only possible in a minority of cases. The incidence of HCC continues to rise world-wide, due in part to the rising number of people who have hepatitis C virus (HCV) infection, infection with hepatitis B virus (HBV), (but not to the same degree as HCV) and non-alcoholic fatty liver disease (NAFLD). NAFLD is now the most rapidly rising cause of cirrhosis in the developed world. The outcome from this disease is poor, with a median survival estimated at around 1-year following diagnosis [2]. In keeping with global trends, the incidence and consequent mortality from HCC in the United Kingdom is also increasing, despite greater awareness for the need for surveillance in patients with cirrhosis, and improvements in and access to imaging. This is thought to be secondary to the persistence of alcohol induced liver disease as a significant cause of CLDs [3], the growing incidence of non-alcoholic fatty liver disease (NAFLD) in the UK, immigration to the UK from HBV-endemic countries and the clinical impact of HCV infected individuals, infected before HCV screening of blood products (in the 1990's).

HCC is unique amongst solid cancers in that the outcome from it depends not only on the performance status of the patient and biological behaviour of the tumour, but also on the degree of liver dysfunction. The current treatment options are surgical (liver resection [LR], liver transplant [LT]), ablative (radiofrequency or microwave ablation [RFA/MCT]), non-surgical (trans-arterial chemo-embolisation, selective internal radiation therapy [yttrium90 spheres]) and medical - in particular the use of the targeted kinase inhibitor, Sorafenib. The only curative treatments are the surgical modalities (LR or LT). However these treatments are not suitable for the majority of patients but can achieve the best outcome in carefully selected patients with early tumours or very early tumours. Sometimes LR and LT are complimentary, particularly when LR is considered as a bridge to transplantation. When the liver parenchyma is normal [5% of the cases in Western countries, and for about 40% in Asia] the treatment of choice is a liver resection (LR) [4]. However most patients also have underlying chronic liver disease and for this group of patients, LT is the treatment of choice as it treats not only the tumour but the underlying chronic liver disease which induces tumourigenesis in the first place. However the relative scarcity of donor organs available for transplantation (NHSBT) and the improved outcomes of LR amongst those with chronic liver disease (CLD) have led to an increased interest in LR for HCC.

For patients with early HCC and CLD who have well-preserved liver function (the vast majority of patients), establishing the best treatment is difficult as there are no well designed randomized controlled trials to guide management. Proposed treatment modalities for individual patients need to take into account not only tumour factors (stage of tumour) but also the degree of underlying chronic liver disease and patient factors (performance status). The Barcelona Clinic Liver Cancer (BCLC) algorithm which incorporates these variables into a decision making process to help choose a specific management option has been found most useful in clinical practice [5].

2. Liver resection as treatment for HCC

2.1. Selection criteria of patients with HCC for Liver Resection (LR)

Clearly extra-hepatic and or distant spread is a contra-indication for LR. This occurs in 60-80% of cases. There is a significant geographical variation in the proportion of patients undergoing surgery with curative intent, varying from 20% in East Asia, through 25-40% in Europe, to 50-70% in Japan. Superior outcomes being related to the implementation of effective screening programs [6].

In addition to the patients overall performance status, the following specific factors need to be considered

1. The Tumour:

a. Stage

b. Size

2. The Liver parenchyma

a. Underlying chronic liver disease (CLD) and portal hypertension (PHT)

b. Quality and volume of the "future functional liver remnant"(FLR)

3. Tumour specific factors

3.1. Staging of HCC

Resection of any cancer is based on pre-operative staging to a large extent. In addition, a proper cancer staging is useful for evaluating prognosis of cancer patients, for tailoring therapy and monitoring therapeutic response. Generally prognosis in solid cancers is solely related to stage. However HCC is unique in that cirrhosis underlies the cancer and thus outcome is related too not only tumor but also to the extent of liver parenchymal damage. Therefore any staging for cirrhotic patients with HCC should take into consideration the severity of the liver disease and the extent of the tumour. Numerous staging systems have been described (at least 8), although none has been universally accepted. The variables used in each classification as well as the populations in which they were derived are different. Only 3 – BCLC, CLIP and JIS have been validated in different cohorts of patients [7]- [12]. The BCLC and Cancer of the Liver Italian Program (CLIP) staging systems have been the most popular in Europe and the USA, and the Japan Integrated Staging Score (JIS) in Japan.

The Okuda staging system includes tumour size, serum albumin, bilirubin and ascites [13]. The Child's classification does not discriminate enough for Child's A or B patients in whom resection is being considered in order to prevent postoperative liver de-compensation. The Cancer of the Liver Italian Program (CLIP) is based on the Child–Pugh class, tumour progression, alpha-fetoprotein (AFP) and presence of portal venous thrombosis. CLIP is the most accurate for prognosis [12] especially in patients with advanced HCC and those undergoing loco-regional therapy [14]. Specifically, a CLIP score of less than 2 predicts better response and longer survival [15]. The BCLC system assesses tumour stage, liver function, physical status and cancer-related symptoms, linking these in a widely used treatment algorithm [16], [17] [18]. The BCLC is the only system that links prognosis with treatment recommendations, and is therefore selected in several major trials of HCC therapy.

Conventional methods like TNM (e.g. TNM) exclude the functional status of the liver, which is an important consideration in these patients. However in patients with intermediate or advanced HCC who undergo surgery the AJCC/UICC system is useful [19]– the parameters include tumour size and number, vascular invasion (micro/macro) and degree of fibrosis Ishak grade. The 7th edition [20] has further refined prognostication for the intermediate/advanced stages of the disease and this continues to be where this staging system is useful but does not really improve discrimination for early HCC.

Other tumour factors known to impact on outcomes after LR include size of lesion, satellite nodules, serum AFP, margin status, vascular involvement and UICC stage 3 or 4 disease. These factors therefore need to be considered carefully prior to consideration of hepatectomy for HCC.

Size of lesion: It is unsurprising that the size of the lesion impacts on outcome after LR. Larger lesions indicating increased tumour load with increased risk of vascular invasion, need increased liver mass to be resected and therefore contribute to a lesser future functional liver remanant (FLR) on a background of underlying CLD. Smaller tumour size is a well-accepted as an important independent prognostic indicator for overall survival [22]- [25] but not disease-free survival. From a multi-institutional cohort of 557 patients, tumour size if less than 5 cm resulted in 43% 5-year survival compared to 32% for larger tumours. HR (95% CI) for recurrent disease and death if lesion more than 5 cm was 1.4 (1.1 – 1.9) [26]. In a series of 12,118 patients from Japan, size less than 2 cm was an independent predictor of survival compared to larger tumours (2 cm, 2-5 cm, 5-10 cm and more than 10 cm; 5 year survival 66%, 53%, 37% and 31%

Okuda staging			
	Negative	Positive	Stage
Tumour size	<50% of Liver	>50% of Liver	I: no positive factors
Ascites	Absent	Present	II: 1-2 positive factors
Bilirubin	<51 mmol/L	>51mmol/L	III: 3-4 positive factors
Serum Albumin	>3g/dL	<3g/dL	

Child-Turcotte-Pugh classification				
	1point	2 points	3 points	Class
Encephalopathy	None	Grade 1-2	Grade 3-4	A 5-6 points
Bilirubin	<2	2-3	>3	B 7-9 points
PT/INR	<1.7	1.7-2	>2	C 10-15 points
Ascites	None	Controlled on Rx	Refractory	
Albumin (g/L)				

CLIP – Cancer of the Liver Italian Program				
Points	CTP	Tumour morphology	AFP	PV thrombosis
0	A	Uninodular ≤50% of Liver		No
1	B	Multinodular ≤50% of Liver		Yes
2	C	Massive>50% of Liver		

BCLC – Barcelona caner of Liver Clinic staging					
Stage	Performance status	Tumour stage	PHT	Bilirubin	Classification
A1	0	Single	No	Normal	Very early
A2	0	Single	Yes	Normal	Early
A3	0	Single	Yes	Raised	
A4	0	3 tumours, <3 cm each	Yes	Raised	
B	0				Intermediate
C	1-2	Vascular invasion			Advanced
D	3-4	Any tumour			Terminal

AJCC TNM 7th edition			
Stage	T	N	M
I	T1 solitary tumour, no vascular invasion	N0	M0
II	T2 Solitary tumor with vascular invasion or multiple tumors, none > 5 cm	N0	M0
IIIA	T3a Multiple tumors > 5 cm	N0	M0
IIIB	T3b Single tumor or multiple tumors of any size involving a major branch of the portal or hepatic vein	N0	M0
IIIC	T4 Tumor(s) with direct invasion of adjacent organs other than gallbladder or with visceral peritoneum	N0	M0
IVA	Any T	N1	M0
IVB	Any T	Any N	M1

Table 1. Table of various staging systems [21]

respectively). In this study on multivariate analysis, tumour size less than 2 cm resulted in a significantly better overall survival. Therefore the Liver Cancer Study Group of Japan (LCSGJ) suggests a tumour cut-off size of 2cm as apposed to the 5 cm suggested by the TNM system [24].

Whilst there is little doubt that the results are superior for small tumours (<5 cm), several studies have indicated that resection for larger tumours (>5 cm) [27], [28] is beneficial. The Memorial Sloan–Kettering Group have analyzed the results of resection in 154 patients (out of total of 412 seen at their institution over a 6 year period) and found that for tumors <5 cm, the overall 5-year survival rate is 57% and the disease-free survival rate is 44%. Even for those with large tumors (>10 cm), the 5-year survival rate was 32%, with disease-free survival rate is only 23% [27]. Therefore they concluded that LR was superior to other forms of treatment for larger tumours and advocated partial hepatectomy as a safe, effective, and potentially curative therapy of choice for HCC >5 cm. For tumors <5 cm, much more relevant is the comparison between LR and ablative options. In a comparative study from China of 1000 small tumours (less than 5 cm) versus 1366 large (more than 5 cm) [28] survival rates after LR at 5 years of 62.7% vs. 37.1% ($p < 0.01$) and at 10 years of 46.3% vs. 29.2% ($p < 0.01$) were seen on univariate analysis. However compared with patients who had large HCC, those with small HCC had a higher percentage of single tumor nodules (82.6% vs. 64.4%), a higher proportion of well encapsulated tumors (73.3% vs. 46.3%), a lower proportion of tumor emboli in the portal vein (4.9% vs. 20.8%) and better differentiation of tumor cells (Edmondson Grade 3–4; 14.9% vs. 20.1%), a higher resection rate (93.6% [1000 of 1068 patients] vs. 55.7% [1366 of 2451 patients]; $P < 0.01$), a higher curative resection rate (80.5% [805 of 1000 patients] vs. 60.7% [829 of 1366 patients]; $p < 0.01$) and a lower operative mortality rate (1.5% [15 of 1000 patients] vs. 3.7% [50 of 1366 patients]; $p < 0.01$). Importantly following multivariate analysis, four independent covariates negatively influenced the survival rate: γ-glutamyl transpeptidase (more than 6IU/mL), presence of cirrhosis, multiple tumors, and emboli in the portal vein. Size of lesion was not an independent predictive factor.

The results of surgery in the so-called giant tumours (>10 cm) which would be exempt from transplantation, are reassuring too; Chen and co-workers [29] reported on 525 patients with tumours >10 cm noting a 2.7% perioperative mortality and a 5-year survival of 16.8%. Yeh and colleagues reported 211 tumours greater than 10 cm in a series of 1196 patients thus representing 17.6% of their patients. They noted resection to be safe and feasible with a reasonable 5-year survival of 16.7% for this cohort although this was significantly lower than the 39.5% documented for tumours less than 10 cm [30]. In a study of 300 patients with tumours >10 cm, the group from MD Anderson reported a 27% 5-year survival [31]. Therefore the value of resecting large and otherwise 'untreatable' tumours was confirmed. It is clear that prognostic indicators such as size can be used as a guide in the decision to operate or not, but cannot be used alone to exclude patients from surgery - such decisions should be based on surgical risk and resectability.

Vascular invasion: Again from the multi-institutional cohorts (vide supra) the presence of vascular invasion appears to be an independent predictor of recurrent disease and death after LR; HR (95% CI) for major vascular invasion – 2.1 (1.4 – 3.3), microvascular invasion – 1.6 (1.2 – 2.1) and 5-year survival with and without macrovascular invasion was 15% versus 41%

respectively [26]. In a cohort of 322 patients undergoing resection for HCC [32] the 5-year survival of those with microscopic venous invasion (n = 140) versus macroscopic venous involvement (n = 50) versus those without any venous invasion (n = 132) was 30.8%, 15% and 50% ($p < 0.05$). Also, larger tumours were associated with higher incidence of venous involvement. Major vascular invasion (macrovascular invasion) into one of the main portal branches or a hepatic vein is associated with a worse prognosis, presumably due to intra-hepatic and systemic dissemination of tumour thrombi. From a multi-institutional study of 102 patients, major portal invasion was associated with 1-, 3- and 5- year survival of 47%, 17% and 10% respectively [31], however in the group which had major vascular involvement but without moderate-severe fibrosis or high nuclear grade 5 year survival was 23% vs 5% and 21% vs 9% respectively. Therefore the MD Anderson data suggests resection in spite of major vascular invasion in the absence of moderate-severe fibrosis in the liver parenchyma and absent high nuclear grade in the tumour. Similarly the incidence of microscopic vascular invasion is increased with tumor size (≤3 cm, 25%; 3.1-5 cm, 40%; 5.1-6.5 cm, 55%; >6.5 cm, 63%) ($p < 0.005$) [33]. Therefore it is clear that tumour size, which can be measured radiologically, is a good surrogate marker for microvascular invasion, which can only be assessed on the resected specimen. It is accepted that larger tumours (especially those more than 7 cm) and certain types of growth patterns (single nodule with extra-nodular growth, contiguous multi-nodular growth patterns) are highly predictive of microvascular invasion (as compared to a single nodular type with clear demarcation) in lesions more than 5 cm in size [34]. However increasing size or number of lesions in the absence of vascular involvement does not impact on survival [26].

3.2. Tumour number, multifocality and satellite nodules

The number of tumours present is another important factor for not only overall survival [35] [31] [36] but for disease-free survival [36]- [39] as well.. The AASLD guidelines recommend LR for a single liver lesion if there is no cirrhosis or significant impairment of liver function [4]. However results from a large multi-institutional cohort study [36] looking at the perioperative and long-term outcomes of 404 patients with single small HCC (<5 cm) as compared to 380 patients with large or multinodular HCC demonstrated overall survival rates were significantly higher in the small HCC group (1 year, 88% vs. 74%; 3 years, 76% vs. 50%; 5 years, 58% vs. 39%; $p < .001$). Among patients with the larger tumours, five independent prognostic factors were identified to be associated with a worse overall survival: namely, symptomatic disease, presence of cirrhosis, multinodular tumor, microvascular tumor invasion, and positive histological margin. Multifocality may be a manifestation of one of 2 differing scenarios: either multiple foci of primary tumour within an at-risk field or the presence of intrahepatic metastases from a primary lesion. It is impossible to determine which scenario is being displayed pre-operatively but the latter carries a significantly worse prognosis.

3.3. Pre-operative Alpha-Fetoprotein (AFP) levels

AFP is a major plasma protein produced by the yolk sac and the liver during fetal development that is thought to be the fetal form of serum albumin. Its levels decrease rapidly after birth and its functions in the fetus are not clearly known. Its levels are raised in HCC and germ cell tumours. Raised AFP levels have been considered to be a marker of poor prognosis both for overall survival [37] [27], [40] and disease-free survival [30], [37], [41], [42]. The relevance of AFP levels has not been addressed specifically in relation to resection although in one study an AFP level more than 100ng/ml was an independent risk factor [OR (95% CI) 2.56 (1.05 – 6.20)] along with microvascular invasion (OR 4.54 (1.86 – 11.09) in a cohort of small HCC who underwent curative resection [43]. AFP levels are probably a reflection of tumour biology and thus a surrogate marker for size/stage of the tumour.

4. Liver specific factors

4.1. Portal hypertension

It is well known that patients with a normal liver tolerate large hepatectomy without significant risk of liver failure. However, in patients with chronic liver disease the tolerance to liver resection and long-term outcome is reduced in parallel to the degree of liver function impairment and appearance of portal hypertension (PHT) [44]. Hemodynamic studies have shown that the presence of a hepatic vein pressure gradient greater than 10 mmHg is associated with a higher risk of postoperative liver decompensation and of poor long-term outcome after liver resection for HCC [45]. Clinically relevant PHT can also be detected by the presence of esophageal varices or splenomegaly associated with reduced platelet count. Assessment of presence or absence of PHT is an important step in not only risk assessment and outcome prediction, but importantly to ascertain suitability for resectional surgery and the extent of such surgery [46]. Indeed a recent study has suggested that this is an essential part of assessment of these patients for resection [47]. HVPG is an invasive test but some interest and success has recently been demonstrated for measurement of liver stiffness by elastography and its correlation with HVPG [48]. While 5-year survival in patients without PHT exceeds 70%, those patients with such adverse profile present a reduction to 50–60%. If liver disease is decompensated (ascites, jaundice), survival is even further decreased. Presence of PHT higher risk does not translate into absolute contraindication for resection [49], as less extensive resection/ablation etc. can be considered but the predicted outcome with surgery has to be weighed against other available treatment options in an individual patient.

4.2. Future liver remnant/ Functional Liver Remnant (FLR)

One of the important limiting factors for LR in HCC is the amount of viable liver parenchyma left behind- future liver remnant or more appropriately called functional liver remnant (FLR). In a normal liver, removal of a part of the liver leads to rapid hypertrophy of the remnant to reach the pre-operative liver-body weight ratio. Adequate FLR is not only an adequate volume of liver remnant but also a remnant of adequate function sufficient to meet post-operative physiological demands. Although the removal of up to 75% of the total liver volume is feasible in a young patient (≤40 years of age) with normal hepatic parenchyma, resection must be more conservative in the presence of underlying liver diseases (steatosis, steato-hepatitis, fibrosis, cirrhosis, cholestasis, chemo-therapy induced liver injury), elderly patients and in the setting of excessive intra-operative blood loss [50]. An adequate FLR is generally considered to be around 25%, 30% and 40% of the pre-operative liver volume in normal [51], steatotic and cirrhotic livers [52] respectively, although it is accepted that volume is a poor correlate of function in livers with chronic disease. Below a certain threshold, a liver remnant cannot sustain metabolic, synthetic and detoxifying functions and liver failure results leading on to the spiral of cholestasis, coagulopathy, sepsis, multiple organ failure and potentially death. Various techniques of assessing the FLR have been described including assessment of volume using axial imaging e.g. triple phase CT Liver, and MR Liver. Dynamic quantitative liver function tests, such as the indocyanine green test and galactose elimination capacity, are more accurate as they measure the elimination process of a substance that is cleared and/or metabolized almost exclusively by the liver. However, these tests only measure global liver function. Nuclear imaging techniques (Tc-galactosyl serum albumin scintigraphy and Tc-mebrofenin hepatobiliary scintigraphy) can measure both total and future remnant liver function and potentially identify patients at risk for post resectional liver failure [53]. A novel technique described has been the utilization of a combination LiMAX test (Liver MAximum capacity) and (triple phase CT, 3-D analysis – MeVIS, CT volumetry and virtual resection) and to successfully predict FLR and postoperative outcome after hepatectomy pre-operatively [54].

Preoperative portal vein embolization of the lobe free of disease may induce compensatory liver growth, allowing resection of larger volumes of tumour bearing liver [55] [56]. Indeed pre-operative selective internal radiotherapy (SIRT/Transarterial radioembolization – TARE) is being used to down-size liver tumors [57] including HCC [58] and increase FLR prior to major hepatectomy.

5. Liver resection for HCC — Technical considerations

Both non-cirrhotic patients and cirrhotics could be subjected to surgical resections as long as liver function was well-preserved and tumor had low burden (ideally single tumor). Usually, best results of surgical approaches are obtained in experienced centers with a perioperative mortality of less than 3% and a 5-year survival rate higher than 50% [6]. The correct selection of candidates is very important for the outcome and all issues discussed above need to be considered. Historically, patients with HCC and cirrhosis had a worse prognosis after LR but those without extrahepatic disease and small tumours had early mortality much lower than that reported for LT. Mortality rate related to LR in non-cirrhotics is approximately 1% [59]. The most common causes of death following LR are postoperative haemorrhage, liver failure and sepsis, even in well-compensated Child's A or B cirrhotics. Extended left and right hepatectomy are well documented in cirrhotic patients with low complication rates, ensuring a sufficient remnant hepatic function. The improvements of surgical techniques (e.g. Pringle's manoeuvre, anterior approach, low CVP anaesthesia), a better Knowledge of Couinaud's segmental anatomy, the development of ultrasonic dissectors and vascular staplers have contributed to reduce postoperative morbidities, including bleeding complications. Therefore LR for HCC should be an important treatment modality in the current era.

5.1. The anterior approach and the hanging manoeuvre

During right hepatic resection for hepatocellular carcinoma (HCC), complete mobilization of the right lobe of liver with the right hepatic vein controlled outside the liver before parenchymal transection had been advised by most surgeons in an effort to reduce blood loss. However, this can be difficult, when resection for large HCC is being performed. The size of the tumor may limit access to the posterior aspect of the right lobe of liver and the anterior surface of the inferior vena cava, where the right hepatic vein and many caval branches are present. Injudicious mobilization and forceful retraction of the liver may cause profuse bleeding from avulsion of the hepatic vein and caval branches, prolonged ischemia of the liver remnant from rotation of the hepatoduodenal ligament iatrogenic tumor rupture, and scatter of tumoural cells into peripheral blood. Alternatively, the anterior approach can be used in the more difficult cases of right hepatic resection for HCC. The technique implies initial completion of parenchymal transection before the right lobe is mobilized. Briefly following laparotomy, intra-operative ultrasonography and hilar dissection to control the right hepatic artery and portal vein, mobilization of the tumor and the right lobe of liver is not performed as in the conventional approach. The plane of parenchymal transection, depending on the extent of hepatic resection, is marked on the Glisson capsule with the help of intraoperative ultrasonography and transection carried out from the anterior surface of the liver down to the right side of liver hilum and down to the anterior surface of the inferior vena cava. The right hepatic vein is then isolated, clamped, divided, and sutured outside the liver parenchyma. When the specimen is completely disconnected from the inferior vena cava, the right hepatic lobe is mobilized from the right abdominal cavity by dividing the triangular ligament and other posterior attachments [25], [60]. This technique pioneered from Hong Kong demonstrated significantly fewer intraoperative haemorrhages and blood transfusions, a lower hospital death rate, a lower incidence of pulmonary metastases, and a better median disease-free survival and median overall cumulative survival in n=54 patients as compared to patients who underwent conventional approach n=106 to major liver resection for HCC more than 5 cm in size [25]. A randomized controlled study from the same institute reported better operative (lower blood loss, lower transfusion requirements, lower plasma albumin mRNA levels) and survival outcomes [lower in-hospital mortality 91/60 vs. 6/60), overall survival but not disease free survival] from anterior approach compared with the conventional approach [61]. However the anterior approach can potentially be dangerous" because "torrential bleeding can occur at the deeper plane of parenchymal transection" and "without prior mobilization of the right liver and the tumor, and control of the right hepatic vein, bleeding can be substantial and difficult to control. Therefore the anterior approach can be an effective alternative when difficulty is encountered during liver mobilization utilizing the conventional technique [62].

5.2. Anatomic (AR) vs. Non-Anatomic Resections (NAR)

Microportal invasion and intrahepatic metastasis were considered to be the most important factors leading to recurrence and were associated with poor prognosis [26], [63], [64]. Therefore anatomic resection [65] (AR), which is the systematic removal of a hepatic segment/s bearing the tumour/s. Theoretically, this procedure may be effective in eradicating intrahepatic metastasis of HCC, leading to more favorable results in HCC patients. Although some authors have reported that AR may prevent hepatic recurrence and prolong survival [7–9], others have failed to detect survival benefits of AR [10–12]. Thus, the superiority of AR compared to non-anatomic resection (NAR) remains controversial. A recent metaanalysis of 16 nonrandomized studies involving 2,917 patients (AR n=1,577 vs NAR n= 1,340) reported that AR was characterized by better survival and lower local recurrence rates than NAR for the treatment of HCC [66]. Patients in the AR group had lower prevalence of cirrhosis and hepatitis virus infection, better liver function, and larger tumor size compared with patients in the NAR group. AR provided a better 5-year overall survival than NAR (OR, 1.63; 95% CI, 1.15-2.32). Local recurrence (OR, 0.28; 95% CI, 0.16-0.50) and early (≤2 years) recurrence (OR, 0.55; 95 CI, 0.34-0.89) were all significantly lower in the AR group. AR improved disease-free survival significantly at 3 years (OR, 2.09; 95% CI, 1.52-2.88) and 5 years (OR, 2.24; 95% CI, 1.85-2.72). There were no differences regarding postoperative morbidity, mortality, and length of hospital stay between two groups. However another metaanalysis reported on nine comparative studies comprising 1,503 patients (833 AR and 670 NAR) [67]. In the combined results, disease-free survival was significantly higher in the AR group than in the NAR group (OR 1.78, 95% CI 1.22-2.59, P = 0.003; heterogeneity P = 0.08). Given the heterogeneity in the studies the authors cautioned against acceptance of the results. Presence of cirrhosis is a well-established risk factor not only for both hepatocellular carcinoma occurrence but also for recurrence after hepatic resection [2, 4, 5] in comparison to chronic hepatitis without cirrhosis. Since most of cirrhotic patients were submitted to NAR to save the liver parenchyma as much as possible to avoid postoperative liver failure, the end result of Zhou et al. is a natural consequence of this fundamental bias of the study population therefore the jury regarding the superiority of AR for HCC is still out [68].

5.3. Laparoscopic liver resection for HCC

Laparoscopic liver resection (LLR) was first reported in the early nineties as a novel procedure and initially adopted for non-anatomical liver wedge resection for peripheral benign tumors [69]. With increasing advances in instrumentation and techniques, LLR has been established as a safe and feasible option for both benign and malignant liver lesions. A world review of laparoscopic liver resection (2804 patients, 127 published papers, both malignant and benign tumours) demonstrated that the procedure in experienced hands carries an acceptable morbidity and mortality for both minor and major hepatectomy [70]. Intuitively it does appear that for patients with a solitary HCC <5 cm in the periphery of the liver i.e. segments 2, 3, 4b, 5, and 6, compensated liver disease in the absence of significant portal hypertension, LLR has an important role. A number of advantages have been recognized when comparing LLR vs LR from case-matched analyses [71], [72] and case series - including reductions in postoperative pain, less blood loss, lower blood transfusion requirements, less operative morbidity [71], and shorter length of hospitalization [71] with similar long-term outcomes [71] especially for cirrhotic patients [72]. However to date there are no randomized trials comparing these 2 modes of surgery.

At least 3 different meta-analyses [73] [74], [75] have been published in the last 20 months comparing available evidence for and against LLR vs LR for HCC. All 3 analyses concluded that LLR results in less blood loss, decreased rate of intraoperative transfusion and shorter lengths of hospital stay with no adverse impact long-term oncologic outcomes or increased risk of tumor recurrence. In fact for tumours in the periphery of the liver, resection can be performed with reduced mortality and morbidity and equivalent oncologic outcomes, disease-free survival, and overall survival when compared with similarly selected cirrhotic patients undergoing open resection [76].

Importantly, because HCC recurrence remains high in the cirrhotic liver, treatment following surgical resection mandates routine surveillance and further treatment of the recurrence either by locoregional therapy, re-resection, or transplantation as appropriate - the latter two of which are facilitated by an initial laparoscopic resection [76], [77].

6. Long-term outcome after liver resection for HCC

The majority of patients presenting with hepatocellular cancer are inoperable, largely due to extent of disease and poor liver function. The overall resection rate is <40% with a long term survival – of no more than 15%, due largely to the high post op mortality rate, intra-hepatic recurrence, distant metastases, progressive liver disease and the lifelong risk of hepatitis – although the new treatment options now available may reduce the risk in the long term.

Reviewing survival after resection for HCC in 17 series reported since 2000, each of which included more than 100 patients Takayama [78] et al. reported median survival rates of 80% (range 63 – 97%) at 1-year, 70% (34 – 78%) at 3 years and 50% (17–69%) at 5 years. Such wide ranges of survival rates are attributed mainly to differences in the HCC stage among the studies, but the survival rate is obviously much better for early-stage HCCs [79].

There is a large variation in the mortality rate following resection due to differences in definitions thus making inter-series comparisons difficult, this being further complicated by the mix of cirrhotic and non-cirrhotic patients, and various distributions of Child-Pugh status. Irrespective of the presence or absence of cirrhosis, the median perioperative mortality rate either 30 day or in-hospital mortality was a median of 4.7% with a range from 0 to 21.1%, with lower rates seen in series with larger volumes irrespective of underlying liver disease [80].

HCC frequently recurs after curative liver resection. The post- operative 5-year recurrence rate is 77–100%, and median survival after recurrence is 7–28 months [81]. Nonetheless, the long-term survival after hepatectomy remains unsatisfactory because of the high incidence of recurrence. Intrahepatic recurrences are the most common and are seen in up to 36.8–78% of patients [82]. About 80% of recurrent tumors develop exclusively within the liver, and only 20% of such tumors are resectable. As a treatment option, repeat liver resection has plays an important role in selected patients, yielding results similar to those after primary resection, with a 5-year survival rate of about 50%. Japanese authors have proposed that repeat resection is indicated for the treatment of recurrence in patients with a single HCC at the first resection, a disease-free interval longer than 1 year and recurrent HCC with no portal invasion [78]. In patients who met these criteria, the 5-year survival rate was 86% after the second resection [83].

Predictors of poor outcomes in HCC are common to all therapeutic approaches and include more than three tumors, a tumor size larger than 5 cm, portal vein invasion, intrahepatic metastases, absence of a tumor pseudocapsule, advanced TNM stage (III or IV), Hepatitis C viral infection [84] and a Child – Pugh class of C [85]. The most important factors appear to be vascular invasion and liver function [86].

7. Liver resection prior to liver transplantation (Salvage liver transplantation)

Resection can be used as a treatment for HCC prior to LT in three different settings. First, resection can be used as a primary therapy, and LT reserved as a ''salvage'' therapy for patients who develop recurrence or liver failure. Second, resection can be used as an initial therapy to select patients who might get benefit from LT, according to detailed pathological examination of the tumor and the surrounding liver parenchyma. Third, resection can be used as a ''bridge'' therapy for patients who have already been enlisted for LT. Salvage LT has been performed for recurrent HCC or deterioration of liver function after primary liver resection.

Resection as the first-line treatment for patients with small HCC with preserved liver function, followed by salvage transplantation only for recurrence or liver failure is an attractive option. Initial resection, which should be preferably an anatomic resection, gives rapid access to an effective therapy, without the need for a donor, and offers 5-year survival rates exceeding 50% with a good quality of life [87]. The main obstacle to this strategy is the risk of ''loss of chance of cure'' in case of rapid and extensive recurrence not amendable to salvage LT. At the time of recurrence, salvage LT is only applicable/gives best results in patients with a tumor within the Milan criteria.

Another justification for resection prior to transplantation is that it helps refine the selection process, giving access to detailed pathological examination of the tumor and the surrounding liver parenchyma. Important prognostic information can be obtained, including differentiation, presence of satellite nodules, and the presence of microvascular and capsular invasions. As a result, resection may help avoid transplantation in patients with tumors apparently within the Milan criteria but with histological features of especially poor prognosis. In contrast, resection may help decide on transplantation in patients with tumors slightly outside the Milan criteria but with histological features of good prognosis.

Resection can also be used as a ''bridge'' therapy in patients already enlisted for LT. TACE and radiofrequency ablation, which are the mainstays of ''bridge'' therapies, can be challenged by resection, which provides the best control of the tumour, allowing accurate histological assessment of both the tumour and the underlying liver status. Although limited resection appears to be sufficient in this setting, it is associated with increased risk and is only appropriate for patients with peripheral tumours and Child A cirrhosis. The subsequent LT may be made more difficult. The use of laparoscopic or transthoracic approaches for peripheral tumours may further contribute to expand this strategy by minimizing technical difficulties during the transplant procedure (vide supra). An important consideration is that significant adhesions and anatomical distortion exist in the abdomen following LR, although LLR seems to have a benefit to facilitate later LT by reducing these (vide supra). Although it has been claimed that prior LR neither increases operative morbidity nor impairs survival following cadaveric LT [88], this strategy is by no means universally acceptable [89]. This is due to LT after liver resection being associated with a higher operative mortality, an increased risk of recurrence, and a poorer outcome than primary LT [89]. In addition, liver resection as a bridge to LT impairs the patient transplantability and the chance of long-term survival of cirrhotic patients with HCC [89]. Indeed a recent comparative analysis of prognostic factors for HCC recurrence in a Western and an Eastern HCC patient cohort revealed on multi-variate analysis that that our independent risk factors for post-LT HCC recurrence: micro- vascular invasion (odds ratio, OR = 4.88; $p = 0.001$), poor tumour grading (OR = 6.86; $p = 0.002$), diameter of the largest tumour (OR = 4.72; $p = 0.05$), and previous liver resection (LR) (OR = 3.34; $p = 0.04$) [90]. It is therefore suggested that primary LT should therefore remain the ideal choice of treatment of a cirrhotic patient with HCC, even when the tumour is resectable. The salvage LT strategy should therefore be restricted to those patients with favourable oncological factors, thereby excluding patients with poor tumour grading, vascular invasion, diameter >3 cm and presence of satellite nodules at pathological examination, as recently suggested by the Belghiti group [91].

8. Liver transplantation for HCC

Liver transplantation (LT) is the treatment of choice for Child B and C patients with HCC but LT is limited by the lack of donor organs (demand exceeds availability) and the therapy cannot be given immediately (at least in the cadaveric LT setting)! One of the consequences of this shortage is that access to transplantation is usually restricted by rules that take into account need, transplant benefit, utility and distributive justice.

Liver transplantation for HCC before 1995 yielded disappointing results; 2-year survivals were 30% or less [92], [93], 3-year survival 3-year survival rates of 21% to 47% and the recurrence rates were high after transplantation (29% to 54%) [94]. These results were due to a bias toward performing transplantation for patients with unrespectable tumours. Through the 1980s and early 1990s, hepatic resection remained the treatment of choice for patients with early HCC and enough hepatic reserve to tolerate resection. Therefore, transplantation was often left to those with unresectable tumours (large, multiple, or both). The disappointing results called into question the value of transplantation for HCC [95]. However, within the total cohort of HCC patients who underwent transplantation, centers also reported on subgroups with early-stage disease that did well [96], [97]. Specifically, it was known that patients who had undergone transplantation and were found to have incidental small HCCs on histological examination of the explanted liver had excellent disease-free survival [98], [99].

In the current era the benchmark for LT in HCC is the Milan criteria. Following years of unrestricted use of LT for HCC with survival post LT being dismal (vide supra), the Milan criteria were introduced [100]. This prospective study included single tumours up to 5 cm or up to 3 tumours each not more than 3 cm and after four years their actuarial survival rate was 75%, the rate of recurrence-free survival was 83% and recurrence was seen in 8%. These results have been duplicated other in large cohorts [101] [102]. The Milan criteria have been widely implemented - the TNM staging system was modified such that T2 corresponds to the Milan criteria, UNOS has adopted these changes into their policy on recipient prioritization for liver transplantation and the BCLC staging system has incorporated the Milan Criteria into tis algorithm.

9. Assessment of candidates for LT

Staging of HCC patients (Table 1) should not only assess the tumour in the liver but also take into account the background liver disease and their performance status [103]. This will improve the accuracy of prognostication and enable selection of specific treatment alternatives.

Despite significant technological advances in cross-sectional imaging techniques (ultrasonography, CT, and MRI), standard imaging methods can underestimate or overestimate the extent of HCC in up to 25% of cases, compared with pathological findings of the explanted liver [104]. Conclusive imaging features rely on the presence of arterial enhancement followed by washout on portal venous or delayed imaging [105]. Dynamic CT or MRI, including unenhanced, arterial, portal venous, and delayed phases, provide improved sensitivity and specificity as compared with standard techniques of the past. Currently, there is no data showing the superiority of either MRI or CT. Dynamic ultrasonography has improved the accuracy of ultra sonography, but is less useful than CT or MRI because of the inability to reliably acquire images of the entire liver during a particular contrast phase. The American Association for the Study of Liver Disease (AASLD) has proposed an algorithm for diagnosis of HCC based on availability of state-of-the-art CT or MRI [106]. Bone scintigraphy has been used for evaluating bone metastases; however, the technique is poor in terms of cost-effectiveness when used routinely. There is insufficient data to propose [18] F-fluorodeoxyglucose (FDG)-PET for staging HCC before liver transplantation although PET scans using other isotopes (carbon-11, Fluorine-18 choline) have been utilized in staging HCC [107].

10. UK guidelines

The criteria first published in 2003 [108] for selection to the transplant list for cases with HCC has recently been revised. The current UK guidelines from May 2008 [109] (UK Guidelines for the management of suspected hepatocellular carcinoma (HCC) in adults) advise the following:

1. Radiological assessment should include both multidetecor (MD) CT and MRI, with size assessed by the widest dimensions of the neoplasm on either modality.

2. A lesion (for the purposes of counting numbers) will require to be identified as an arterialised focal abnormality with portal phase washout on MDCT or Gd enhanced MR. Other lesions are considered indeterminate.

3. Tumour rupture and an AFP > 10,000 IU/l are absolute contraindications to transplantation, as are extrahepatic spread and macroscopic vascular invasion.

4. The following are criteria for listing for transplantation; standard Milan criteria or the new UK criteria, which include: up to 5 lesions all < 3 cm single lesion > 5 cm < 7 cm diameter where there has been no evidence of tumour progression (volume increase by <20%; no extrahepatic spread; no new nodule formation) over a 6 month period. Locoregional +/- chemotherapy may be given during that time. Their waiting list place may be considered from the time of their first staging scan.

5. Locoregional therapy should be considered for all transplant list cases.

6. Cases outwith current proposed selection criteria will not be selectable on to the transplant list after their tumour has been downsized by surgical or loco-regional treatments.

When utilising staging systems; clinical based systems are probably of greater use rather than the TNM (pathological classification) or the upto-7 criteria [110] (which relies on micro-vascular invasion) given that clinical decisions can be made more appropriately and prognostic information can be provided in counselling patients for such treatment. This is where the BCLC treatment algorithm becomes useful and indeed has been validated in cohorts outside of spain for this purpose. The International consensus report [103] recommended the use of BCLC staging system when considering treatment options (Evidence level 2b Strong recommendation) and the TNM system to assess prognosis after transplantation (Evidence level 2b Strong recommendation).

11. Role of tumour biopsy

A tissue diagnosis of a suspicious liver lesion would be an ideal guide to appropriate treatment in the setting of equivocal imaging and serology. Increasing advances in imaging (scanning machines and techniques) resulting in better discrimination of hypervascular lesions into HCC or other tumours has resulted in a decreasing need for pre-listing biopsy of tumours suspected of being HCC. The accuracy of cross-sectional imaging in diagnosing small malignant liver tumours (less than 2 cm), especially in the cirrhotic liver, however, remains problematic with sensitivities for MRI detection of such lesions being 13–67% and approaching 100% for lesions more than 3 cm [111] [112] [113]. Therefore the European Association for the Study of the Liver (EASL) permitted needle biopsy of lesions ranging from 10 to 20 mm in diameter in patients with cirrhosis [114] this has however been updated in 2012. Tumour biopsy is not required in cirrhotic patients considered for liver transplantation who have high-quality dynamic CT or MRI findings typical for HCC and a lesion larger than 1 cm according to current AASLD guidelines [106]; and for patients with lesions smaller or equal to 10 mm or atypical findings, non-invasive imaging does not allow an accurate diagnosis, and should not be used to make a decision for or against transplantation. These recommendations were incorporated into the 2012 International consensus conference report [103] and EASL endorses these guidelines [115].

A systematic review [116] of 8 studies (none were RCT) revealed a needle track risk of seeding of 2.7% (CI 1.8 – 4) overall or 0.9% per year with a median time of about 17 (IQR 7- 48) months. However whether this risk does impact on treatment delivery and outcome from it is open to question [117]. In addition tumour biopsy has other limitations: The specificity of liver biopsy is close to 100%, but sensitivity varies depending on location of the tumour, needle size (86–90% with an 18 gauge cutting needle, 67% with 21–22 gauge needle), and tumour size (>90% for nodules >1 cm *vs* 83% for nodules <1 cm) [103] [118], [119]. A positive tumour biopsy is clinically relevant to rule in a diagnosis of HCC, but a negative biopsy is less useful. It is however clear that in the presence of unequivocal evidence i.e. AFP levels greater than 400 ng/L and imaging characteristics in a patient with known cirrhosis, there is no need for tumour biopsy according to the UNOS recommendations.

The recently updated European clinical practice guidelines for the management of HCC [115], referred to above, highlight the importance of preventive strategies and implementation of surveillance in those at risk. Surveillance with either USS or a combination of USS with serum alpha-fetoprotein is widely adopted with the intention of detecting early tumours in patients fit enough for surgical treatment. The diagnostic criteria for HCC as referred to in the consensus document are summarised in Table 2.

Size of nodule	Cirrhotic patient only
Nodule <1cm	4 month recall
Nodule 1-2cm	Non-invasive criteria i.e. typical features on one imaging technique, or biopsy
Nodule >2cm	Non-invasive criteria, with biopsy if atypical radiological features or uncertainty.

Table 2. Table for Diagnosis of HCC

Non-invasive criteria can only be applied to cirrhotic patients and should be based on triple or 4-phase CT scan or dynamic contrast enhanced MRI. The typical radiological hallmark of HCC is a hypervascular lesion relative to non-tumour liver in the arterial phase of a scan, with subsequent washout in venous or delayed phases. If features are suboptimal on one imaging modality, especially for small lesions, a second imaging technique (i.e. MRI + CT, not contrast enhanced USS) is recommended. In pathological diagnosis, in addition to assessment by an expert liver histopathologist, immunostaining for glypican-3, glutamine synthase are recommended to differentiate high grade dysplastic nodules from early HCC. In non-cirrhotic patients with a suspicious liver nodule (s), biopsy of non-tumour and tumour liver should be performed to confirm the diagnosis in patients who are candidates for treatment.

12. MELD prioritization points

Following publication of the Milan criteria, the suitability of certain patients with HCC for LT led to an increasing number of patients being put forward for this procedure during the 1990s and early 2000s. Increasing demand and shortage of available organs led to long waiting times and stage progression for these patients with HCC whilst on the W/L leading them becoming unsuitable for Tx; in Spain the wait time increased from 62 to 162 days [44] and in the USA 25% of HCC patients dropped off the list every year [120]. When the MELD-based prioritization system for liver transplantation replaced the Child-Pugh system in February 2002, patients with HCC were given prioritization points as the MELD was not affected by the presence of HCC. Earlier under the CTP system patients with T2 or lower HCC were moved into a higher-priority group (status 2B), but waiting time within the group remained a significant factor and that was perceived as a significant injustice to HCC patients. Under the MELD prioritization the system initially gave additional points (up to 24 for T1 HCC and 29 for patients with T2 HCC) with extra points being added every 90 days spent on the waiting list - to represent a 10% increase in mortality. Although the average waiting time decreased from 2.28 years before the MELD system to 0.69 years under MELD, and >85% of HCC patients waited less than 90 days for transplantation and Tx for HCC tripled it went too far. Non-HCC patients with MELD scores of 24 to 29 had a higher chance of dying or dropping off the list because they often had more significant hepatic decompensation than HCC patients with MELD plus points. Also, the increase in transplantations for HCC had an adverse effect on organ allocation [121]. Fourteen percent of transplants performed for HCC had no HCC on explant histology in the first 8 months of MELD system [122]. This pre-transplantation false-positive diagnosis occurred more often for small, single lesions (e.g., T1). Moreover, data from the pre-MELD era indicated that patients with T1 lesions had less than a 10% risk of dropout in the first year listed. Conversely, patients with T2 lesions were responsible for much of the poor intention-to-treat outcomes under the old system [123]. Because of these data, the assigned MELD scores for patients with HCC were decreased to 20 and 24 for T1 and T2 lesions, respectively, in April 2003. Therefore the assigned MELD scores for patients with HCC were decreased to 20 and 24 for T1 and T2 lesions, respectively, in April 2003. This change decreased the proportion of transplantations performed for HCC from 21% to 14% [122]. Before MELD, the rate was 8%. More recently, the score upgrade for T1 lesions (20 points) was eliminated, so that now only patients with T2 lesions may receive a score upgrade (initially 24 points and now 22 points). The effects of these changes are not yet known.

Expansion of Milan criteria: Proponents of expanding the current criteria are driven by the increasing number of HCC patients in need of treatment and the observation that some patients with tumour burdens exceeding the Milan criteria do have long, disease-free survival after transplantation. Several studies have reported a good outcome for some patients transplanted outside these conventional criteria and the nature of these criteria has been challenged for being too strict, because they exclude specific subgroups with meaningful, although lower, chances to benefit from transplantation. Furthermore, some patients might be excluded from transplantation as a result of the improvement in the accuracy of imaging techniques that enable the identification of very small lesions (<1 cm), which were undetectable a decade ago. Most of the studies on patients exceeding Milan criteria, however, are retrospective, with only a small number of patients, disease of variable severity, and short follow-up [124] [6], [125] [126].

In the context of shortage of available grafts, decisions have to take into account the collective benefit of all potential liver recipients, in addition to the benefit for the individual patient. Even though a survival opportunity considerably lower than that achieved in non-HCC patients might be considered worth the risk of surgery for some patients with HCC, the negative effects on others on the donor list must be taken into consideration. The international consensus group [103] recommended that liver transplantation should be reserved for HCC patients who have a predicted 5-year survival comparable to non-HCC patients.

Milan criteria	**5-year survival**
Single tumour ≤ 5cm	85%
Not more than 3 tumours, largest ≤ 3 cm	
UCSF	
Single lesion ≤ 6.5 cm	80%
Multiple lesions ≤ 3 cm	
Largest tumour diameter if multiple ≤ 4.5 cm	
Total tumour diameter if multiple ≤ 8 cm	
UK criteria	
Single lesion lesion > 5 cm < 7 cm diameter where there has been no evidence of tumour progression (volume increase by <20%; no extrahepatic spread; no new nodule formation) over a 6 month period.	
If multiple, up to 5 lesions all < 3 cm	
Metro-ticket (up-to 7 criteria)	
Single tumour 7 cm	71%
Multiple tumours seven as the sum of the size of the largest tumour [in cm] and the number of tumours	

* All survival figures depend on absence of vascular invasion. The metroticket model can predict for 3- and 5-year survival with and without vascular invasion (http://www.hcc-olt-metroticket.org/calculator/)

Table 3. Liver Transplantation criteria for HCC

The UCSF group found that patients who had undergone transplantation with single tumours up to 6.5 cm or no more than 3 tumours with maximum sum of diameters up to 8 cm and no tumour larger than 4.5 cm had acceptable disease-free survival, similar to that of patients who met Milan criteria [126]. This data was based on explant histology sizing and not on pretransplantation imaging. A follow-up study on a larger number of patients confirmed an acceptable 5-year disease-free survival of 88.5%, compared with 93.8% for those who met Milan criteria [123]. These findings have been subsequently prospectively validated based on pre-operative imaging too [127]. Numerous other expansions of Milan have been proposed including single lesions - 6 cm or up to 3 tumours, but none more than 5 cm where recurrence-free survival was 70% at 3 years [128], and the Up-to-seven criteria (Metroticket prognostication model - hepatocellular carcinomas with seven as the sum of the size of the largest tumour [in cm] and the number of tumours with or without vascular invasion) where a 5-year overall survival of 71 2% (64 3–77 0) was seen [110]. But these have not been validated prospectively. Therefore the international consensus group [103] recommended only modest expansion of the Milan criteria (in line with UCSF recommendations) but emphasised that this should occur on the background of an individual centres waiting list of non-HCC patients, waiting list mortality and the loco-regional scarcity/abundance of donor organs.

13. Role of downstaging

An attractive strategy to improve the results of liver transplantation for expanded criteria HCC is downstaging to within Milan criteria using loco-regional therapy. The goal of downstaging using therapy, as alcohol injection, radiofrequency ablation (RFA), transarterial chemoembolization (TACE), transarterial radioembolisation/selective internal radiotherapy (TARE/SIRT), or liver resection, is to decrease the tumour size and number in patients initially presenting with tumours that do not meet locally acceptable criteria for liver transplantation.

Theoretically, a downstaged tumour may carry a reduced risk of posttransplant recurrence comparable to that of one initially within the Milan criteria. More importantly, downstaging may allow selection of tumours with more favourable biology that respond well to treatment and also do well after liver transplant.

Two prospective studies showed that survival after liver transplantation in patients with large tumour burden successfully treated by downstaging was similar to survival in patients who initially met the criteria for transplantation. Pinna et al. compared the outcome of patients down-staged from outside Milan (n=48) to those within Milan (n=129) and reported similar LT rates (67 vs 68%), 1- and 3-year survival rates (71% vs 80% and 71% vs 78% respectively) between the 2 groups with no significant difference in actuarial intention to treat survival between the 2 groups (56.3% vs 62.8%) [129]. Forty-three patients were downstaged to meet the Milan criteria with a combination of liver resection, local ablation or TACE. Ten patients dropped out before transplantation due to liver failure (n = 2) or tumour progression (n = 8) and 32 underwent liver transplantation. The rate of dropout due to cancer progression was, as expected, higher in the downstaging group (27.1% vs. 11.6%) with more advanced HCC and the dropout should be regarded as a part of the selection process in order to achieve an acceptable posttransplant outcome in these patients. The authors rightly stated in the discussion, 'we clinically selected the HCCs with a more favourable biology'. Interestingly in this series nearly 70% of the patients in this series of expanded criteria recipients had serum alphafetoprotein < 30 ng/mL. Serum alphafetoprotein has been found to be an important prognostic indicator for patients with HCC after liver transplantation and the incorporation of serum alphafetoprotein into a scoring system [130] as selection criteria can help to identify the high-risk, high-volume HCC for exclusion and the low-risk, low-volume HCC [131] for LT after down-staging. It is likely that downstaging may simply provide another mode of selection but its advantage over more simple selection criteria such as tumour size and number, histologic features or serum alphafetoprotein remains to be confirmed by further studies.

In another prospective study [132], 43/61 (70.5%) patients were downstaged (TACE and RFA) to UNOS criteria (vide supra) and after 3-months of progression free interval, 35(57.4%) underwent LT. Treatment failure was observed in 18 patients (29.5%), primarily due to tumour progression. In the explant of 35 patients who underwent LT, 13 had complete tumour necrosis, 17 met T2 criteria, and five exceeded T2 criteria and none demonstrated microvascular invasion or poorly differentiated disease. The Kaplan-Meier intention-to-treat survival at 1 and 4 years after down staging were 87.5% and 69.3%, respectively. The 1-year and 4-year post transplantation survival rates were 96.2% and 92.1%, respectively. No patient had HCC recurrence after a median post transplantation follow-up of 25 months. The only factor predicting treatment failure was pre-treatment alpha-fetoprotein >1,000 ng/mL. The main thrust of this study appears to suggest that using response to locoregional therapy to select transplant recipients provides an attractive alternative to simply expanding the existing criteria.

14. Managing patients on wait-list for LT

One of the consequences of waiting for transplantation is that during this time, the disease may change or in other words allow the true biological nature of the neoplasm to be expressed thereby aiding improved selection of patients for LT. Also the waiting time in which the disease can evolve allows treatment strategies, which can be implemented to influence its course. The seminal article of the BCLC study group [44] which compared the intention- to-treat (ITT) outcomes of resection and transplantation for HCC, identified that the concept of dropout on the waiting list was crucial, and it has become the equivalent of the risk of pretransplant mortality addressed by the Model for End-Stage Liver Disease (MELD) priority system for non-HCC patients. Therefore managing patients involves minimizing the drop-out rate and successfully "bridging" patients to a LT.

The term "bridging" is for strategies that are implemented in patients who already qualify for LT according to the accepted selection criteria so that they can wait until a graft is available. A bridging strategy can be effective because (1) it allows candidates to wait for a longer time or more candidates to wait for the same time (or both) or (2) it improves the results of transplantation by excluding patients whose disease will recur or by stopping the progression of a tumour before extrahepatic spread has occurred. The word "down-staging" refers to the reduction of the clinical stage of a disease from any initial stage (e.g., from T2 to T1), down-staging in the context of LT for HCC is used for strategies allowing the transplantation of patients who at first do not qualify for OLT because their tumours are outside the accepted criteria (T3 or higher). Down-staging strategies may use the same neoadjuvant treatments that are used in bridging strategies.

Therefore the aims of managing patients whilst on a wait-list i.e. bridging strategies are

1. For patients to remain good candidates until a graft is available.

2. For the transplant program and society to exclude poor candidates even though on entry they fulfilled restrictive selection criteria.

3. To improve the results after transplantation.

4. To be compatible with a treatment other than transplantation in the case of dropout.

5. To have an optimal cost and complication/effectiveness ratio.

Managing patients while they are waiting for a liver graft to become available involves monitoring not only the tumour but also the background liver disease. With increases in waiting times for liver transplantation, it is common practice to monitor patients with HCC to ensure that they remain within the acceptability criteria for liver transplantation. Both imaging and measurement of AFP levels are commonly utilised. There is no agreement about specific timing or optimum imaging methods (dynamic CT, dynamic MRI, or contrast-enhanced ultrasonography). In our Unit a 3-month interval between surveillance scans whilst on the wait-list is adopted.

Locoregional therapies represent bridging strategies for patients on the waiting list, because they can decrease tumour-related dropout rates and the incidence of recurrences after liver transplantation, above all for patients that have to wait 6 months or longer [133]. There is, however, no evidence that bridging strategies could be helpful in patients with United Network for Organ Sharing (UNOS) T1 tumours (<2 cm). Bridging strategies might be appropriate for patients with UNOS T2 lesions (one nodule 2–5 cm or three or fewer nodules each ≤3 cm) who are likely to wait 6 months or longer. Therefore a recent consensus conference [103] (clavien PA Lancet Oncol 2012) concluded that in patients with UNOS T2 (one nodule 2–5 cm or three or fewer nodules each ≤3 cm) HCC (Milan criteria) and a likely waiting time of longer than 6 months, locoregional therapy may be appropriate. However no one particular type of treatment was found superior although pathologically RFA was found to cause more tumour necrosis [133]. They also recommended that patients found to have progressed beyond criteria acceptable for listing for liver transplantation should be placed on hold and considered for downstaging, if this was not appropriate/not effective, they should be removed from the waiting list. Liver resection before transplantation in patients with well preserved liver function, and newer strategies such as a combination of TACE with RFA and use of 90-yttrium radioembolisation or targeted therapies, have shown some benefits in preliminary studies.

Two well-documented cohort studies - Rochester (54 patients) [134] and Innsbruck (116 patients) [135] have confirmed that TACE allows long waiting times [median 211 days (range 28-1099 days) in the Rochester study; median 274 days (range 36-1037 days) in the Innsbruck study] with relatively low total dropout rates (9% and 14%, respectively). Recurrences were rare in both studies and were not higher than what would be expected for T2 patients.

However a multicenter case-control study compared matched patients with TACE (100) and without TACE (100) and the survival rates 5 years after OLT were similar (59.3% versus 59.4%) [136]. Nevertheless, there were fewer recurrences in the TACE group (13 versus 23) but more non–tumour-related deaths (15 patients versus 7 patients). Therefore TACE may allow patients to wait longer than would otherwise be possible, and is not associated with more recurrences (which may in fact be less frequent). If the option of TACE is chosen, it should be pursued (if needed with multiple treatments) until the best possible effect on tumour necrosis is obtained [133].

RFA was not at first sight an appealing treatment in pretransplant patients because of the risk of local spread, and there were early reports of RFA in which seeding was frequent. Experience with the technique and a well-conducted cohort study have shown that seeding and recurrence are rare when patients and contraindications are selected carefully (i.e., subcapsular tumours and direct nodule puncture) [137]. Other confirmatory studies have shown that the technique can be used safely in pretransplant patients and that the percutaneous route is as safe as the laparoscopic approach and less cumbersome [138], [139]. In pathological studies, the results for RFA appear to be superior to those for TACE [140] [141] and RFA appears to be associated with less tumour progression [142]. Therefore RFA appears to be safe and can be used as a bridging strategy if this is indicated. Its ability to reduce dropout rates and its effects on post-transplant results need to be proven in a prospective, comparative study. In some anatomical situations – subcapsular lesions and very large lesions (more than 5-6 cm in diameter) optimal treatment is difficult to achieve with RFA, however this can be overcome with use of probes which can cause larger burns and those designed for use on the surface of the liver.

Although resection appears to be safe before transplantation (in terms of operative results and long- term outcomes) and to have a place in decision analysis when the waiting time is longer than 1 year, resection is very rarely used at the moment as a bridging strategy. This is further discussed in the salvage transplantation section.

Radioembolization with yttrium-90 represents 5% to 10% of bridging LRT procedures in the OPTN registry, but data on its impact are scanty. In a study that reported the correlation between radiological and pathological findings in patients with HCC who underwent radioembolization with yttrium-90 microspheres before transplantation, all target lesions demonstrated some degree of histological necrosis, and 23 of 38 (61%) showed complete pathological necrosis [143]. A recent study retrospectively analyzed transarterial radioembolization (TARE) and TACE in similar patients (122 and 123, respectively); 44 TARE patients and 46 TACE patients were at stage T2 [144]. Although there was no survival benefit for TARE, the time to disease progression and the AFP responses were significantly more favourable with TARE, and this suggests that this treatment could be a promising modality before LT but current data are too scanty to recommend the use of TARE for this, but this technique may be an appropriate one to use and should be the object of further investigation.

Conformal radiotherapy (CRT) is known as a feasible and efficient therapeutic option for HCC patients who are ineligible for a curative treatment (i.e., surgical resection or transplantation). However, minimal data exists for the use of CRT as a bridging option for patients on the waiting list and although CRT may be a safe and potent local bridging therapy for patients with advanced HCC who are on the waiting list for LT [145]. Further studies are warranted to compare the effectiveness of CRT and other local therapeutic options in this setting.

It is important to emphasize that proof that bridging treatments does not result in more recurrences and worse outcomes after transplantation is not yet available (the above quoted studies may have a strong selection bias in the allocation of patients to treatment and no-treatment arms). Therefore a RCT with a no-treatment arm is the suggestion from a recent consensus conference [133] but the ethical and logistical problems in implementing such a trial can be substantial.

15. Role of LDLT

Living-donor liver transplantation (LDLT) using the right or left hemiliver of a healthy donor is the best therapeutic strategy for liver transplantation in some countries, especially in Asia, because of limited availability of deceased-donor organs. LDLT has also been used in other countries with well established programmes for organ donation from brain dead or non-heart-beating donors for organ shortage, long waiting times associated with deaths on the waiting list, drop-out due to medical reasons, or progression of tumours beyond acceptable criteria.

The main issue in LDLT is donor safety, because of the risk of complications or death, even if small. The concept of double equipoise was proposed to describe the balance between the recipient's survival benefit with LDLT and the risk of a complication or death of a healthy donor [146]. The physicians might discuss probable risks and benefits with their patients and meet the test of equipoise.

Six studies compared deceased-donor liver transplantation (DDLT) and LDLT for HCC, including a report from a multicentre US consortium of LDLT centres [147] [148] [149] [150]-[152]. No convincing difference in outcome could be identified according to type of graft, although a higher risk of recurrence was noted in fast-tracked patients, since a short delay between diagnosis and liver transplantation might not allow enough time for the biological behaviour of the tumour to manifest. Therefore the recent consensus conference [103] suggested a period of observation (e.g., 3 months) when offering LDLT in recipients with HCC although it is not included in their recommendations. They did recommend that LDLT is acceptable for HCC patients who have an expected 5-year survival similar to comparably staged patients receiving a deceased-donor liver. However a more recent meta-analysis of 12 studies which provided information on disease free survival on a total of n=633 LDLT and n=1232 DDLT concluded lower disease free survival for LDLT [153]. This result could no doubt occur due to reporting bias but the fact that the boundaries of criteria for LDLT are more relaxed as compared to DDLT. Most centres would transplant HCC without macrovascular invasion and absence of extra-hepatic disease in the setting of LDLT whilst the same tumour load would not be considered for DDLT and this practice has been cautioned against [154].

16. Post-LT management

The role of immunosuppression in HCC patients after liver transplantation is still controversial, because experimental models would have shown oncogenic properties of immunosuppressive drugs. Currently, most programmes are careful to balance the inherent risks of rejection and tumour recurrence. However, there are no RCTs that have shown that lowering immunosuppression reduces the risk of HCC recurrence after liver transplantation. One class of immunosuppressive drugs, the mTOR inhibitors, might be useful for patients with HCC who receive a liver transplantation, since experimental studies have shown that this drug has strong immunosuppressive effects with concomitant anti-neoplastic properties [155]. Uncontrolled pilot trials and retrospective analyses have suggested that sirolimus, an mTOR inhibitor, was associated with lower tumour recurrence and improved survival after liver transplantation [156], [157], these results have not been confirmed in an RCT. At present, therefore, the type or dose of immunosuppression therapy influencing the incidence of HCC recurrence or its prognosis are still much debated [103].

There is also no evidence to support the use of adjuvant treatment to decrease risk of post LT recurrence [103]. Numerous uncontrolled studies and 4 RCTs (n=213) [158]- [162] do suggest some benefit but the variety of drugs used and the varied inclusion criteria and end-points make interpretation difficult. Sorafenib (multitargeted tyrosine-kinase inhibitor) and Licartin [159] (131I-radiolabelled murine monoclonal antibody that specifically binds HCC cells) show some promise but are not recommended for adjuvant use after transplantation at present.

The main problem after liver transplantation for HCC is the risk of tumour recurrence, which occurs in 8–20% of recipients. HCC recurrence occurs usually during the first 2 years after liver transplantation, and is associated with a median survival of less than 1 year (IQR 7–18 months) from the time of diagnosis [163]. The routine use of imaging and α-fetoprotein monitoring has allowed earlier detection of recurrence, with a likelihood of cure with ablation therapies in up to a third of cases [164]. However no particular protocol for surveillance has been proven and individual centres like ours tailor their imaging frequency based on AFP levels.

The treatment of HCC recurrence after liver transplantation is much debated. Retransplantation is not appropriate since during most recurrences there is often systemic dissemination of tumour cells [165]. Locoregional therapy for HCC recurrence, including liver resection [166], radiofrequency ablation, or TACE, has been successfully used in selected patients with limited disease, and might be considered when technically feasible. Sorafenib has been used after liver transplantation recurrence, sometimes in conjunction with mTOR inhibitors with success and with limited side-effects [167].

17. Concluding statements

The best results for liver resection are obtained in patients with small solitary tumours. While multifocal disease may not impede resection as regards technical feasibility, most of the data suggests that long-term survival even in the absence of portal hypertension is poor with a high rate of disease recurrence [44]. This is the major drawback of surgical resection (as well as of ablation) and is due to two mechanisms. The most frequent is cell dissemination prior to treatment. This gives rise to metastatic nests and its incidence is higher in tumours exhibiting microscopic vascular invasion and/or satellites [168]. More than 80% of the patients with this profile will suffer recurrence within the first two years of follow-up and their prognosis is negatively affected. The second mechanism for recurrence is related to the oncogenic capacity of the background liver parenchyma which is diseased that can give rise to metachronous tumours [168]. They are more prevalent after the two years of follow- up and their potential to be successfully treated is higher as compared with early recurrence that is usually multifocal. Since the prevalence of vascular invasion/satellites increases along with tumour size, it is clear that the larger the tumour, the higher the risk of these and of recurrence. However, there are some infrequent patients with large solitary HCC in whom the expansive tumour growth has not been associated with development of additional tumour sites. Hence, if after proper staging of a large HCC there is no proven dissemination, surgery should not be contraindicated, but physicians and patients should be aware of the statistics showing that the likelihood of microscopic vascular invasion (and hence, early recurrence after surgery) parallels tumour size. Indeed, intraoperative ultrasound may disclose additional tumour sites not detected preoperatively and abort the proposed resection. Careful evaluation of the non-tumoural liver parenchyma to be resected and of the expected remaining volume is mandatory prior to operation.

Interestingly, the risk of HCC recurrence after transplantation is less than after resection or ablation even if stratifying for the same pathology risk profile. Hence, with similar survival and less recurrence, it would appear reasonable to consider transplantation as the first option as it would solve HCC and the underlying oncogenic liver. This consideration has to be tempered by the fact that liver transplantation is not a simple procedure. Morbidity and death rate in the early and intermediate follow-up period are higher than after resection surgery in optimal candidates. Also, while recurrence of hepatitis B and alcoholic liver disease may be prevented, the status in patients infected with hepatitis C virus is not so encouraging [169] [170]. Effective viral eradication is not common in cirrhotics (the underlying disease in most HCC), treatment pre and post-transplantation may have severe side effects, reinfection of the graft is the rule and the long-term outcome is significantly impaired as compared to the other populations. All these facts have maintained surgical resection as the first line surgical option in patients with optimal profile as defined by solitary HCC in a liver without clinically relevant portal hypertension. Operative risk is very low and analysis of the resected tumour will allow the classification of the tumor as at low risk for recurrence (no vascular invasion or satellites) or as at high risk because of adverse pathology profile [171]. If this is the case recurrence will impair prognosis and if the patient had been transplanted the risk and survival would have been significantly better. Based on this, the recommendation in these high-risk patients is to propose transplantation because of high risk of recurrence and not delay the decision to the appearance of recurrence as at that time multifocality will be the rule and transplantation will be contraindicated. By contrast, if the resected tumour does not have an invasive phenotype, the patient can avoid liver transplantation and the associated risks, while being under strict surveillance. Recurrence will likely correspond to a metachronous tumour and benefit again of the same decision making process for treatment allocation [5].

Because of the lack of donor livers for transplantation, strict selection criteria were introduced in order to achieve acceptable outcomes. Since the introduction of these Milan criteria in 1993, LT for HCC has been associated with an overall 70% 5-year survival. Although the Milan criteria have been criticised in recent years for being too restrictive, recent data has shown them to have stood the 'test of time' and are as relevant today as they were 20 years ago. Therefore any expansion of these criteria such as the UCSF or 'Metro-ticket' criteria must be critically assessed.

Author details

R Lochan, HL Reeves and DM Manas

Department of HPB Surgery and Institute of Transplantation, Freeman Hospital, Newcastle upon Tyne, UK

References

[1] Parkin DM, Bray F, Ferlay J, Pisani P. Global cancer statistics, 2002. CA Cancer J Clin. 2005; 55(2): 74-108.

[2] Nguyen VT, Amin J, Law MG, Dore GJ. Predictors and survival in hepatitis B-related hepatocellular carcinoma in New South Wales, Australia. J Gastroenterol Hepatol. 2009; 24(3): 436-42.

[3] Jewell J, Sheron N. Trends in European liver death rates: implications for alcohol policy. Clin Med. 2010; 10(3): 259-63.

[4] Bruix J, Sherman M. Management of hepatocellular carcinoma: an update. Hepatology. 2011; 53(3): 1020-2.

[5] Tremosini S, Reig M, de Lope CR, Forner A, Bruix J. Treatment of early hepatocellular carcinoma: Towards personalized therapy. Dig Liver Dis. 2010; 42 Suppl 3: S242-8.

[6] Llovet JM, Schwartz M, Mazzaferro V. Resection and liver transplantation for hepatocellular carcinoma. Semin Liver Dis. 2005; 25(2): 181-200.

[7] Cillo U, Bassanello M, Vitale A, Grigoletto FA, Burra P, Fagiuoli S, et al. The critical issue of hepatocellular carcinoma prognostic classification: which is the best tool available? J Hepatol. 2004; 40(1): 124-31.

[8] Rabe C, Lenz M, Schmitz V, Pilz T, Fimmers R, Sauerbruch T, et al. An independent evaluation of modern prognostic scores in a central European cohort of 120 patients with hepatocellular carcinoma. Eur J Gastroenterol Hepatol. 2003; 15(12): 1305-15.

[9] Giannini E, Risso D, Botta F, Romagnoli P, Malfatti F, Fumagalli A, et al. Prognosis of hepatocellular carcinoma in anti-HCV positive cirrhotic patients: a single-centre comparison amongst four different staging systems. J Intern Med. 2004; 255(3): 399-408.

[10] Ueno S, Tanabe G, Sako K, Hiwaki T, Hokotate H, Fukukura Y, et al. Discrimination value of the new western prognostic system (CLIP score) for hepatocellular carcinoma in 662 Japanese patients. Cancer of the Liver Italian Program. Hepatology. 2001; 34(3): 529-34.

[11] Farinati F, Rinaldi M, Gianni S, Naccarato R. How should patients with hepatocellular carcinoma be staged? Validation of a new prognostic system. Cancer. 2000; 89(11): 2266-73.

[12] Levy I, Sherman M. Staging of hepatocellular carcinoma: assessment of the CLIP, Okuda, and Child-Pugh staging systems in a cohort of 257 patients in Toronto. Gut. 2002; 50(6): 881-5.

[13] Okuda K, Ohtsuki T, Obata H, Tomimatsu M, Okazaki N, Hasegawa H, et al. Natural history of hepatocellular carcinoma and prognosis in relation to treatment. Study of 850 patients. Cancer. 1985; 56(4): 918-28.

[14] Llovet JM, Bruix J. Prospective validation of the Cancer of the Liver Italian Program (CLIP) score: a new prognostic system for patients with cirrhosis and hepatocellular carcinoma. Hepatology. 2000; 32(3): 679-80.

[15] Miraglia R, Pietrosi G, Maruzzelli L, Petridis I, Caruso S, Marrone G, et al. Predictive factors of tumor response to trans-catheter treatment in cirrhotic patients with hepatocellular carcinoma: a multivariate analysis of pre-treatment findings. World J Gastroenterol. 2007; 13(45): 6022-6.

[16] Llovet JM, Burroughs A, Bruix J. Hepatocellular carcinoma. Lancet. 2003; 362(9399): 1907-17.

[17] Bruix J, Llovet JM. Prognostic prediction and treatment strategy in hepatocellular carcinoma. Hepatology. 2002; 35(3): 519-24.

[18] Llovet JM, Bru C, Bruix J. Prognosis of hepatocellular carcinoma: the BCLC staging classification. Semin Liver Dis. 1999; 19(3): 329-38.

[19] Poon RT, Fan ST. Evaluation of the new AJCC/UICC staging system for hepatocellular carcinoma after hepatic resection in Chinese patients. Surg Oncol Clin N Am. 2003; 12(1): 35-50, viii.

[20] Sobin LH, Compton CC. TNM seventh edition: what's new, what's changed: communication from the International Union Against Cancer and the American Joint Committee on Cancer. Cancer. 2010; 116(22): 5336-9.

[21] El-Serag HB, Marrero JA, Rudolph L, Reddy KR. Diagnosis and treatment of hepatocellular carcinoma. Gastroenterology. 2008; 134(6): 1752-63.

[22] Huang YH, Wu JC, Chau GY, Lui WY, King KL, Chiang JH, et al. Supportive treatment, resection and transcatheter arterial chemoembolization in resectable hepatocellular carcinoma: an analysis of survival in 419 patients. Eur J Gastroenterol Hepatol. 1999; 11(3): 315-21.

[23] Yeh CN, Chen MF, Lee WC, Jeng LB. Prognostic factors of hepatic resection for hepatocellular carcinoma with cirrhosis: univariate and multivariate analysis. J Surg Oncol. 2002; 81(4): 195-202.

[24] Ikai I, Arii S, Kojiro M, Ichida T, Makuuchi M, Matsuyama Y, et al. Reevaluation of prognostic factors for survival after liver resection in patients with hepatocellular carcinoma in a Japanese nationwide survey. Cancer. 2004; 101(4): 796-802.

[25] Liu CL, Fan ST, Lo CM, Tung-Ping Poon R, Wong J. Anterior approach for major right hepatic resection for large hepatocellular carcinoma. Ann Surg. 2000; 232(1): 25-31.

[26] Vauthey JN, Lauwers GY, Esnaola NF, Do KA, Belghiti J, Mirza N, et al. Simplified staging for hepatocellular carcinoma. J Clin Oncol. 2002; 20(6): 1527-36.

[27] Fong Y, Sun RL, Jarnagin W, Blumgart LH. An analysis of 412 cases of hepatocellular carcinoma at a Western center. Ann Surg. 1999; 229(6): 790-9; discussion 9-800.

[28] Zhou XD, Tang ZY, Yang BH, Lin ZY, Ma ZC, Ye SL, et al. Experience of 1000 patients who underwent hepatectomy for small hepatocellular carcinoma. Cancer. 2001; 91(8): 1479-86.

[29] Chen XP, Qiu FZ, Wu ZD, Zhang BX. Chinese experience with hepatectomy for huge hepatocellular carcinoma. Br J Surg. 2004; 91(3): 322-6.

[30] Yeh CN, Lee WC, Chen MF. Hepatic resection and prognosis for patients with hepatocellular carcinoma larger than 10 cm: two decades of experience at Chang Gung memorial hospital. Ann Surg Oncol. 2003; 10(9): 1070-6.

[31] Pawlik TM, Poon RT, Abdalla EK, Zorzi D, Ikai I, Curley SA, et al. Critical appraisal of the clinical and pathologic predictors of survival after resection of large hepatocellular carcinoma. Arch Surg. 2005; 140(5): 450-7; discussion 7-8.

[32] Tsai TJ, Chau GY, Lui WY, Tsay SH, King KL, Loong CC, et al. Clinical significance of microscopic tumor venous invasion in patients with resectable hepatocellular carcinoma. Surgery. 2000; 127(6): 603-8.

[33] Pawlik TM, Delman KA, Vauthey JN, Nagorney DM, Ng IO, Ikai I, et al. Tumor size predicts vascular invasion and histologic grade: Implications for selection of surgical treatment for hepatocellular carcinoma. Liver Transpl. 2005; 11(9): 1086-92.

[34] Nagano Y, Shimada H, Takeda K, Ueda M, Matsuo K, Tanaka K, et al. Predictive factors of microvascular invasion in patients with hepatocellular carcinoma larger than 5 cm. World J Surg. 2008; 32(10): 2218-22.

[35] Nonami T, Harada A, Kurokawa T, Nakao A, Takagi H. Hepatic resection for hepatocellular carcinoma. Am J Surg. 1997; 173(4): 288-91.

[36] Ng KK, Vauthey JN, Pawlik TM, Lauwers GY, Regimbeau JM, Belghiti J, et al. Is hepatic resection for large or multinodular hepatocellular carcinoma justified? Results from a multi-institutional database. Ann Surg Oncol. 2005; 12(5): 364-73.

[37] Lise M, Bacchetti S, Da Pian P, Nitti D, Pilati PL, Pigato P. Prognostic factors affecting long term outcome after liver resection for hepatocellular carcinoma: results in a series of 100 Italian patients. Cancer. 1998; 82(6): 1028-36.

[38] Hasegawa K, Kokudo N, Imamura H, Matsuyama Y, Aoki T, Minagawa M, et al. Prognostic impact of anatomic resection for hepatocellular carcinoma. Ann Surg. 2005; 242(2): 252-9.

[39] Sasaki Y, Yamada T, Tanaka H, Ohigashi H, Eguchi H, Yano M, et al. Risk of recurrence in a long-term follow-up after surgery in 417 patients with hepatitis B- or hepatitis C-related hepatocellular carcinoma. Ann Surg. 2006; 244(5): 771-80.

[40] Poon RT, Fan ST, Ng IO, Wong J. Prognosis after hepatic resection for stage IVA hepatocellular carcinoma: a need for reclassification. Ann Surg. 2003; 237(3): 376-83.

[41] Wu CC, Cheng SB, Ho WM, Chen JT, Liu TJ, P'Eng F K. Liver resection for hepatocellular carcinoma in patients with cirrhosis. Br J Surg. 2005; 92(3): 348-55.

[42] John AR, Khan S, Mirza DF, Mayer AD, Buckels JA, Bramhall SR. Multivariate and univariate analysis of prognostic factors following resection in HCC: the Birmingham experience. Dig Surg. 2006; 23(1-2): 103-9.

[43] Zhou YM, Yang JM, Li B, Yin ZF, Xu F, Wang B, et al. Risk factors for early recurrence of small hepatocellular carcinoma after curative resection. Hepatobiliary Pancreat Dis Int. 2010; 9(1): 33-7.

[44] Llovet JM, Fuster J, Bruix J. Intention-to-treat analysis of surgical treatment for early hepatocellular carcinoma: resection versus transplantation. Hepatology. 1999; 30(6): 1434-40.

[45] Bruix J, Castells A, Bosch J, Feu F, Fuster J, Garcia-Pagan JC, et al. Surgical resection of hepatocellular carcinoma in cirrhotic patients: prognostic value of preoperative portal pressure. Gastroenterology. 1996; 111(4): 1018-22.

[46] Kanematsu T, Furui J, Yanaga K, Okudaira S, Kamohara Y, Eguchi S. Measurement of portal venous pressure is useful for selecting the optimal type of resection in cir-

rhotic patients with hepatocellular carcinoma. Hepatogastroenterology. 2005; 52(66): 1828-31.

[47] Boleslawski E, Petrovai G, Truant S, Dharancy S, Duhamel A, Salleron J, et al. Hepatic venous pressure gradient in the assessment of portal hypertension before liver resection in patients with cirrhosis. Br J Surg. 2012; 99(6): 855-63.

[48] Llop E, Berzigotti A, Reig M, Erice E, Reverter E, Seijo S, et al. Assessment of portal hypertension by transient elastography in patients with compensated cirrhosis and potentially resectable liver tumors. J Hepatol. 2012; 56(1): 103-8.

[49] Cucchetti A, Ercolani G, Vivarelli M, Cescon M, Ravaioli M, Ramacciato G, et al. Is portal hypertension a contraindication to hepatic resection? Ann Surg. 2009; 250(6): 922-8.

[50] Clavien PA, Petrowsky H, DeOliveira ML, Graf R. Strategies for safer liver surgery and partial liver transplantation. N Engl J Med. 2007; 356(15): 1545-59.

[51] Schindl MJ, Redhead DN, Fearon KC, Garden OJ, Wigmore SJ. The value of residual liver volume as a predictor of hepatic dysfunction and infection after major liver resection. Gut. 2005; 54(2): 289-96.

[52] Kubota K, Makuuchi M, Kusaka K, Kobayashi T, Miki K, Hasegawa K, et al. Measurement of liver volume and hepatic functional reserve as a guide to decision-making in resectional surgery for hepatic tumors. Hepatology. 1997; 26(5): 1176-81.

[53] Hoekstra LT, de Graaf W, Nibourg GA, Heger M, Bennink RJ, Stieger B, et al. Physiological and Biochemical Basis of Clinical Liver Function Tests: A Review. Ann Surg. 2012.

[54] Stockmann M, Lock JF, Riecke B, Heyne K, Martus P, Fricke M, et al. Prediction of postoperative outcome after hepatectomy with a new bedside test for maximal liver function capacity. Ann Surg. 2009; 250(1): 119-25.

[55] Farges O, Belghiti J, Kianmanesh R, Regimbeau JM, Santoro R, Vilgrain V, et al. Portal vein embolization before right hepatectomy: prospective clinical trial. Ann Surg. 2003; 237(2): 208-17.

[56] Tanaka H, Hirohashi K, Kubo S, Shuto T, Higaki I, Kinoshita H. Preoperative portal vein embolization improves prognosis after right hepatectomy for hepatocellular carcinoma in patients with impaired hepatic function. Br J Surg. 2000; 87(7): 879-82.

[57] Gulec SA, Pennington K, Hall M, Fong Y. Preoperative Y-90 microsphere selective internal radiation treatment for tumor downsizing and future liver remnant recruitment: a novel approach to improving the safety of major hepatic resections. World J Surg Oncol. 2009; 7: 6.

[58] Inarrairaegui M, Pardo F, Bilbao JI, Rotellar F, Benito A, D'Avola D, et al. Response to radioembolization with yttrium-90 resin microspheres may allow surgical treatment

with curative intent and prolonged survival in previously unresectable hepatocellular carcinoma. Eur J Surg Oncol. 2012; 38(7): 594-601.

[59] Fan ST, Lo CM, Liu CL, Lam CM, Yuen WK, Yeung C, et al. Hepatectomy for hepatocellular carcinoma: toward zero hospital deaths. Ann Surg. 1999; 229(3): 322-30.

[60] Lai EC, Fan ST, Lo CM, Chu KM, Liu CL. Anterior approach for difficult major right hepatectomy. World J Surg. 1996; 20(3): 314-7; discussion 8.

[61] Liu CL, Fan ST, Cheung ST, Lo CM, Ng IO, Wong J. Anterior approach versus conventional approach right hepatic resection for large hepatocellular carcinoma: a prospective randomized controlled study. Ann Surg. 2006; 244(2): 194-203.

[62] Ishizawa T, Kokudo N, Makuuchi M. Right hepatectomy for hepatocellular carcinoma: is the anterior approach superior to the conventional approach? Ann Surg. 2008; 247(2): 390-1; author reply 1-2.

[63] Adachi E, Maeda T, Kajiyama K, Kinukawa N, Matsumata T, Sugimachi K, et al. Factors correlated with portal venous invasion by hepatocellular carcinoma: univariate and multivariate analyses of 232 resected cases without preoperative treatments. Cancer. 1996; 77(10): 2022-31.

[64] Park JH, Koh KC, Choi MS, Lee JH, Yoo BC, Paik SW, et al. Analysis of risk factors associated with early multinodular recurrences after hepatic resection for hepatocellular carcinoma. Am J Surg. 2006; 192(1): 29-33.

[65] Makuuchi M, Hasegawa H, Yamazaki S. Ultrasonically guided subsegmentectomy. Surg Gynecol Obstet. 1985; 161(4): 346-50.

[66] Zhou Y, Xu D, Wu L, Li B. Meta-analysis of anatomic resection versus nonanatomic resection for hepatocellular carcinoma. Langenbecks Arch Surg. 2011; 396(7): 1109-17.

[67] Chen J, Huang K, Wu J, Zhu H, Shi Y, Wang Y, et al. Survival after anatomic resection versus nonanatomic resection for hepatocellular carcinoma: a meta-analysis. Dig Dis Sci. 2011; 56(6): 1626-33.

[68] Bigonzi E, Cucchetti A, Pinna AD. Meta-analysis of anatomic resection versus nonanatomic resection for hepatocellular carcinoma: are they comparing apples with oranges? Langenbecks Arch Surg. 2012; 397(1): 141-2; author reply 2.

[69] Gagner M, Rheault M, Dubuc J. Laparoscopic partial hepatectomy for liver tumor (abstract). Surg Endosc. 1992; 6: 99.

[70] Nguyen KT, Gamblin TC, Geller DA. World review of laparoscopic liver resection-2,804 patients. Ann Surg. 2009; 250(5): 831-41.

[71] Lee KF, Chong CN, Wong J, Cheung YS, Lai P. Long-term results of laparoscopic hepatectomy versus open hepatectomy for hepatocellular carcinoma: a case-matched analysis. World J Surg. 2011; 35(10): 2268-74.

[72] Truant S, Bouras AF, Hebbar M, Boleslawski E, Fromont G, Dharancy S, et al. Laparoscopic resection vs. open liver resection for peripheral hepatocellular carcinoma in patients with chronic liver disease: a case-matched study. Surgical endoscopy. 2011; 25(11): 3668-77.

[73] Yin Z, Fan X, Ye H, Yin D, Wang J. Short- and Long-term Outcomes after Laparoscopic and Open Hepatectomy for Hepatocellular Carcinoma: A Global Systematic Review and Meta-analysis. Ann Surg Oncol. 2012.

[74] Li N, Wu YR, Wu B, Lu MQ. Surgical and oncologic outcomes following laparoscopic versus open liver resection for hepatocellular carcinoma: A meta-analysis. Hepatol Res. 2012; 42(1): 51-9.

[75] Fancellu A, Rosman AS, Sanna V, Nigri GR, Zorcolo L, Pisano M, et al. Meta-analysis of trials comparing minimally-invasive and open liver resections for hepatocellular carcinoma. J Surg Res. 2011; 171(1): e33-45.

[76] Kluger MD, Cherqui D. Laparoscopic resection of hepatocellular carcinoma. Recent Results Cancer Res. 2013; 190: 111-26.

[77] Laurent A, Tayar C, Andreoletti M, Lauzet JY, Merle JC, Cherqui D. Laparoscopic liver resection facilitates salvage liver transplantation for hepatocellular carcinoma. J Hepatobiliary Pancreat Surg. 2009; 16(3): 310-4.

[78] Takayama T. Surgical treatment for hepatocellular carcinoma. Jpn J Clin Oncol. 2011; 41(4): 447-54.

[79] Takayama T, Makuuchi M, Hirohashi S, Sakamoto M, Yamamoto J, Shimada K, et al. Early hepatocellular carcinoma as an entity with a high rate of surgical cure. Hepatology. 1998; 28(5): 1241-6.

[80] Morris-Stiff G, Gomez D, de Liguori Carino N, Prasad KR. Surgical management of hepatocellular carcinoma: is the jury still out? Surg Oncol. 2009; 18(4): 298-321.

[81] Takayama T, Sekine T, Makuuchi M, Yamasaki S, Kosuge T, Yamamoto J, et al. Adoptive immunotherapy to lower postsurgical recurrence rates of hepatocellular carcinoma: a randomised trial. Lancet. 2000; 356(9232): 802-7.

[82] Zhou Y, Sui C, Li B, Yin Z, Tan Y, Yang J, et al. Repeat hepatectomy for recurrent hepatocellular carcinoma: a local experience and a systematic review. World J Surg Oncol. 2010; 8: 55.

[83] Minagawa M, Makuuchi M, Takayama T, Kokudo N. Selection criteria for repeat hepatectomy in patients with recurrent hepatocellular carcinoma. Ann Surg. 2003; 238(5): 703-10.

[84] Sogawa H, Shrager B, Jibara G, Tabrizian P, Roayaie S, Schwartz M. Resection or transplant-listing for solitary hepatitis C-associated hepatocellular carcinoma: an intention-to-treat analysis. HPB (Oxford). 2012.

[85] Poon RT, Fan ST, Lo CM, Ng IO, Liu CL, Lam CM, et al. Improving survival results after resection of hepatocellular carcinoma: a prospective study of 377 patients over 10 years. Ann Surg. 2001; 234(1): 63-70.

[86] Poon RT, Ng IO, Fan ST, Lai EC, Lo CM, Liu CL, et al. Clinicopathologic features of long-term survivors and disease-free survivors after resection of hepatocellular carcinoma: a study of a prospective cohort. J Clin Oncol. 2001; 19(12): 3037-44.

[87] Poon RT, Fan ST. Resection prior to liver transplantation for hepatocellular carcinoma: a strategy of optimizing the role of resection and transplantation in cirrhotic patients with preserved liver function. Liver Transpl. 2004; 10(6): 813-5.

[88] Belghiti J, Cortes A, Abdalla EK, Regimbeau JM, Prakash K, Durand F, et al. Resection prior to liver transplantation for hepatocellular carcinoma. Ann Surg. 2003; 238(6): 885-92; discussion 92-3.

[89] Adam R, Azoulay D, Castaing D, Eshkenazy R, Pascal G, Hashizume K, et al. Liver resection as a bridge to transplantation for hepatocellular carcinoma on cirrhosis: a reasonable strategy? Ann Surg. 2003; 238(4): 508-18; discussion 18-9.

[90] Lai Q, Avolio AW, Lerut J, Singh G, Chan SC, Berloco PB, et al. Recurrence of hepatocellular cancer after liver transplantation: The role of primary resection and salvage transplantation in East and West. J Hepatol. 2012; 57(5): 974-9.

[91] Fuks D, Dokmak S, Paradis V, Diouf M, Durand F, Belghiti J. Benefit of initial resection of hepatocellular carcinoma followed by transplantation in case of recurrence: an intention-to-treat analysis. Hepatology. 2012; 55(1): 132-40.

[92] Iwatsuki S, Gordon RD, Shaw BW, Jr., Starzl TE. Role of liver transplantation in cancer therapy. Ann Surg. 1985; 202(4): 401-7.

[93] Ismail T, Angrisani L, Gunson BK, Hubscher SG, Buckels JA, Neuberger JM, et al. Primary hepatic malignancy: the role of liver transplantation. Br J Surg. 1990; 77(9): 983-7.

[94] Bismuth H, Majno PE, Adam R. Liver transplantation for hepatocellular carcinoma. Semin Liver Dis. 1999; 19(3): 311-22.

[95] Olthoff KM, Millis JM, Rosove MH, Goldstein LI, Ramming KP, Busuttil RW. Is liver transplantation justified for the treatment of hepatic malignancies? Arch Surg. 1990; 125(10): 1261-6; discussion 6-8.

[96] Pichlmayr R, Weimann A, Steinhoff G, Ringe B. Liver transplantation for hepatocellular carcinoma: clinical results and future aspects. Cancer Chemother Pharmacol. 1992; 31 Suppl: S157-61.

[97] Pichlmayr R, Weimann A, Oldhafer KJ, Schlitt HJ, Klempnauer J, Bornscheuer A, et al. Role of liver transplantation in the treatment of unresectable liver cancer. World J Surg. 1995; 19(6): 807-13.

[98] Adham M, Oussoultzoglou E, Ducerf C, Bancel B, Bizollon T, Rode A, et al. Results of orthotopic liver transplantation for liver cirrhosis in the presence of incidental and/or undetected hepatocellular carcinoma and tumour characteristics. Transpl Int. 1998; 11 Suppl 1: S197-200.

[99] Sama C, Morselli Labate A, Barbara L. The role of liver transplantation in the treatment of hepatocellular carcinoma. Ital J Gastroenterol. 1992; 24(3): 139-43.

[100] Mazzaferro V, Regalia E, Doci R, Andreola S, Pulvirenti A, Bozzetti F, et al. Liver transplantation for the treatment of small hepatocellular carcinomas in patients with cirrhosis. N Engl J Med. 1996; 334(11): 693-9.

[101] Registry ELT. European Liver Transplant Registry Results [cited 7/08/2012]; Available from: http://www.eltr.org/spip.php?rubrique37

[102] Network OPaT. OPTN/SRTR Annual Report. 2012 [cited 7/08/2012]; Available from: http://www.ustransplant.org/annual_reports

[103] Clavien PA, Lesurtel M, Bossuyt PM, Gores GJ, Langer B, Perrier A. Recommendations for liver transplantation for hepatocellular carcinoma: an international consensus conference report. Lancet Oncol. 2012; 13(1): e11-22.

[104] Kneteman N, Livraghi T, Madoff D, de Santibanez E, Kew M. Tools for monitoring patients with hepatocellular carcinoma on the waiting list and after liver transplantation. Liver Transpl. 2011; 17 Suppl 2: S117-27.

[105] Freeman RB, Mithoefer A, Ruthazer R, Nguyen K, Schore A, Harper A, et al. Optimizing staging for hepatocellular carcinoma before liver transplantation: A retrospective analysis of the UNOS/OPTN database. Liver Transpl. 2006; 12(10): 1504-11.

[106] Bruix J, Sherman M. Management of hepatocellular carcinoma. Hepatology. 2005; 42(5): 1208-36.

[107] Treglia G, Giovannini E, Di Franco D, Calcagni ML, Rufini V, Picchio M, et al. The role of positron emission tomography using carbon-11 and fluorine-18 choline in tumors other than prostate cancer: a systematic review. Ann Nucl Med. 2012; 26(6): 451-61.

[108] Ryder SD. Guidelines for the diagnosis and treatment of hepatocellular carcinoma (HCC) in adults. Gut. 2003; 52 Suppl 3: iii1-8.

[109] Gimson A, Neuberger J, O'Grady J. Guidelines for Liver Transplantation for hepatocelullar carcinoma: NHSBT; 2008.

[110] Mazzaferro V, Llovet JM, Miceli R, Bhoori S, Schiavo M, Mariani L, et al. Predicting survival after liver transplantation in patients with hepatocellular carcinoma beyond the Milan criteria: a retrospective, exploratory analysis. Lancet Oncol. 2009; 10(1): 35-43.

[111] Hecht EM, Holland AE, Israel GM, Hahn WY, Kim DC, West AB, et al. Hepatocellular carcinoma in the cirrhotic liver: gadolinium-enhanced 3D T1-weighted MR imaging as a stand-alone sequence for diagnosis. Radiology. 2006; 239(2): 438-47.

[112] Monzawa S, Ichikawa T, Nakajima H, Kitanaka Y, Omata K, Araki T. Dynamic CT for detecting small hepatocellular carcinoma: usefulness of delayed phase imaging. AJR Am J Roentgenol. 2007; 188(1): 147-53.

[113] Obuz F, Oksuzler M, Secil M, Sagol O, Karademir S, Astarcioglu H. Efficiency of MR imaging in the detection of malignant liver lesions. Diagn Interv Radiol. 2006; 12(1): 17-21.

[114] Bruix J, Sherman M, Llovet JM, Beaugrand M, Lencioni R, Burroughs AK, et al. Clinical management of hepatocellular carcinoma. Conclusions of the Barcelona-2000 EASL conference. European Association for the Study of the Liver. J Hepatol. 2001; 35(3): 421-30.

[115] EASL-EORTC clinical practice guidelines: management of hepatocellular carcinoma. J Hepatol. 2012; 56(4): 908-43.

[116] Silva MA, Hegab B, Hyde C, Guo B, Buckels JA, Mirza DF. Needle track seeding following biopsy of liver lesions in the diagnosis of hepatocellular cancer: a systematic review and meta-analysis. Gut. 2008; 57(11): 1592-6.

[117] Young AL, Lodge JP. Needle-track seeding following biopsy of liver lesions in the diagnosis of hepatocellular cancer: a systematic review and meta-analysis. Gut. 2009; 58(6): 887-8.

[118] Bret PM, Sente JM, Bretagnolle M, Fond A, Labadie M, Paliard P. Ultrasonically guided fine-needle biopsy in focal intrahepatic lesions: six years' experience. Can Assoc Radiol J. 1986; 37(1): 5-8.

[119] Guo Z, Kurtycz DF, Salem R, De Las Casas LE, Caya JG, Hoerl HD. Radiologically guided percutaneous fine-needle aspiration biopsy of the liver: retrospective study of 119 cases evaluating diagnostic effectiveness and clinical complications. Diagn Cytopathol. 2002; 26(5): 283-9.

[120] Yao FY, Bass NM, Nikolai B, Davern TJ, Kerlan R, Wu V, et al. Liver transplantation for hepatocellular carcinoma: analysis of survival according to the intention-to-treat principle and dropout from the waiting list. Liver Transpl. 2002; 8(10): 873-83.

[121] Hayashi PH, Trotter JF, Forman L, Kugelmas M, Steinberg T, Russ P, et al. Impact of pretransplant diagnosis of hepatocellular carcinoma on cadveric liver allocation in the era of MELD. Liver Transpl. 2004; 10(1): 42-8.

[122] Freeman RB. Liver allocation for HCC: a moving target. Liver Transpl. 2004; 10(1): 49-51.

[123] Yao FY, KInkhabwala M, J. L, Bass NM, Kerlan R, Roberts JP. The impact of expansion of conventional tumor criteria and pre-operative loco-regional treatments on

survival following liver transplantation for hepatocellular carcinoma results from two centers. Hepatology. 2003; 38(4 Suppl): 157.

[124] Majno P, Mazzaferro V. Living donor liver transplantation for hepatocellular carcinoma exceeding conventional criteria: questions, answers and demands for a common language. Liver Transpl. 2006; 12(6): 896-8.

[125] Schwartz M, Roayaie S, Konstadoulakis M. Strategies for the management of hepatocellular carcinoma. Nat Clin Pract Oncol. 2007; 4(7): 424-32.

[126] Yao FY, Ferrell L, Bass NM, Watson JJ, Bacchetti P, Venook A, et al. Liver transplantation for hepatocellular carcinoma: expansion of the tumor size limits does not adversely impact survival. Hepatology. 2001; 33(6): 1394-403.

[127] Yao FY, Xiao L, Bass NM, Kerlan R, Ascher NL, Roberts JP. Liver transplantation for hepatocellular carcinoma: validation of the UCSF-expanded criteria based on preoperative imaging. Am J Transplant. 2007; 7(11): 2587-96.

[128] Herrero JI, Sangro B, Quiroga J, Pardo F, Herraiz M, Cienfuegos JA, et al. Influence of tumor characteristics on the outcome of liver transplantation among patients with liver cirrhosis and hepatocellular carcinoma. Liver Transpl. 2001; 7(7): 631-6.

[129] Ravaioli M, Grazi GL, Piscaglia F, Trevisani F, Cescon M, Ercolani G, et al. Liver transplantation for hepatocellular carcinoma: results of down-staging in patients initially outside the Milan selection criteria. Am J Transplant. 2008; 8(12): 2547-57.

[130] Vibert E, Azoulay D, Hoti E, Iacopinelli S, Samuel D, Salloum C, et al. Progression of alphafetoprotein before liver transplantation for hepatocellular carcinoma in cirrhotic patients: a critical factor. Am J Transplant. 2010; 10(1): 129-37.

[131] Toso C, Trotter J, Wei A, Bigam DL, Shah S, Lancaster J, et al. Total tumor volume predicts risk of recurrence following liver transplantation in patients with hepatocellular carcinoma. Liver Transpl. 2008; 14(8): 1107-15.

[132] Yao FY, Kerlan RK, Jr., Hirose R, Davern TJ, 3rd, Bass NM, Feng S, et al. Excellent outcome following down-staging of hepatocellular carcinoma prior to liver transplantation: an intention-to-treat analysis. Hepatology. 2008; 48(3): 819-27.

[133] Majno P, Lencioni R, Mornex F, Girard N, Poon RT, Cherqui D. Is the treatment of hepatocellular carcinoma on the waiting list necessary? Liver Transpl. 2011; 17 Suppl 2: S98-108.

[134] Maddala YK, Stadheim L, Andrews JC, Burgart LJ, Rosen CB, Kremers WK, et al. Drop-out rates of patients with hepatocellular cancer listed for liver transplantation: outcome with chemoembolization. Liver Transpl. 2004; 10(3): 449-55.

[135] Millonig G, Graziadei IW, Freund MC, Jaschke W, Stadlmann S, Ladurner R, et al. Response to preoperative chemoembolization correlates with outcome after liver

transplantation in patients with hepatocellular carcinoma. Liver Transpl. 2007; 13(2): 272-9.

[136] Decaens T, Roudot-Thoraval F, Bresson-Hadni S, Meyer C, Gugenheim J, Durand F, et al. Impact of pretransplantation transarterial chemoembolization on survival and recurrence after liver transplantation for hepatocellular carcinoma. Liver Transpl. 2005; 11(7): 767-75.

[137] Mazzaferro V, Battiston C, Perrone S, Pulvirenti A, Regalia E, Romito R, et al. Radiofrequency ablation of small hepatocellular carcinoma in cirrhotic patients awaiting liver transplantation: a prospective study. Ann Surg. 2004; 240(5): 900-9.

[138] Martin AP, Goldstein RM, Dempster J, Netto GJ, Katabi N, Derrick HC, et al. Radiofrequency thermal ablation of hepatocellular carcinoma before liver transplantation--a clinical and histological examination. Clin Transplant. 2006; 20(6): 695-705.

[139] Lu DS, Yu NC, Raman SS, Lassman C, Tong MJ, Britten C, et al. Percutaneous radiofrequency ablation of hepatocellular carcinoma as a bridge to liver transplantation. Hepatology. 2005; 41(5): 1130-7.

[140] Pompili M, Mirante VG, Rondinara G, Fassati LR, Piscaglia F, Agnes S, et al. Percutaneous ablation procedures in cirrhotic patients with hepatocellular carcinoma submitted to liver transplantation: Assessment of efficacy at explant analysis and of safety for tumor recurrence. Liver Transpl. 2005; 11(9): 1117-26.

[141] Riaz A, Lewandowski RJ, Kulik L, Salem R. Yttrium-90 radioembolization using TheraSphere in the management of primary and secondary liver tumors. Q J Nucl Med Mol Imaging. 2009; 53(3): 311-6.

[142] Huo TI, Huang YH, Su CW, Lin HC, Chiang JH, Chiou YY, et al. Validation of the HCC-MELD for dropout probability in patients with small hepatocellular carcinoma undergoing locoregional therapy. Clin Transplant. 2008; 22(4): 469-75.

[143] Riaz A, Kulik L, Lewandowski RJ, Ryu RK, Giakoumis Spear G, Mulcahy MF, et al. Radiologic-pathologic correlation of hepatocellular carcinoma treated with internal radiation using yttrium-90 microspheres. Hepatology. 2009; 49(4): 1185-93.

[144] Salem R, Lewandowski RJ, Kulik L, Wang E, Riaz A, Ryu RK, et al. Radioembolization results in longer time-to-progression and reduced toxicity compared with chemoembolization in patients with hepatocellular carcinoma. Gastroenterology. 2011; 140(2): 497-507 e2.

[145] Sandroussi C, Dawson LA, Lee M, Guindi M, Fischer S, Ghanekar A, et al. Radiotherapy as a bridge to liver transplantation for hepatocellular carcinoma. Transpl Int. 2010; 23(3): 299-306.

[146] Cronin DC, 2nd, Millis JM. Living donor liver transplantation: The ethics and the practice. Hepatology. 2008; 47(1): 11-3.

[147] Di Sandro S, Slim AO, Giacomoni A, Lauterio A, Mangoni I, Aseni P, et al. Living donor liver transplantation for hepatocellular carcinoma: long-term results compared with deceased donor liver transplantation. Transplant Proc. 2009; 41(4): 1283-5.

[148] Fisher RA, Kulik LM, Freise CE, Lok AS, Shearon TH, Brown RS, Jr., et al. Hepatocellular carcinoma recurrence and death following living and deceased donor liver transplantation. Am J Transplant. 2007; 7(6): 1601-8.

[149] Hwang S, Lee SG, Joh JW, Suh KS, Kim DG. Liver transplantation for adult patients with hepatocellular carcinoma in Korea: comparison between cadaveric donor and living donor liver transplantations. Liver Transpl. 2005; 11(10): 1265-72.

[150] Kulik L, Abecassis M. Living donor liver transplantation for hepatocellular carcinoma. Gastroenterology. 2004; 127(5 Suppl 1): S277-82.

[151] Lo CM, Fan ST, Liu CL, Chan SC, Ng IO, Wong J. Living donor versus deceased donor liver transplantation for early irresectable hepatocellular carcinoma. Br J Surg. 2007; 94(1): 78-86.

[152] Vakili K, Pomposelli JJ, Cheah YL, Akoad M, Lewis WD, Khettry U, et al. Living donor liver transplantation for hepatocellular carcinoma: Increased recurrence but improved survival. Liver Transpl. 2009; 15(12): 1861-6.

[153] Grant RC, Sandhu L, Dixon PR, Greig PD, Grant DR, McGilvray ID. Living vs. deceased donor liver transplantation for hepatocellular carcinoma: a systematic review and meta-analysis. Clin Transplant. 2012.

[154] Bhangui P, Vibert E, Majno P, Salloum C, Andreani P, Zocrato J, et al. Intention-to-treat analysis of liver transplantation for hepatocellular carcinoma: living versus deceased donor transplantation. Hepatology. 2011; 53(5): 1570-9.

[155] Soll C, Clavien PA. Inhibition of mammalian target of rapamycin: two goals with one shot? J Hepatol. 2011; 54(1): 182-3.

[156] Chinnakotla S, Davis GL, Vasani S, Kim P, Tomiyama K, Sanchez E, et al. Impact of sirolimus on the recurrence of hepatocellular carcinoma after liver transplantation. Liver Transpl. 2009; 15(12): 1834-42.

[157] Toso C, Merani S, Bigam DL, Shapiro AM, Kneteman NM. Sirolimus-based immunosuppression is associated with increased survival after liver transplantation for hepatocellular carcinoma. Hepatology. 2010; 51(4): 1237-43.

[158] Sun J, Hou BH, Jian ZX, Ou YL, Ou JR. [Value of perioperative adjuvant therapy in liver transplantation for advanced hepatocellular carcinoma]. Nan Fang Yi Ke Da Xue Xue Bao. 2007; 27(4): 471-3.

[159] Xu J, Shen ZY, Chen XG, Zhang Q, Bian HJ, Zhu P, et al. A randomized controlled trial of Licartin for preventing hepatoma recurrence after liver transplantation. Hepatology. 2007; 45(2): 269-76.

[160] Soderdahl G, Backman L, Isoniemi H, Cahlin C, Hockerstedt K, Broome U, et al. A prospective, randomized, multi-centre trial of systemic adjuvant chemotherapy versus no additional treatment in liver transplantation for hepatocellular carcinoma. Transpl Int. 2006; 19(4): 288-94.

[161] Pokorny H, Gnant M, Rasoul-Rockenschaub S, Gollackner B, Steiner B, Steger G, et al. Does additional doxorubicin chemotherapy improve outcome in patients with hepatocellular carcinoma treated by liver transplantation? Am J Transplant. 2005; 5(4 Pt 1): 788-94.

[162] Li N, Zhou J, Weng D, Zhang C, Li L, Wang B, et al. Adjuvant adenovirus-mediated delivery of herpes simplex virus thymidine kinase administration improves outcome of liver transplantation in patients with advanced hepatocellular carcinoma. Clin Cancer Res. 2007; 13(19): 5847-54.

[163] Zimmerman MA, Ghobrial RM, Tong MJ, Hiatt JR, Cameron AM, Hong J, et al. Recurrence of hepatocellular carcinoma following liver transplantation: a review of preoperative and postoperative prognostic indicators. Arch Surg. 2008; 143(2): 182-8; discussion 8.

[164] Roberts JP. Tumor surveillance-what can and should be done? Screening for recurrence of hepatocellular carcinoma after liver transplantation. Liver Transpl. 2005; (11 Suppl 2): S45-6.

[165] Escartin A, Sapisochin G, Bilbao I, Vilallonga R, Bueno J, Castells L, et al. Recurrence of hepatocellular carcinoma after liver transplantation. Transplant Proc. 2007; 39(7): 2308-10.

[166] Valdivieso A, Bustamante J, Gastaca M, Uriarte JG, Ventoso A, Ruiz P, et al. Management of hepatocellular carcinoma recurrence after liver transplantation. Transplant Proc. 2010; 42(2): 660-2.

[167] Yoon DH, Ryoo BY, Ryu MH, Lee SG, Hwang S, Suh DJ, et al. Sorafenib for recurrent hepatocellular carcinoma after liver transplantation. Jpn J Clin Oncol. 2010; 40(8): 768-73.

[168] Imamura H, Matsuyama Y, Tanaka E, Ohkubo T, Hasegawa K, Miyagawa S, et al. Risk factors contributing to early and late phase intrahepatic recurrence of hepatocellular carcinoma after hepatectomy. J Hepatol. 2003; 38(2): 200-7.

[169] Carrion JA, Navasa M, Garcia-Retortillo M, Garcia-Pagan JC, Crespo G, Bruguera M, et al. Efficacy of antiviral therapy on hepatitis C recurrence after liver transplantation: a randomized controlled study. Gastroenterology. 2007; 132(5): 1746-56.

[170] Berenguer M, Palau A, Aguilera V, Rayon JM, Juan FS, Prieto M. Clinical benefits of antiviral therapy in patients with recurrent hepatitis C following liver transplantation. Am J Transplant. 2008; 8(3): 679-87.

[171] Sala M, Fuster J, Llovet JM, Navasa M, Sole M, Varela M, et al. High pathological risk of recurrence after surgical resection for hepatocellular carcinoma: an indication for salvage liver transplantation. Liver Transpl. 2004; 10(10): 1294-300.

Chapter 14

Viral Hepatitis

Ahmad Ali Asadi Noghabi,
Fatameh Bahramnejad and Mitra Zandi

Additional information is available at the end of the chapter

http://dx.doi.org/10.5772/55915

1. Introduction

Main objective patients and families know about the ways of monitoring, controlling and managing the disease on completion of this chapter it is expected that a patient with hepatitis:

- Describe the process of hepatitis
- Identify the various types of hepatitis
- Identify the transmission routs of hepatitis
- Describe diagnostic tests
- Define treatment measures
- Identify medication regimen
- Explain the medication's side effects
- Describe the prevention rules to prevent hepatitis from being transmitted to the households and community
- Identify the precipitating factors of hepatitis
- Describe the required preparations related to the diagnostic test
- Explain the ways of managing sexual problems and its prevention measures
- State the importance of follow-up plan
- Discuss measures to manage complications

- Explain the measures to protect liver
- Identify the involvement of other body organs
- Explain the pregnancy related issues in a patients with Hepatitis
- Identify the alternative and Complementary medicine to manage the condition

At the end of this chapter, it is expected that the family of patients with Hepatitis:

- Describe the process of hepatitis
- Identify the various types of hepatitis
- Identify the transmission routs of hepatitis
- Describe hepatitis diagnostic tests
- Name different treatment plans for hepatitis
- Identify safety measures to prevent transmission
- Describe the measures for providing
- Describe the measures for providing psychological to patients with hepatitis

2. What is hepatitis?

It is a systemic and viral infection, in which the inflammation of liver cells and necrosis occur and these changes lead to biochemical and cellular clinical alterations. Literally, hepatitis means the "inflammation of liver"[1]. The most important factors causing it are viruses. Alcoholic drinks, medicines, poisons and some hereditary diseases also bring about hepatitis [2]. Hepatitis is divided into two kinds of chronic and acute [3].

In acute hepatitis, the diseases lasts for less than 6 months and finally leads to the complete removal of liver damage and the return of liver structure and function to normal level or leads to the immediate progression of acute damage toward extensive necrosis and the demise of patient. However, in chronic hepatitis, the process of disease lasts more than 6 months and patients does not have clinical symptoms [4].

Most patients suffering from viral hepatitis do not have any symptoms and their disease is diagnosed by doing medical tests. Nonetheless, the acute symptoms of disease exist in some patients[5]. Following the contact with the virus causing hepatitis and going through a period, which varies from a week to a few months and is called the latent period, the acute symptoms of suffering from viral hepatitis would emerge, which include: lack of appetite, excessive fatigue, exhaustion and vomit, abdominal pain, darkening of urine, paling of stool and turning of skin into yellow [6]. The symptoms of the disease usually last for days or weeks and its symptoms would be eradicated automatically. It must be attended that symptoms resembling influenza could be seen as muscular pain, exhaustion, and slight fever days or weeks before the emergence of the disease acute symptoms [2].

http://dx.doi.org/10.5772/55915

3. Acute hepatitis symptom

Pain at the right and the upper abdominal area is due to the exposure of liver capsule to traction and it is removed by the amelioration of the disease. Getting jaundiced means the yellowness of the skin and eyes. It must be attended that most patients suffering from hepatitis A and C do not have any symptoms of acute hepatitis, esp. jaundice. Some patients complain of bodily irritation which could be rooted in liver damage. Joint-related pain is also a part of acute hepatitis syndromes [7]. In case of the progression of hepatitis, there is the likelihood of swell in stomach and inflammation of feet which could lead to digestive bleeding.

Five types of hepatitis have been found; A, B, C, D, and E. types A and E are akin with regard to the way of transmission (the stool-oral path). Types B, C and D are also similar to each other [8].

4. Viral hepatitis, type A

What is hepatitis A?: This type is more common in developing countries or in crowded places with poor hygienic conditions. Its transmission way is through oral-stool path. Individuals are afflicted with it by having water and seafood tainted with sewage. This disease is not transmitted through blood but it is likely to be transmitted via sexual contact and having oral-anal contact [9].

Duration: The common course of the disease is 15 to 150 days and it could lat from 4 to 8 weeks. This disease does not have chronic and carrier courses. In case of the emergence of jaundice, the disease is not probably infectious [2].

Diagnosis: The diagnosis method is based on symptoms, signs, physical examination and blood tests. Blood test usually remains as positive 5 days prior to the onset of symptoms up to 6 months after infection [10,11].

Treatment: Individuals must be reminded that this type of hepatitis does not have any treatment, although most individuals might recuperate by supportive treatments. A person with hepatitis A virus requires in-hospital treatment for liver functioning. The patient must be trained to start walking slowly and progressively at once after feeling recuperated and to take rest after each time of walking [2,12]. The food for these patients mustn't be kept more than 2 hours at the level of room temperature.

Cautions: It is better for individuals who travel to endemic areas to get injected by vaccine in form of prophylaxis [8]. Hands ought to be washed thoroughly after bath taking, going to toilet or nay kind of contact with body liquids (blood, phlegm, semen).

The suffering patient must not prepare any food for family members. Also, she/he must not participate in carrying food to table (work prohibition at restaurants and fast food outlets)[13].

There ought not to be any sharing of bathroom toiletries between the suffering individual and other family members. The individual suffering from hepatitis is detected through symptoms, signs, physical examination and blood tests. A positive blood test usually pops up 5 days before the emergence of symptoms and remains unchanged up to 6 months after infection. There is no treatment for hepatitis A, although most individuals recuperate by supportive treatments. The individuals must be trained not to refer back to their work office or school until they have fever or jaundice or their appetite returns. Throughout the recuperation period, it is mandatory to refrain from drinking alcohol or taking non-prescribed medications.

There are two vaccines available for preventing Hepatitis A-related infection, namely as VAQTA and HAVRIX. Those who receive two dosages of these vaccines would be immune [14, 15].

5. Hepatitis E

What is hepatitis A? This type is transferred via the oral-stool tract and mostly due to polluted water in areas that have weak and inappropriate sewage systems.

Duration: It common period is variable and lasts between 15 to 65 days.

Symptoms: It is akin to Hepatitis A with regard to clinical symptoms and transferring ways. Jaundice almost always exists and avoidance from virus is made possible through rinsing hands as the main prevention method of this disease. The effectiveness of immune globins in creating immunity against Hepatitis E is unknown. The clinical symptoms of hepatitis A and E are like influenza, appetite loss, indigestion, epigastria pain, vomiting, and irritation of stomach and acidity of abdomen alongside hatred of cigarette smoke [2,16].

Treatment: It is better for these patients to use a diet full of protein (beans, meat, dairy, etc), high calorie (cereals, potato, etc), balanced fat (at the chronic courses of the disease with a low-protein diet), enough taking of liquids, eating food in several meals with low volume, avoiding to drink alcohol at the chronic courses of the disease and 6 months after that.

Patients must have enough rest at the chronic phase of the disease. Patients can gradually resume their activities after feeling healthy and examining their laboratorial tests. However, after being active, they ought to rest and avoid taking part in drudgeries [14].

Caution: It is necessary to prevent these two types of hepatitis by training individuals about the correct way of dumping sewage of houses and cities, exact observance of individual health, correction and refining the process of food provision and distribution, community health training programs, legal reporting of cases of hepatitis A and E to local health centers, vaccinating the travelers going to developing countries, application of non-permitted medications (injective and non-injective), homosexual individuals and those suffering from chronic liver diseases, and injection of immune globins for family members and sexual partners suffering from hepatitis A [8,14]

Rinsing and disinfecting fruits and vegetables, not using polluted water and foods (boiling water for one minute deactivates hepatitis virus) and not using personal things of others [16].

6. Hepatitis B

What is Hepatitis B? This type is transferred via blood (sub-phlegm and endodermal ways). Its virus could be found in blood, saliva, semen and vaginal discharges and can be transferred via the phlegmatic membrane and damaged skin. Also, pregnant mothers could be afflicted through sexual contact after or during delivery [9].

Duration: Its common course lasts from 1 to 6 months [2].

Symptom: The symptoms and signs of hepatitis B might be quite arcane, deceitful and variable. Respiratory and fever-related symptoms are rare. Some patients suffer from rash and joint pain. Patients might lose their appetite and suffer from indigestion, abdominal pain, general pain, ill health and weakness. Jaundice might occur or not. In case of its occurrence, it would be accompanied by light color stool and dark urine. Clinically, it has a lot of similarities with hepatitis A but its common course is longer [13]. More than 90 percent of infections can be prevented in women suffering from HBV and their infants can receive the hepatitis B vaccine and immune globins B in prophylaxis manner for preventing infection. Babies must undergo serological test within 9 to 15 months of age [1].

It must be mentioned that at-risk individuals might be afflicted with the virus of hepatitis B via using polluted blood products, contact of polluted blood with eyes, mouth, bleeding or damaged skin of healthy people, transfer from mother to fetus, tattooing and cupping, sexual contact, non-sterile dental and medical devices, esp. shared and non-sterile syringe, razorblade or toothbrush. This virus is not transferred through shaking hand, kissing or going to pool [17].

Cautions: Therefore, individual hygiene is the basis of infection control. Disinfection must be done on a daily basis at related laboratories. Gloves must be worn when contacting with patient's blood or discharges and smoking and eating must be refrained at work site. Patients and their families must be reminded that this disease is contagious and the pre-awareness of this disease is chronic. It is essential that family members and health personnel receive the hepatitis B vaccine in three dosages intravenously within a one-month interval from the second dosage and 6 months for the third dosage within six months after the first dosage injection. Such immunization leads to the protection of patient for at least 5 to 10 years [18,19]. These patients must be to have insight about their disease and to know the transmission ways of this disease. Knowing this disease affects the quality of life among individuals and their families [20].

The infant born from a mother infected with hepatitis virus B ought to receive immune globins within 12hours after birth [9].

An individual who has been at exposure to hepatitis virus B and has not ever been afflicted with hepatitis and has not received vaccine must receive the immune globins injection at most 24 hours after contact with the virus [8].

Patient must take rest till the ebbing of hepatitis symptoms like liver inflammation, jaundice, and decrease in high liver enzymes (sometimes up to 3 to 4 months).

At the chronic phase of the disease, which entails a limit on protein and fat intake, patient must at several meals with a low volume of food intake.

In case of vomiting, taking of all medications must be avoided. If it is not stopped, patient must refer to doctor and avoid drinking alcohol, refrain from sexual intercourse or in case of having sex, condom must be used [2,8].

In case of need, medications must be taken only with doctor's prescription. After recuperation (usually 18 months afterward), patient must refer to doctor for undergoing checkups and laboratorial tests. It is recommended to healthy carriers to undergo the required checkups and laboratorial tests once every six months at the first year of the disease and after that once every year. In case of going to dentist's, doctor's, laboratory or anywhere in which the possibility for the transmission of the virus exists, it is recommended to patient to inform the health personnel there about the positive nature of their disease and show their special card [17]. Patient must be trained not to use bathroom toiletries in a shared manner. Toothbrush, nail clipper, shaving machine, thermometer and cosmetics must be absolutely personal.

7. Hepatitis C

What is Hepatitis C? A significant percentage of hepatitis cases are neither A, B nor D. Consequently, they are referred to as hepatitis type C. Hepatitis C is transmitted through blood, sexual contact, using septic syringe by the applicators of injective, intravenous medications, the abrupt penetration of needle head and other kinds of injuries among health care personnel [15] and also cutaneously (breathing in narcotics like cocaine) [17,21].

This virus is not transmitted through nestling, breastfeeding, sneeze, water, food, sudden contact and shared dishes.

Duration: The latent course of this disease varies from 2 to 26 weeks. Most patients do not show any overt symptoms. In case the virus exists in the individual's body for more than 6 months and gradually damages the tissues of liver, the chronic hepatitis C emerges [17].

Symptoms: Patient might complain about slight to severe lethargy and weakness, decrease in appetite, spew and vomit, having pain at the upper and right sides of abdomen (below ribs), fever and pain in joints [22,23]

Besides, they are recommended to drink abundant liquids (8 liters daily) and to eat foods that have a lot of vitamin and minerals, like fresh fruit juices (without food limitations). In addition, they are advised to eat foods at several meals in low volume and to use ginger for relieving vomit [9,22].

Treatment: One of the main treatments about hepatitis C is taking the medication group of interferon. Throughout undergoing treatment with interferon, patients must be examined closely by virtue of the possible side effects. Therefore, immediate monitoring while undergoing treatments is viable for reducing these side effects to some extent. These treatments inevitably entail some degrees of side effects like fatigue, muscular pain, flu-like symptoms

http://dx.doi.org/10.5772/55915

and change of mood and reduction in sexual desire which might bear negative effects on patients' lives, their social interactions and their abilities for doing work and different activities. The significance of the side effects emanating from treatments forms the basis of decision making by patient and doctor for commencing with or quitting treatment before thoroughly completing the treatment course. Stopping the treatment before completing the course indicates patients' lack of tolerance. Hair loss, annihilation of bone morrow and psycho-physiological impacts (depression, cognitive changes and apathy) are among the side effects. The side effects of interferon group continue from a few hours after prescription and patients get used to it after a few weeks of consumption [2,14,24,25].

Cautions: The hepatitis virus type C is transmitted through using septic blood products, the contact of septic blood with eyes, healthy individuals' mouth and injured skin, toothbrush, shaving machine and all septic personal things, tattooing and cupping, sexual contact, using septic dental and medical devices, esp. non-sterile and shared syringe. Hence, it is recommended to observe the personal hygienic points including of sterilizing the devices used in ear perforation and tattooing, using gloves and rinsing hands and not using others' personal devices. It is also recommended that individuals use condom when having sexual contact with the afflicted person [22]. The family members of the suffering individual and also the members of society in which they live must be informed that there are no vaccines for hepatitis C. With regard to injective addicts, they ought to use new injection tools in every injection in case of being unable to withdraw from their addiction and they are advised not use needle, syringe, swap, filter, spoon, toothbrush and shaving razorblade and hair clipper in a shared manner. Besides, they must be trained about the correct way of dumping the applied tools. By virtue of breastfeeding women who suffer from hepatitis, it is advised that they examine their breast tips each time before breastfeeding since Hepatitis C is a disease that can be transmitted through blood. In case of having a crack, bleeding or any kind of blood at breast tips, breastfeeding must be stopped temporarily and all the milk must be thrown away. It is also recommended to these mothers to wean their infants once they start to grow teeth and feed them by bottle [14,15].

The individuals who are afflicted with Hepatitis C are recommended to inform the personnel at medical centers, dentist's, laboratories or nay other places which entails the possibility of virus transmission [22]. It must be explained to patient to refrain from taking acetaminophen, anti-convulsion medications, alcohol, etc. In case of having dry mouth, they are recommended to drink water frequently in a sipping manner and to chew sugar-free gums.

They are also advised to follow the hygiene of mouth and teeth. Cutting down on sugary drinks and foods, using florid supplements once a day, using floss, snit-microbe mouthwash, reducing cigarette and quitting it, regular examination of teeth, their whitening and taking care of false teeth are among the tips given to these patients [9].

8. Hepatitis D

What is the hepatitis D? : In some cases, hepatitis B takes place due to the fact that its virus is at exposure with the superficial antigen and risk of hepatitis D. Anti-delta antibodies within the antigen in the blood sample ascertains the existence of hepatitis B. hepatitis D is prevalent among the users of injective, intravenous medications, hem dialysis patients and receivers of various blood donations.

Duration: Its common course is between 21 to 40 days.

Symptom: The symptoms of hepatitis D are akin to hepatitis B and its treatment is similar to all other forms of hepatitis [2,9].

9. Cirrhosis

What is Cirrhosis? It is a chronic disease that is identified by the replacement of fibrosis instead of the natural tissue of liver and consequently the deformation of liver's structure and performance. There are three kinds of Cirrhosis of liver: alcoholic Cirrhosis, post-necrosis Cirrhosis and bilious Cirrhosis [2].

Among the most important causes of Cirrhosis are chronic hepatitis B and C, excessive consumption of alcoholic drinks, disturbances in the exiting tract of blood from liver, increase of iron in liver, etc.

Symptoms: The symptoms of Cirrhosis at initial stages are fatigue, lethargy, loss of appetite, vomit, weight loss, enlarging of blood vessels in shape of spiders under the skin, hair loss, enlarging of nipples in men, accumulation of liquids in abdomen and feet, reduction in sexual desire and potency in men, malodorous smell, oily diarrhea, emergence of dead blood cells under skin, irritation and bloody vomit [17].

Treatment: Patient must be trained to use sufficient amount of fruit and vegetables.

They are also recommended to use all other proteins except red meat, including of herbal protein, fish, chicken, etc. and also to refrain from drinking alcohol and take vitamins, esp., A, C and K.

Eating foods in several mealtimes with low volume (instead of 3 meals, having six meals) and having a nutritional diet full of calorie and average amounts of protein (1 gram per each kilogram of protein) with limitations for using salt are among other tips [26,27]

Using ice cubes is conducive for relieving vomit and constipation alongside taking liquids and exercising are also recommended. Skincare is possible through changing lifestyle, using alcoholic soaps and liquids for cleansing the skin and applying softeners for massaging the skin while exercising the joints and limbs.

They are also advised to go to doctor in case of having blood (clot, nasal or gum bleeding and the existence of blood in stool) and to use soft-bristle toothbrush. Patients must gently clean their nose and use cold compress for decreasing their bleeding. Eating foods full of vitamin C is also recommended. Supportive measures are also recourse to for preventing deterioration.

Patients must measure their stomach with a meter on a daily basis and observe the limitation on using salt and liquids, they ought to report any symptoms to doctor. There are no limitations

http://dx.doi.org/10.5772/55915

on activities but in case of having fever, bleeding and all other problems, caution must be exercised. Since the metabolism of most medicines is carried out through liver, it is recommended to avoid wishful consumption of medicines [25,26].

10. Sexual functioning training

Chronic hepatitis infection brings about changes in the hormone levels of body. In short, these patients experience the following conditions:

- disturbance in the function of testicles
- body hair loss
- increase in breast size (genichomasty)
- improper distribution of fat in body (fat accumulation in special parts of body).
- disturbance in erection
- Irrespective of patients' gender, these patients experience sexual disturbances at different dimensions and in case of consuming alcohol by these patients, they become susceptible in sexual issues which require more serious and costly measures. The continuation of sexual disturbances brings about effect on the quality of life among these individuals.

Hepatitis C information Center It is necessary to train these patients to consult with doctor or nurse in case of having sense of stimulation, pain at the time of stimulation, incapability in erection, incapability in maintaining erection for making sexual contact, delay in ejaculation or lack of ejaculation despite having enough stimulants, lack of ability in controlling or scheduling ejaculation and finally reaching to sexual climax. A good sexual partner has a significant role in solving sexual problem [28,29].

Author details

Ahmad Ali Asadi Noghabi, Fatameh Bahramnejad and Mitra Zandi

Tehran University of Medical Sciences, Iran

References

[1] Smith, G, & Watson, R. (2005). Gastrointestinal Nursing. Blackwell Sciences.

[2] Smeltzer, F, Bare, B, Hinkel, L, & Cheever, H. (2010). *Brunner & suddarth's Text book of Medical- surgical Nursing*. International:.Lippincot, Williams & Wilkins.

[3] Moradman Badie BSeyde Ali naghi M, Chaman R, Hosseni M, Hasibis M, Moharami B. ((2011). Frequency and correlation hepatitis C and hepatitis B with HiV. Knowledge and health. , 6(31), 40-43.

[4] Carpenter CJCFlanigan TP,Lederman MM. ((2001). HIV infection and the acquired immunodeficiency syndrome. In: Cecil Essential of medicine. USA: W.B Saunders company.

[5] Alavian, S. M. (2012). On the Occasion of the World Hepatitis Day: World Hepatitis Day and Our Achievements and Responsibilities in Iran. International Journal of Preventive Medicine, 3(7).

[6] Kalantari, H. (2011). Viral hepatitis. Journal of Isfahan Medical school.29(128).

[7] Gothomas, H, Lemon, S, & Zuckerman, A. (2005). Viral hepatitis. Blackwell Publishing L.td.

[8] Neighbors, M, Sands, J, Monhan, F, Marek, J, & Green, C. (2007). Phipps Medical Surgical Nursing. Mosby, Elsevire.

[9] Black, J, & Hawaks, J. (2009). *Medical- Surgical Nursing*. International: Sanders Elsevier.

[10] Chord, L. A. J. ((2002). Forgeneral readers a comprehensive discussion of the causes of hepatitis and of the treatment. University press of Mississipi.

[11] Lankarani, M, Alavian, S. M, & Johbari, M. (2004). Anti HAV body in HBV carriers. Govaresh.9(4).

[12] Saffa, M. J, Abedini, O, Ajami, A, Abedini, F, Mirabi, A, Khalilian, A, & Saffa, H. (2012). Age-specific sero prevalence of Anti-Hepatitis a anti body among years old population of Savadkuh Mazandaran. Hapatitis Monthly. 12(5)., 1-30.

[13] Osborn, K. Wrach Ch, Watson A. ((2010). Medical-Surgical Nursing preparation for practice. International,Pearson.

[14] Ignatavicius, D, & Workman, L. (2006). Medical- Surgical Nursing Critical thinking for collaborative care. International W.B. Saunders Company.

[15] Lewis ShHeitkemper M, Dirkseh Sh, O'Brien Medical- Surgical Nursing assessment and management of clinical problems. Mosby : Elsevire., 2007.

[16] Alavian, S. M, Ahmadzadeh, A. L, Lankarani, K. B, & Shahabaie, M. A. Bahrami Ahmadi A. (2008). Hepatitis E, C infection in Iran: a systematic review. Hept mon. 8(4).

[17] Mehrvarz, A. (2006). liver and bilious tract diseases adapted from Green Books Collection; Tehran, Hayan Publication.

[18] Alavian, S. M, & Hajarizadeh, B. Ahmadzadeh Asl M, Kabir A. (2008). Hepatitis B virus infection in Iran:a systematic review. Hept mon. 8(5).

[19] Alavian, S. M. Tehran,Arjomand Publication.

[20] Samiei, S, Monjamed, Z, Mehran, A, & Taheri, Z. (2005). Investigation quality of self care in patients member of family wich have simplex and multiplex hepatitis B. HAYAT.11(3-4).

[21] Alavian, S. M, Adibi, P, & Zali, M. R. (2005). Hepatitis C Virus in Iran: Epidemiology of an emerging infection. AVCH Iran Med.8

[22] Hajrasooliha, H. (2004). The manual for patient about the special aspects of hepatitis C, Tehran; Rezvan Publications in cooperation with the artistic group of Chakameh

[23] Alavian, S. M. (2004). The comprehensive manual of liver and hepatitis diseases. Tehran. Noor Danesh Publication.

[24] Asadi Noghabi AAZAndi M, Mehran A, Hassan pour dehkordi A. (2010). The Effect of Education on Quality of Life in Patients under Interferon Therapy. Hepat Mon: 10(3).

[25] The group of compilers at Iran Nutrition Associationspecial therapeutic manual) (2003). Tehran, Salemi Publication.

[26] Ghafari, F, & Fotokian, Z. (2009). Patient and Family Training.Tehran: Bashari Publication.

[27] Holly, R, & Wilson, M. H. and You: A Patient Education Resource for Pregnant Women and New Mothers. Journal of women's health: 12(5).

[28] Nicole, M, Loo, M, & Douglas, P. (2012). Exploring Hepatitis B A Neglected Disease. Minnesota Medicine. 37

[29] Musavi GhAsad Noughani AA. (2008). Exploring the relationship between sexual function disturbance and blood biochemical parameters and level of depression among the male patients suffering from chronic hepatitis referring to the Research Center of Digestion and Liver of Baghiatollah University of Medical Sciences (2007-2008).